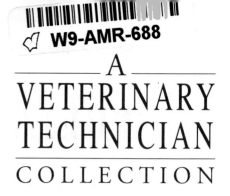

NURSING CARE IN VETERINARY PRACTICE

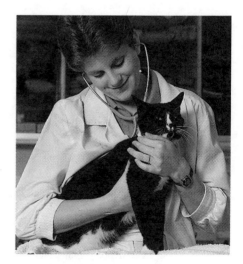

PREFACE

The Veterinary Technician Collection is a compilation of the best articles from past issues of *Veterinary Technician*. This edition, *Nursing Care in Veterinary Practice*, is the first in a series of collections. Each of the articles has been carefully reviewed by the authors and, when appropriate, updates have been added. In this way, the articles remain timely and useful. We trust that you will find this book a valuable addition to your reference library.

Published by Veterinary Learning Systems
Trenton, New Jersey

ISBN 1-884254-04-7

CONTENTS

The Problem-Oriented Medical Record*

Fred Freeland, DVM
Division of Agriculture, Home Economics,
   and Forestry
Abraham Baldwin Agricultural College
Tifton, Georgia

The problem-oriented medical record offers veterinarians a systematic format to use in order to arrive at a specific diagnosis and to formulate follow-up care. The medical record used in trying to reach a diagnosis must list all relevant observations, diagnostic tests with results, treatments, and the patient's responses to treatments. The use of the problem-oriented medical record system can improve patient care, facilitate the training of medical personnel, and provide a good means of auditing the proficiency of the health care team.

The problem-oriented method of medical recordkeeping involves four orderly steps: collecting the data base; defining the problems; formulating the initial plan; and, at necessary intervals during care, formulating follow-up plans. The initial plan includes diagnostic plans, therapeutic plans, and client education plans. Although the veterinary technician will be more involved in some of these steps than in others, the technician's knowledge of the whole process is vital to providing good patient care and critical for completing those steps for which the technician may be primarily responsible.

Collecting the Data Base

The *data base* is the collection of information that is the basis for defining problems. The term *base* may be taken

---

*The problem-oriented method of medical recordkeeping described here was developed for medical doctors by Lawrence Weed, MD, and adapted to veterinary medicine by veterinarians at the University of Georgia. This article is derived from the article "The Transition of Quality Patient Care from an Art to a Science: The Problem Oriented Concept" by Carl A. Osborne, DVM, PhD (*JAAHA*, May-June, 1975, pp 250-260). Comments about the veterinary technician's role in this recordkeeping system have been added.

literally; this collection is the information needed to construct a logical, defensible initial plan. The data base always includes the patient history and the results of the physical examination; it also commonly includes laboratory data, especially urinalysis, complete blood cell counts, and serum chemistries.

Patient History

The keys to a valuable patient history are accuracy and thoroughness. Accuracy may be compromised by accepting owners' statements as accurate observations or facts when the owners are giving their interpretations of events.

The following provides some examples of interpretations that owners may give (on the left side) and the observations that may be the justification for those interpretations:

"My dog has worms."	The dog scoots on its rear.
"My dog vomits up water but not solid food."	The paper covering the floor of the cage is soaked every morning.
"My horse is on a deworming program."	The horse is wormed once a year.

It is often recommended that the veterinarian take the patient history, as the veterinarian may more easily recognize the difference between observation and interpretation than the technician would. When taking a history, the veterinary technician should be careful to record the owner's words accurately and completely to allow the veterinarian to follow up the history later with the appropriate further questions. Collecting the history in this two-stage manner may actually be an advantage, because the veterinarian can ask the owner to elaborate on comments recorded by the technician and the results could be a much clearer communication.

Questions asked as part of the history should be very precise; they should be requests for information and should be worded carefully to avoid suggesting any desired response. Giving the owner a comfortable chance to answer, ''I don't know,'' could avoid eliciting inaccurate responses owners may give to please the history taker or to hide their lack of knowledge.

A well-designed patient history form can help to increase the accuracy and thoroughness of the history and can reduce variations that might be seen in information gathered by different history takers. The veterinary technician can contribute greatly to a practice by developing customized forms and being alert for ways to refine them. Figure 1 is one example of a patient history form; others can be found in veterinary textbooks or may be obtained from colleagues and veterinary schools.

The best history takers are knowledgeable about veterinary medicine, are good communicators, and are careful observers of human behavior.

Physical Examination

A routine and systematic method of performing a physical examination can help to ensure that important findings are not overlooked. A physical examination form with a checkoff list can be very helpful (Figure 2). Following the initial general examination, many veterinarians use specialized detailed examination forms in cases of neurologic, ophthalmologic, dermatologic, and other specialized problems.

Having the owner present during the physical examination is advantageous because unsuspected problems that require additional questioning of the owner may be discovered.

Some preliminaries of the initial physical examination may be carried out by the veterinary technician, especially in uncomplicated cases in which only a brief examination is required; such preliminaries may consist of taking a rectal temperature and determining the heart and respiratory rates. The technician does not judge the significance of the findings but records them for further evaluation by the veterinarian. The skills required to perform a good physical examination are developed through practice. The technician that has become proficient at assisting the veterinarian in performing an efficient and accurate examination often accumulates a mental data bank of what constitutes normal and abnormal in appearances and in basic physical findings; this accumulation of skill and knowledge can have great value in other aspects of the veterinary practice. Veterinary technicians may become expert in carrying out certain portions of specialty examinations; in many cases, they are responsible for equipment preparation and patient preparation and conduct major portions of some examinations, such as taking electrocardiograms.

Initial Laboratory Data

Many veterinarians are adopting a standard data base of laboratory data that are collected on any patient that is admitted for surgery or that has an undetermined illness. The data collected often include the complete blood count, serum chemistry, urinalysis, and fecal analysis.

Veterinary technicians are often responsible for collecting and processing laboratory samples. Maintaining the inventory of equipment and supplies needed for the procedures is another area in which technicians can contribute to the smooth operation of the clinic.

Defining the Problems

After collecting the patient history, performing the physical examination, and evaluating the information obtained from initial laboratory tests, the veterinarian will formulate the initial or temporary problem list (Figure 3). The initial problem list includes all problems identified by the data base, even problems that are not going to be treated immediately; the list is not a list of tentative diagnoses.

Each problem is stated in a way that reflects the highest current level of understanding the problem. The different levels of understanding, or refinements in the definition of the problem, are listed as follows from lowest to highest, with examples:

1. A clinical sign (e.g., vomiting, polydipsia)
2. An abnormal physical finding (e.g., abdominal mass, heart murmur)
3. An abnormal laboratory finding (e.g., leukocytosis, proteinuria)
4. A pathophysiologic syndrome (e.g., renal failure, nephrotic syndrome, heart failure)
5. A diagnostic entity (e.g., cirrhosis, bacterial endocarditis).

When possible, related problems may be grouped under the heading of a single problem name that encompasses them. Also, the problem list may be subdivided into major and minor problems, depending on their priority for evaluation. The initial problem list is usually formulated and discussed with the owners at the time of the initial office visit.

Because clients will often ask technicians questions they neglected to ask or were embarrassed to ask the veterinarian, it is advised that technicians know and be able to interpret what is on the initial problem list. Technicians who are questioned by clients should answer questions with

ABRAHAM BALDWIN VETERINARY TECHNOLOGY PROGRAM
PATIENT HISTORY

Date/Time __11-13-87 / 1:10 pm__

Owner ___SMITH, LYNN (MRS.)___

Address ___1234 HOMETOWN ST., TIFTON, GA 31794___

Phone ___386 - 5678___

Patient Species/Breed/Sex/Color/Coat ___K-9 / MIN. SCHNAUZ. / M / SILVER___

Patient Name/Birthdate ___MAX / 9-84___

Regular Veterinarian's name/city ___DR. JAMES BRUNCH / TIFTON___

Presenting Complaint or Request
___INCREASED DRINKING AND URINATION, VOMITING___

Vacc. Hist. (Types/Dates)	Diet and Feeding
DA₂ PL 9-86	PURINA DOG CHOW — FREE CHOICE
RABIES 12-8	INFREQUENT TABLE SCRAPS

Vacc. Hist. (Types/Dates)	Diet and Feeding
$DA_2 PL$ 9-86	PURINA DOG CHOW — FREE CHOICE
RABIES 12-8	INFREQUENT TABLE SCRAPS

Parasite control	Previous Problems Incl. adverse drug reactions
HEARTGARD SINCE 4-87	— ALLERGIC TO PENICILLIN
	— DOG FIGHT INJURIES 10-86

History (Include all problems noticed, location of lesions, duration and/or frequency, and owner's descriptions where applicable. Use back if necessary.)

— VOMITING YELLOW FOAMY FLUID 3-5 TIMES/DAY FOR PAST WEEK; VOMITS FOOD IF JUST EATEN

— DRINKS A LOT OF WATER, OFTEN VOMITS IT BACK UP

Signature _Brenda Frydl RVT_   **Continued on back** ___NO___

PATIENT HISTORY

Figure 1—Example of a patient history form.

ABRAHAM BALDWIN VETERINARY TECHNOLOGY PROGRAM
PHYSICAL EXAMINATION

Date/Time 11-13-87 / 1:10 pm

Owner SMITH, LYNN (MRS.)

Address 1234 HOMETOWN ST., TIFTON, GA 31794

Phone 386 - 5678

Patient Species/Breed/Sex/Color/Coat K-9 / MIN. SCHNAUZ / M / SILVER

Patient Name/Birthdate MAX / 9-84

Regular Veterinarian's name/city DR. JAMES BRUNCH / TIFTON

Presenting Complaint or Request

INCREASED DRINKING AND URINATION, VOMITING

N = Normal
ABN = Abnormal
NE = Not Examined

1) GEN (N) ABN NE	2) INTE N (ABN) NE	3) MUS (N) ABN NE	4) CIRC (N) ABN NE	5) RESP (N) ABN NE	6) DIG N (ABN) NE
7) GU N (ABN) NE	8) EYES (N) ABN NE	9) LYM (N) ABN NE	10) NS N ABN (NE)	11) EARS (N) ABN NE	12) MM (N) ABN NE

T 101^5 P 68   R 40   WT 25 lb

Describe abnormalities (Use the number above.)

2 — 1cm x 1cm PEDUNCULATED MASS ON RIGHT ELBOW; PRESENT
       FOR 6 MO., NO CHANGE NOTICED

6 — HISTORY OF VOMITING; VOMITED ~ 100ml WHITE FOAMY
       FLUID IN EXAM ROOM

7 — HISTORY OF POLYURIA / POLYDIPSIA

Signature *Fred Freeland* DVM

PHYSICAL EXAMINATION

Figure 2—Example of a physical examination form.

TEMPORARY PROBLEM LIST
INITIAL PLAN

Problem	Dx:	Rule outs, Procedures	Rx:	CE
ELBOW MASS;	ASPIRATE CYTOLOGY;	R/O BENIGN TUMOR ☐		DISCUSS RESULTS
VOMITING;	R/O	LIVER DIS., RENAL DIS., DIABETES		
		MELLITUS, ADRENAL DYSFUNCTION		
		— EDTA BLOOD FOR CBC ☒		
		— SERUM FOR CHEMISTRY PANEL INCL. ELECTROLYTES ☒		
		— URINE FOR UA ☒		
POLYURIA;	R/O	AS ABOVE; URINARY TRACT INFECTION		
POLYDIPSIA.		— CYSTOCENTESIS FOR CULTURE IF INDICATED		
		BY SEDIMENT ON UA ☐		
		— HOSPITALIZE TO QUANTITATE WATER INTAKE		
		AND URINE OUTPUT ☒		

Signature *Fred Freeland* DVM

Figure 3—The temporary problem list.

ABRAHAM BALDWIN VETERINARY TECHNOLOGY PROGRAM
PROGRESS RECORD

OWNER SMITH, LYNN

PATIENT MAX

	CODES	
Appetite		**Bowel Movement**
N = Normal		N = Normal
F = Fair		A = Abnormal
P = Poor		(Specify)
O = None		O = None

Date	App	BM	Temp	Pr#	
1-14-87	O	O	101.²	3	TUMOR ON ELBOW
					S — OWNER REPORTS NO CHANGE OVER 6 MO. PERIOD,
					ASPIRATE CYTOLOGY REVEALS NO MALIGNANT FEATURES
					A — BENIGN TUMOR
					P — DISCUSS WITH OWNER, OWNED DECLINED REMOVAL
				4	VOMITING
					S — BRIGHT ALERT, NO CLINICAL DEHYDRATION
					O — VOMITED 3X IN 18 HRS, TOTAL ~200ml. HYPERGLYCEMIA
					(320 mg/dl), HYPERCHOLESTEROLEMIA (250 mg/dl), GLUCOSURIA
					(4+), USG 1.034, NO BACTERIA
					A — VOMITING 2° TO DIABETES MELLITUS
					P — DISCUSS D.M. WITH OWNER; SEE PROBLEM #5
				5	POLYURIA, POLYDIPSIA
					S — NO DEHYDRATION
					O — DRANK 3.5 L IN 18 HRS; URINE OUTPUT ~1L;
					GLUCOSURIA (4+)
					A — PU/PD 2° TO DIABETES MELLITUS
					P — DISCUSS WITH OWNER; OWNER WISHES TO TREAT
					— REGULAR INSULIN 0.1u/lb/hr I.M., CHECK BLOOD
					GLUCOSE q hr UNTIL READING ~200 mg/dl THEN
					GIVE 0.25u/lb q6h, CHECK BLOOD GLUCOSE q 24h
					F. Freeland

Page No. 1

PROGRESS RECORD

Figure 4—Follow-up examinations are recorded in the progress notes.

ABRAHAM BALDWIN VETERINARY TECHNOLOGY PROGRAM
HEALTH RECORD

Owner ___SMITH, LYNN (MRS.)___

Address ___1234 HOMETOWN ST., TIFTON, GA 31794___

Home phone ___386 - 5678___   Business phone ___386 - 3535___

Patient species ___CANINE___   Breed ___MIN. SCHNAUZ.___ Sex ___M___   Color ___SILVER___ Coat ___SHORT___

Patient name ___MAX___   Birthdate ___9-84___

Year	1984	1985	1986	1987	1988					
DHLPP	11-6-84	9-20-85	9-10-86	9-15-87						
FVRCP										
RABIES	12-12-84	12-10-85								
FELV										
Heartworm		6-10-85 NEG	4-12-86 NEG	4-10-87 NEG						
Fecal	11-6-84 NEG	9-20-85 NEG	9-10-86 NEG	9-15-87 NEG						

MASTER PROBLEM LIST

PROB. NO.	ACTIVE DATE	PROBLEM	RESOLVED DATE DX	RX
1	10-12-86	DOG FIGHT LACERATIONS	10-12-86	10-20-86
2	10-14-86	ALLERGIC TO PENICILLIN ✱		
3	11-13-87	TUMOR ON ELBOW 11-13-87▷ BENIGN CYTOLOGY	11-13-87	
		11-14-87▷ INACTIVE		
4	11-13-87	VOMITING 11-14-87▷ DIABETES MELLITUS, SEE PROBLEM #5	11-14-87	
5	11-13-87	POLYURIA, POLYDIPSIA 11-14-87▷ DIABETES MELLITUS	11-14-87	

HEALTH RECORD

Continued on back _____

Figure 5—The master problem list includes summaries of key diagnoses and problems based on the patient's known medical history.

which they feel comfortable and should seek answers from the veterinarian for more complicated questions. Technicians should report to the veterinarian questions that have been asked by the client for the following reasons: (1) it is important that any of the client's misunderstandings be discovered; and (2) these communications between the technician and the veterinarian will help determine which questions the technician can answer in the future and which questions the veterinarian would prefer to answer. The veterinary technician should avoid making statements that may be interpreted by the client as a diagnosis or prognosis.

Formulating the Initial Plan

From the initial problem list, the veterinarian will formulate the initial plan (Figure 3). A diagnostic plan is formulated to investigate problems on the initial problem list according to their priority. Each problem is considered separately, and specific tests and procedures are listed along with the reason for performing them.

The veterinary technician often obtains and processes the laboratory samples or participates in other ways in carrying out the diagnostic plan. Understanding the reasons for each step of the diagnostic plan can help in obtaining the necessary data. For example, the technician who understands the diagnostic plan would realize that, in a given case, multiple tests were to be conducted in sequence, with each test depending on interpretation of the previous test, and thus would not discard samples prematurely.

In addition to the diagnostic plan, the veterinarian will also formulate a therapeutic plan. In the ideal situation, therapy is withheld until the diagnosis is reached; however, this is often not possible. In these cases, before beginning therapy, all diagnostic samples should be collected and properly preserved for later analysis. The proper preservation of samples may be the duty of the technician.

Formulating Follow-up Plans

Ideally, all the steps in the problem-oriented medical investigation discussed so far—taking the history, completing the physical examination, and formulating the initial diagnostic and therapeutic plans—have been accomplished on the first day the patient is seen. In life-threatening emergencies, all the previous steps may be covered within a few minutes.

Every unresolved problem is reevaluated by the veterinarian at appropriate intervals, depending on the significance of the problem and the rate at which changes occur. These periodic reevaluations are recorded as progress notes and the resulting follow-up plans (Figure 4).

Each time a problem is reevaluated, the medical record should be amended and organized by dividing progress notes into four sections referred to as the *SOAP format*. The four categories of notes, in the order in which they are written into the record, are as follows:

- S, that is, subjective, wherein subjective clinical information is recorded (e.g., information about the patient's alertness, appetite, and activity level)

- O, that is, objective, wherein the progress of objective clinical data is recorded (e.g., laboratory data, body temperature, and body weight)
- A, that is, assessment, wherein the significance of the subjective and objective observations is interpreted
- P, that is, the plan, which is the section wherein updated diagnostic, therapeutic, and client education plans for each problem are listed.

If nothing has changed in a particular category between evaluations, that section may be omitted or it can be written that no changes have occurred since the previous entry.

The veterinarian formulates the follow-up plans and makes the assessment of the case and therefore usually makes the entries under the A and P sections of the record. In many situations, the veterinary technician may be responsible for recording the subjective and objective findings in the record. It is important that the terms used be clear and that entries be written legibly and signed by the person making the entry. Abbreviations that are not commonly recognized in veterinary medicine should not be used. It is wise to double-check numeric data transferred from laboratory sheets onto the record. In most cases, the original laboratory sheet will remain with the record.

Many parts of the diagnostic and therapeutic plans are carried out by veterinary technicians. When a treatment, procedure, or diagnostic sample is requested under the P section, the technician must understand what is to be done and who is to do it. If the technician is responsible for carrying out any part of the diagnostic or therapeutic plan, he or she must also assume responsibility for writing in the record that the step is completed and, if appropriate, for entering the results.

The client education plan may be written by the veterinarian or by the technician, depending on the complexity of the case. In many cases, the client education plan is carried out by the veterinary technician.

Master Problem List

The veterinarian should maintain a master problem list in the front of the patient's record. This is a numbered list of every problem the patient has (active problem) or has had (inactive or resolved problem). The master problem list is created or amended according to information on the initial problem list, usually within 24 hours for hospitalized patients and as soon as possible for outpatients. The master problem list will grow throughout the patient's lifetime and serves as a brief overview of the current episode of illness and the patient's entire medical history (Figure 5). It also serves as an index to the medical record.

Conclusions

The problem-oriented medical record is most useful as an aid in providing good patient care when those using it understand the overall structure. Because technicians will be writing entries for many sections as well as carrying out the prescribed plans, it is especially important that they be familiar with the system.

BIBLIOGRAPHY

Osborne CA: The problem-oriented medical system: Improved knowledge, wisdom, and understanding of patient care. *Vet Clin North Am* 13(4):745–790, 1983.

Osborne CA: The transition of quality patient care from an art to a science: The problem oriented concept. *JAAHA* 11:250–260, 1975.

Guide to Fluid Therapy and Intravenous Catheter Placement

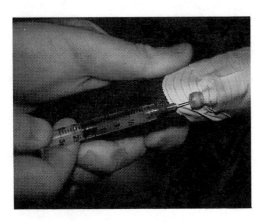

David B. Joseph, AHT
Northridge, California

Fluid therapy is indicated if metabolic disease, dehydration, trauma, or shock occurs in small animals. An understanding of the basic concept of how fluid is distributed in the body and an understanding of the placement and care of intravenous catheters are essential for veterinary technicians in small animal practice. A technician who is proficient in placing intravenous catheters quickly and efficiently is a great asset to the veterinary medical team.

BASIC CONCEPTS OF FLUID

Water represents approximately 70% of the total body weight in an adult animal. Total body water (TBW) is divided into intracellular fluid (ICF) and extracellular fluid (ECF). Each fluid constitutes approximately 50% of total body water. Extracellular fluid is subdivided into plasma and interstitial fluid volumes. Plasma volume represents approximately 5% of body weight; interstitial fluid volume makes up 25% to 30% of body weight.

Cerebrospinal, gastrointestinal, and bile fluids are considered as transcellular fluid and are approximately 5% of

Originally published in Volume 13, Number 5, June 1992

total body water. These fluids are not taken into account when calculating fluid replacement volumes.

Intracellular fluid volume is maintained by osmotic forces generated by intracellular potassium and magnesium. The kidneys are responsible for the regulation of extracellular fluid. Routes of water loss in healthy animals include sensible and insensible losses. Sensible losses consist of urinary and gastrointestinal fluid losses and constitute more than two thirds of maintenance fluid requirements. Insensible losses, such as cutaneous (sweat) and pulmonary (i.e., breathing) fluid losses, are quantitatively less important but must be included in computations for fluid replacement therapy. If dehydration or metabolic changes occur and the fluid status is altered in the body, fluid must be administered via an oral, subcutaneous, or intravenous route.

INDICATIONS FOR FLUID THERAPY

Several factors must be considered in determining whether fluid therapy is necessary. In most cases, the patient is presented for an examination. The technician can obtain a careful and accurate history before the veterinarian arrives. The most common method for assessing hydration status is by skin turgor. The technician grasps the patient's skin over the lumbar area between the thumb, index finger, and middle finger and gently pulls upward. If the skin returns to normal quickly after release, noticeable dehydration is absent. If the skin does not return quickly, some degree of dehydration is present.

Using this method, a technician can estimate the percentage of dehydration. The method works well only if the patient is more than 5% to 6% dehydrated. As dehydration progresses, skin turgor increases substantially. The skin remains elevated at 10% to 12%. At 12% to 15%, death is imminent. Obese animals may appear well hydrated because of excessive subcutaneous fat. In contrast, emaciated animals may appear excessively dehydrated because of the lack of subcutaneous fat.

Other parameters that are evaluated during the physical examination and that indicate dehydration are prolonged capillary refill time, decreased body weight, sunken eyes, and dry mucous membranes. Body weight can be an accurate indication of hydration status if the patient's weight has been previously recorded. A loss of one pound of body weight indicates a loss of 500 milliliters of fluid. The following facts also must be considered before the institution of fluid therapy:

- Dehydration affects young animals faster than adults.
- Old animals with chronic disease (especially azotemia) require more fluids than other animals.
- Drugs, such as corticosteroids and diuretics, can alter fluid and electrolyte requirements.
- Animals that have received various forms of anesthesia may require additional fluids for several days.

ROUTES FOR FLUID THERAPY

There are several routes by which fluids may be administered. The best method is oral administration. If a large amount of hypertonic or high-calorie fluids is needed, the technician can pass a stomach tube via the mouth to administer the fluids. The oral route is unacceptable if vomiting or severe dehydration is present.

As dehydration progresses, blood flow is diverted from the extremities and to the internal organs; fluids thus are not distributed throughout the body. Subcutaneous administration is a convenient route for isotonic fluids only (i.e., lactated Ringer's solution or 0.9% sodium chloride). Disadvantages of this route are (1) the relatively small quantity of fluids that can be administered because of skin elasticity and (2) the fact that the route should not be used in extremely dehydrated patients because of constriction of the vasculature in the skin.

Intraperitoneal administration of fluids is used most often in small kittens and puppies. Use of this route requires advance training. Only isotonic fluids that have been warmed to body temperature should be administered. To avoid secondary infections, asepsis should be strictly enforced. Disadvantages of the route are the small quantity of fluids that can be administered, possible organ laceration or puncture, and required restraint of the animal. The route should not be used in severely dehydrated animals.

Intraosseous fluid administration should only be performed by the veterinarian. Rectal administration of isotonic fluids is an often overlooked route of administration. The route works well in very young puppies and kittens. Warm water, sodium, potassium, and chloride are well absorbed via this route. Disadvantages include retention of the fluids given, especially if there are gastrointestinal disturbances.

Intravenous fluid administration is the quickest and preferred route. All types of fluids can be administered via this route. Intravenous fluids are extremely useful in treating patients with severe dehydration, hypovolemic shock, or extensive fluid or blood loss.

PLACEMENT OF INTRAVENOUS CATHETERS

The proper placement of intravenous catheters can be among the most challenging tasks that a veterinary technician performs. Intravenous catheters come in various sizes and styles. The technician should select a catheter that he or she feels comfortable placing. Catheter size should correspond to the vein size of the patient; placing a catheter that is too large can damage the vein and decrease the patency of the catheter.

Before placing an intravenous catheter in a peripheral vein, the technician should be sure that the following supplies are readily available:

- Electric clippers with a No. 40 blade
- Several gauze pads saturated with povidone-iodine or chlorhexidine scrub
- Several gauze pads saturated with 70% alcohol
- Dry gauze
- Intravenous catheter
- 3-cc syringe filled with heparinized saline
- Selected warmed intravenous fluids and an administration set
- Antibiotic ointment and a cotton-tipped applicator
- Sterile pad
- Tape.

The technician should select an appropriate catheter and open it, being careful to avoid contamination of the catheter. It is advisable to break the seal between the catheter and needle hub before insertion. An assistant restrains the patient by having it sit and then placing one arm around the patient's neck; the other arm is used to extend the leg into which the intravenous catheter will be placed. The leg is prepared. In clipping the patient's fur, the technician must not irritate the skin or cause clipper burns; a skin reaction may cause an undesirable effect.

Preparation of the leg for the insertion of an indwelling intravenous catheter should be identical to surgical preparation. The technician should not use a back-and-forth motion but rather start at the center of the shaved area and proceed in a circular outward motion. This prevents contaminants from crossing the site at which the catheter will enter the body. The scrub procedure should be repeated three times; each scrub is followed by an alcohol rinse. The alcohol should be completely dry before insertion of the catheter; otherwise the tape will adhere poorly to the patient or catheter.

The assistant should hold off the vein by grasping the leg with one hand and rolling the vein outward with the thumb. This elevates the vein and positions it for catheter placement. If the vein is standing up poorly or if a greater increase in blood pressure is desired, a tourniquet can be applied. The tourniquet must not be tight enough to cause discomfort to the patient. In patients with severe dehydration or thick skin, it is helpful to lift the skin next to the vein gently with an 18-gauge needle and make a small opening in the skin with the needle tip. This must be done close to the vein but without puncturing it.

When this has been accomplished, the technician can move the opening over the vein and insert the intravenous catheter. The catheter is grasped in one hand so that the bevel on the needle is up. Placing the thumb of the other hand next to the vein adds stability in case the vein begins to roll. A 5° to 25° angle allows the needle to penetrate the skin and enter the vein (Figure 1). When the vein is entered, a pop is felt and a flash of venous blood is seen in the hub. Once blood flow has been determined, the catheter and stylet are slightly advanced further into the vein. While the stylet is held, the catheter is advanced all the way into the vein (Figure 2).

For best results, the catheter should enter the vein smoothly and be advanced to the hub. The assistant then releases the thumb or tourniquet from the vein but retains support of the elbow so the patient's leg stays extended. The stylet is removed, and the catheter is capped quickly. Excess blood, which may prevent the adhesive tape from adhering to the skin, is wiped off. The catheter is flushed with sterile saline to prevent obstructive clot formation.

The technician places one strip of tape, adhesive side down, on the leg and then lays the catheter on top and wraps the piece of tape around the leg in a clockwise motion, making sure that the tape sticks securely to the leg and catheter (Figure 3). A small amount of antibiotic ointment is placed on a sterile pad, which is placed over the site where the catheter entered the body. A second piece of tape is positioned over the gauze and wrapped in a clockwise manner. The third piece of tape is placed, adhesive side down, under the hub of the catheter. Both sides of the tape should point upward in a counterclockwise direction, thus anchoring the catheter.

The cap is removed from the catheter, and the end of the administration set is placed into the catheter hub. A small piece of one-inch tape is placed between the junction of the hub of the catheter and the administration set (Figure 4). This prevents separation of the administration set from the catheter. A small loop is made with the administration set tubing and taped in place (Figure 5). Depending on the practitioner's preference, the leg may be left unwrapped or wrapped with one of several coverings to prevent swelling of the foot. In wrapping the leg, the technician should start at the bottom of the foot and work upward, being careful to avoid taping over the injection port on the administration set.

FLUID ADMINISTRATION SETS AND MONITORING OF ADMINISTRATION

In administering fluids, good clinical judgment must be exercised. For patients that are severely dehydrated or in

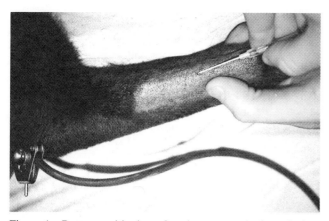

Figure 1—Proper positioning of an intravenous catheter before entering the vein. The bevel faces upward.

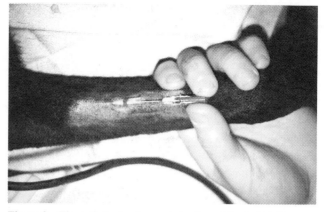

Figure 2—The catheter is advanced slowly and kept straight.

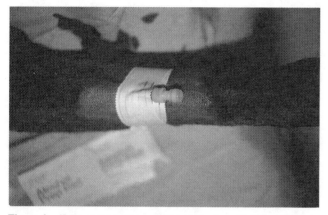

Figure 3—Tape secures the catheter to the leg. Pinching the tape around the catheter holds it more securely.

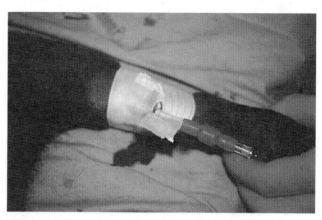

Figure 4—Tape secures the catheter to the administration set. Making tabs on both ends facilitates removal.

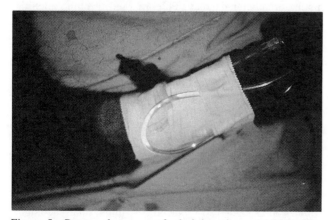

Figure 5—Proper placement of administration set tubing. The tube is not kinked when the loop is made.

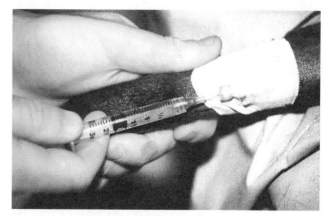

Figure 6—Flushing the catheter with heparinized saline. Blood in the syringe indicates catheter patency.

shock, it is nearly impossible to give fluids too quickly. Calculation of replacement fluids is based on normal fluid use plus replacement of abnormal losses. Normal fluid turnover is 65 ml/kg/day for mature animals and 130 ml/kg/day for immature animals. An intravenous fluid administration rate of 10 to 16 ml/kg/hr during the first hour of therapy is adequate.

Administration sets that provide 10, 15, 20, and 60 drops/ml are available. Burettes should be used to deliver small quantities of fluid precisely to small puppies and kittens. The technician should select an administration set that allows maximum rehydration without adding stress to the patient.

For patients that weigh less than 15 pounds, a microdrip (60 drops/ml) should be used. For patients that weigh more than 15 pounds, the administration set should allow adequate rehydration without overloading the patient's system. In patients with heart disease, pulmonary edema, or ascites, careful monitoring of the quantity of fluids is vital to prevent fluid overload.

Periodic, systematic monitoring of patients receiving fluid therapy is essential. Packed cell volume, total plasma protein, and body weight should be monitored daily. The patient should be weighed on the same scale every day if possible. A gain or loss of 0.5 kilograms reflects a gain or loss of 500 milliliters of fluid. The value of renal function in dehydrated animals cannot be overemphasized. Normal urine output is 1 to 2 ml/kg/hr.

If renal function is questionable, an intravenous injection of 1 to 25 milliliters (depending on the size of the patient) of 50% dextrose may be prescribed. The bladder is catheterized; urine is checked every five minutes for the presence of glucose, which indicates glomerular filtration.

There are several ways to monitor fluid administration. A piece of one-inch white tape with the starting date and time can be placed on the bottle of fluids and marked in sections as to where the fluid should be at given times during the day. This method of monitoring fluid intake is satisfactory but allows error (i.e., improper rate setting or occlusion of the vein caused by bending of the leg); close monitoring of the patient and fluid level thus is essential. Use of an automated infusion device is the preferred method of administering fluids during long periods. Such a device can be programmed to deliver fluids accurately to a patient. Regardless of how the patient rests in the cage, proper fluid therapy is administered.

MAINTENANCE AND CARE OF INTRAVENOUS CATHETERS

Proper nursing care of indwelling intravenous catheters is an important responsibility of the veterinary technician. Poor care of catheters can lead to bacteremia and septicemia. Strict asepsis must be maintained when placing an intravenous catheter or giving injections through the catheter. Before giving injections through the catheter or injection port on the venoset, the injection site should be wiped with 70% isopropyl alcohol.

The venoset should be crimped before the intravenous injection; this allows the drug to enter the patient and not be distributed throughout the administration set. Intravenous injections should be given slowly. To prevent irritation of the vein, drugs should be diluted if possible by periodically allowing fluids to run through the line.

Patients with indwelling intravenous catheters should be monitored daily for signs of infection at the venipuncture site, phlebitis, and thrombophlebitis. Every eight hours, the leg should be examined for signs of swelling or erythema and the bandage material should be checked. This allows visual inspection of the catheter and venipuncture site for signs of phlebitis and thrombophlebitis as well as an opportunity to palpate the lymph nodes above or around the catheter site. If the bandage material is soiled or wet, it should be changed promptly. Patients that are vomiting should be monitored more closely.

The maximum period that an intravenous catheter can be left in place is three days. Beyond this time, the patency of the catheter decreases and the risk of infection increases. At the end of three days, the catheter is removed and a new catheter is placed if necessary. If swelling or erythema is present, the catheter should be removed regardless of how long it has been in place. Intravenous tubing should be kept off the cage floor and replaced every 48 hours or when soiled.

If there is discharge from the catheter site or if the patient becomes febrile, the catheter should be removed and culture samples of the discharge and the tip of catheter should be taken. Both samples should be submitted for culture identification and antibiotic sensitivity testing to determine whether a pathogen is present.

To prevent phlebitis and thrombophlebitis, 0.05% to 0.1% heparin–saline solution should be flushed through the catheter every eight hours (Figure 6). Such low-dose heparin is used to decrease fibrin-clot formation and thus maintain catheter patency. Phlebitis and thrombophlebitis are among the most common problems associated with fluid therapy. After removal of the catheter, warm compresses should be applied to the area for approximately 10 minutes twice daily. No other venipuncture should be performed on the leg. Antibiotic therapy may be indicated.

ADDITIVES COMPATIBLE WITH INTRAVENOUS FLUIDS

Patients that receive intravenous fluid therapy often require supplementation with certain pharmacologic agents, which can be added to replacement fluids. Pharmacologic agents must be checked to determine whether they are compatible with the fluid to which they will be added. Table I provides a quick reference guide to common agents and their compatibility with intravenous solutions.

To add an agent into a liter of fluid, it is necessary to draw the proper amount of the agent into a sterile syringe, wipe the injection port of the fluid container with 70% isopropyl alcohol, and inject the agent into the fluid container. Thorough mixing ensures proper distribution in the container. After the agent is added to the container, the container must be labeled with the name of the agent, number

TABLE I
Physical Compatibility of Parenteral Admixtures

Agent	Lactated Ringer's Solution	0.9% Sodium Chloride	5% Dextrose in Water
Antimicrobial Agents			
Ampicillin	Unknown	Unknown	Compatible
Chloramphenicol	Compatible	Compatible	Compatible
Penicillin sodium or potassium (1,000,000 U)	Compatible	Compatible	Compatible
Oxytetracycline	Unknown	Unknown	Compatible
Tetracycline	Compatible	Compatible	Compatible
Anesthetic Agents			
Diazepam	Incompatible	Unknown	Unknown
Doxapram hydrochloride	Unknown	Unknown	Unknown
Edrophonium	Unknown	Unknown	Unknown
Fentanyl	Unknown	Unknown	Unknown
Meperidine hydrochloride (100 mg)	Compatible	Compatible	Compatible
Morphine (16.2 mg)	Compatible	Compatible	Compatible
Oxymorphone	Unknown	Unknown	Unknown
Pentobarbital sodium	Compatible	Compatible	Compatible
Phenobarbital	Compatible	Compatible	Compatible
Phenothiazines	Compatible	Compatible	Compatible
Procaine	Compatible	Compatible	Compatible
Thiopental	Incompatible	Compatible	Compatible
Intravenous Solutions and Ions			
Calcium chloride or glucoheptonate	Compatible	Compatible	Compatible
Insulin	Compatible	Compatible	Compatible
Mannitol	Unknown	Compatible	Compatible
Potassium chloride	Compatible	Compatible	Compatible
Sodium bicarbonate	Compatible (color change)	Compatible	Compatible
Cardiovascular Drugs			
Amophylline	Compatible	Compatible	Compatible
Antihistamines	Compatible	Compatible	Compatible
Digitalis (class)	Incompatible	Incompatible	Incompatible
Dopamine or dobutamine	Unknown	Compatible	Compatible
Dexamethasone	Compatible	Compatible	Compatible
Epinephrine	Compatible	Color change	Compatible
Ephedrine (50 mg)	Compatible	Compatible	Compatible
Hydrocortisone sodium succinate	Compatible	Compatible	Compatible
Isoproterenol	Unknown	Compatible	Compatible
Lidocaine (2 mg)	Compatible	Compatible	Compatible
Phenylephrine (10 mg)	Compatible	Compatible	Compatible
Procainamide	Unknown	Unknown	Unknown

of milligrams, time of the addition, date, and technician's initials. Such labeling is especially important if potassium is added to fluids. Fluid containers with additives should be discarded when treatment is complete, even if fluid remains in the container.

Several common conditions in hospitalized patients can be corrected with proper drug therapy. These conditions include hyponatremia, metabolic acidosis, and hypokalemia.

Hyponatremia results from gastrointestinal losses, hypoadrenocorticism (Addison's disease), diuretic therapy, and sodium-losing renal disease. Clinical signs of hyponatremia include weakness, vomiting, abdominal pain, seizures, and anorexia. Hyponatremia is easily corrected by infusion of sodium-containing fluids (e.g., 0.9% sodium chloride). Therapy for metabolic acidosis includes sodium bicarbonate at 2.2 mEq/kg for a 15-minute treatment.

Hypokalemia is usually associated with decreased potassium intake; such drugs as diuretics or amphotericin B; overuse of laxatives; and such metabolic conditions as anorexia, vomiting, and diarrhea related to parvoviral infection. In cats, hypokalemia can be a life-threatening condition that requires immediate potassium supplementation. Supplementation must be slow; sudden changes in serum potassium levels can lead to arrhythmia, bradycardia, and death.

The following are the recommended amounts of potassium chloride to be supplemented to fluids based on the patient's serum potassium level (figures derived from 250 cc of 0.9% normal saline):

- Less than 2.0—20 mEq/L
- 2.1 to 2.5—15 mEq/L
- 2.6 to 3.0—10 mEq/L
- 3.1 to 3.5—7 mEq/L.

The infusion rate must not exceed 0.5 mEq/kg/hr.

NUTRITIONAL SUPPORT

The need for proper nutrition is often overlooked in patients that are receiving fluid therapy. This omission can cause the body to catabolize fat and muscle for energy. Approximately 7 cal/kg/day are necessary to prevent most body protein catabolism; 25 cal/kg/day are required to prevent body protein and fat catabolism. Supplying patients with the proper number of calories can speed recovery and reduce client cost.

Before any type of dietary supplementation therapy can be implemented, current body weight should be determined to assess the progress of nutritional therapy. Therapy for normal adult dogs and cats is based on normal calorie and protein requirements. An average-sized dog requires 50 kcal/kg/day. Protein requirements are best met by providing protein as a percentage of the daily caloric intake. An adult dog requires 8% to 12% of its daily calories as protein; an adult cat requires 15% to 20%.

There are several ways to implement proper nutritional supplementation in a patient that is receiving intravenous fluid therapy. If the patient is not vomiting, the preferred way is the oral route. Small amounts of food (e.g., baby food or a prescription diet) fed two or three times daily help to supplement caloric requirements. If vomiting is present, the addition of 50% dextrose is often the first step in caloric supplementation. Adding this solution to fluids provides 1700 kcal/L or 1.7 kcal/ml (55 cc of 50% dextrose is added to a liter of fluids to make a 2.5% dextrose solution, and 110 cc is added to make a 5% solution).

Patients hospitalized for long periods for burns, septic shock, or chronic metabolic conditions must have more substantial caloric supplementation than the addition of dextrose to intravenous fluids. Dogs can be maintained on a mixture of equal volumes of 8.5% amino acids and 50% glucose solution. This mixture contains approximately 0.85 kcal/ml. Such solutions are infused slowly via a central vein.

For the first day's feeding, an 8.5% amino acid solution is mixed with an equal part of 25% glucose solution. If there are no complications, the second day's feeding is made by mixing equal parts of 8.5% amino acid solution and 50% glucose solution. Urinary glucose values should be monitored to avoid hyperglycemia (greater than 200 mg/dl). The technician should only mix enough of the solution for one feeding; the diet is a excellent medium for bacterial growth, which can lead to systemic sepsis.

Several parameters (e.g., body weight; temperature; pulse; respiration; plasma glucose concentration; urine glucose concentration; and plasma concentrations of sodium, potassium, chloride, bicarbonate, calcium, and phosphorus) should be monitored daily until stabilization occurs. If a patient receives intravenous caloric replacement therapy for a long time, periodic evaluation of the hemogram is beneficial. Blood must not be drawn from the catheter that is used to administer intravenous caloric therapy; fibrin clots that may be present in the catheter can produce false values.

SUMMARY

Fluid therapy plays a major role in the recovery of sick animals. Proper technique in placing intravenous catheters and strict attention to asepsis help to alleviate catheter-related problems. A basic understanding of fluid therapy and nutritional support enables the veterinary medical team to benefit the patient and leads to greater client satisfaction. The technician who understand this process and becomes proficient in the placement of intravenous catheters will be an asset to any veterinary practice.

ACKNOWLEDGMENTS

The author is grateful to Catherine R. Grinstead, BA, AHT, Chief Surgical Technician, Veterinary Medical Unit, Veterans Administration, Los Angeles, California, for her assistance in preparing this article and to Ramon Joseph for his photographic help.

■

BIBLIOGRAPHY

Bell FW, Osborne C: Maintenance fluid therapy, in *Current Veterinary Therapy. X*. Philadelphia, WB Saunders Co, 1989, pp 37–43.

DiBartola SP, Muir W: Fluid therapy, in *Current Veterinary Therapy. VIII*. Philadelphia, WB Saunders Co, 1983, pp 28–40.

Gross DR: General concepts of fluid therapy, in *Veterinary Pharmacology and Therapeutics*. Ames, IA, Iowa State University Press, 1988, pp 544–550.

Lewis LD, Morris ML: Anorexia, inanition and critical care nutrition, in *Small Animal Clinical Nutrition*. Topeka, KS, Mark Morris Associates, 1987, pp 5-1–5-41.

Short CE: Fluid and electrolyte therapy, in *Current Veterinary Therapy. VII*. Philadelphia, WB Saunders Co, 1980, pp 49–53.

An Update on Fluid Administration for Veterinary Technicians

Fluid administration is a dynamic treatment that requires careful and continuous monitoring and adjustments as the requirements of the patient change.

Travis Bradley, LVT*
The Animal Medical Center
New York, New York

*Mr. Bradley is currently affiliated with Coast Pet Clinic/Animal Cancer Center, Hermosa Beach, California.

Fluid administration, which is a critical part of veterinary medicine, can make the difference between life and death in some patients. Veterinary technicians play a very important role in fluid administration because they usually place the intravenous catheter, administer the fluids, and monitor the patient under the direction of a veterinarian (Figure 1). In addition, in emergency situations, veterinary technicians assist the veterinarian by administering fluids to acutely traumatized patients.

Sixty percent of the adult body weight of an animal is water.[1] This can be converted to liter volume: one liter of water weighs one kilogram. In a neonate, as much as 80% of body weight is water, which, compared with an adult, makes dehydration in a neonate even more significant.[1] Obese animals tend to have less body water than do thin animals.

Body water can be divided into two components: intracellular fluid (ICF) and extracellular fluid (ECF) (see Components of Body Water). Most intracellular fluid is located in skeletal muscle and skin. Twenty-five percent of extracellular

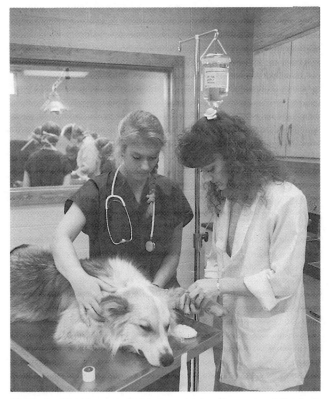

Figure 1—Veterinary technicians assist in all aspects of fluid administration.

fluid is located in plasma, and 75% bathes interstitial tissues. Sodium and chloride are the major electrolytes in extracellular fluid, and potassium and phosphorus are the major electrolytes in intracellular fluid.

Fluid therapy is necessary to replace dehydration deficits, maintain normal hydration, replace essential electrolytes and nutrients, and serve as a vehicle for certain intravenous medications.[1] To help assess a patient, an accurate patient history must be taken; the history should include frequency and amount of fluid loss (e.g., via vomiting, salivating, or diarrhea); body weight before dehydration occurred; and determination of whether polyuria, polydipsia, adipsia, anorexia, pyrexia, or tachypnea is present.

After the patient history has been taken, a physical examination should be performed. Important factors that are linked to fluid status should be assessed; these factors include body weight, skin turgor, pulse rate and quality, capillary refill time, mucous membrane moistness, and enophthalmos (Table I). Geriatric and cachectic animals lose skin elasticity even though they are not dehydrated. Obese animals can have normal skin turgor when they are dehydrated. Pale mucous membrane color may indicate anemia, whereas increased capillary refill time may suggest dehydration or shock. A sunken eyeball is also an indication of dehydration. A rapid, weak pulse rate may re-

---

Components of Body Water[1]

- 60% of an adult animal's weight is water.
- Two thirds of the total 60% body water (or 40% of the body weight) is intracellular fluid.
- One third of the total 60% body water (or 20% of the body weight) is extracellular fluid.
  — Extracellular fluid is further divided into plasma and interstitial fluid.
  — 75% of the extracellular fluid is interstitial water, and 25% is plasma water.

---

flect dehydration in association with decreased cardiac output. Plasma volume can be assessed by pulse rate, pulse quality, and capillary refill time. Interstitial fluid volume can be assessed by the presence or absence of edema, degree of skin turgor, and moistness of mucous membranes.

In addition to the history and physical examination, results of laboratory tests may be of assistance in assessing dehydration. Table II[2] presents some common laboratory findings associated with dehydration.

An increased microhematocrit and increased total serum protein may indicate plasma water depletion. Special attention should be given, however, to anemic or hypoproteinemic animals because they may have normal microhematocrits and normal total serum protein values even in the presence of dehydration. Thus, it is always important to interpret the clinical findings together with the patient history.

ROUTES OF FLUID ADMINISTRATION

After establishing that fluids must be administered, a method of fluid administration must be selected. Fluids can be administered by several routes, including rectal, oral, subcutaneous, intraperitoneal, intravenous, and intraosseous. Each route has advantages and disadvantages. The best method can be determined by assessing the patient's needs, the materials available, and the skill of the health care team. Currently, the preferred route for sick or dehydrated patients is intravenous fluid administration. When a patient is mildly dehydrated and is not vomiting or in need of intravenous medication, however, oral water consumption may be adequate.

TABLE I
Estimating the Level of Dehydration Based on Physical Examination Findings[1]

Dehydration	Physical Examination Findings
<5%	History of vomiting or diarrhea but no physical examination abnormalities
5%	Dry mucous membranes
6%–8%	Mild to moderate decrease in skin turgor; dry oral mucous membranes
10%–12%	Marked degree of decreased skin turgor; dry mucous membranes; weak and rapid pulse; slow capillary refill time; moderate to marked mental depression, enophthamlos

Rectal. Rectal administration of fluids is not recommended in veterinary medicine because the uptake of fluids has not been proven to be very effective.[1]

Oral. Oral (per os or PO) administration may be used for short-term illness and/or anorexia in animals weighing less than 20 kilograms.[1] It is a particularly good method in neonates because other routes of fluid administration may not be feasible. If the animal is not drinking freely, water may be administered by stomach tube, pharyngostomy tube, dose syringe, or baby bottle. The condition of the patient dictates the preferred method. Fluid volumes may be offered free choice or given forcibly through one of the previously described methods. If fluids are to be force-fed, the fluid volume should be similar to that given during intravenous administration (as described later) and, depending on the patient's needs, either tap water or commercially prepared oral electrolyte solutions may be used. A possible complication of force-feeding is aspiration pneumonia. If the patient is vomiting or in shock, oral fluid administration is not advised. A more detailed description of oral fluid administration is provided in the literature.[3]

Subcutaneous. Subcutaneous (SQ or SC) fluid administration may be used in mildly to moderately dehydrated patients or in patients that are not critical and that require maintenance fluids. In critical patients, absorption of fluids from the subcutaneous space takes too long to be readily effective. Subcutaneous fluid administration is not practical in patients weighing more than 10 kilograms.[1]

When administering fluids subcutaneously, it is important to use isotonic fluids to assure proper absorption. Fluid is deposited subcutaneously in the dorsal area of loose skin around the shoulders. An 18- to 20-gauge needle connected to an administration set and fluid bag for large volumes or to a syringe for smaller volumes should be used. No more than 10 to 12 ml/kg at each injection site should be administered. The recommended fluid volume for a 5- to 6-kilogram cat is 150 to 200 milliliters subcutaneously once or twice daily.[1] Possible complications are sepsis and irritation. Subcutaneous fluid administration cannot be used if the animal has devitalized skin in the area of administration or if the animal is being treated for severe dehydration or shock.

Intraperitoneal. Intraperitoneal (IP) fluid administration may be an acceptable route when intravenous access is not available. This route of administration allows greater volumes of fluid to be delivered than does the subcutaneous route and has a faster rate of absorption. Isotonic fluids must be used to assure proper absorption. The injection site—halfway between the umbilicus and the pelvic brim, extending from the midline laterally—must be surgically prepared. A 16- to 20-gauge needle attached to an administration set and fluid bag for large volumes or to a syringe for small volumes should be used; the needle should be inserted into the abdomen at an angle parallel to the skin to avoid hitting abdominal organs. Before injecting the fluids, aspiration should be done to make sure that an organ or blood vessel has not been hit. Fluid volumes are similar to those administered intravenously. Possible complications include abdominal sepsis and laceration of abdominal organs. Intraperitoneal fluid administration should not be used if the patient is scheduled for abdominal surgery or if the patient has abdominal sepsis, ascites, or peritonitis.

Intravenous. Intravenous (IV) fluid administration is the preferred method in dehydrated, hypovolemic, and hypotensive patients. When vascular volume is compromised or when the circulatory system is collapsed, peripheral and splanchnic vasoconstriction occur to preserve core blood pressure and circulation to the internal organs. These events make absorption of fluids and medications from the gastrointestinal tract or subcutaneous and peritoneal space difficult and irregular.[4] Intravenous administration offers the advantages of quick uptake into the vasculature and precise administration of specific doses.

To deliver fluids intravenously, a sterile intravenous catheter must be placed and managed throughout the duration of fluid administration. An indwelling jugular catheter is preferred because it provides continuous access to the vascular space for administration of fluids and medications. In addition, there usually is a good venous return, which simplifies repeated blood sampling. A jugular vein is the vein of choice; but when it is unavailable, a lateral saphenous vein in dogs or a medial femoral vein in cats may be used.

TABLE II
Laboratory Findings Associated with Dehydration[2]

Parameter	Normal Values		Laboratory Findings and Diagnosis
	Dogs	*Cats*	
Urine (volume)	24–40 ml/kg/day	22–30 ml/kg/day	If urine volume is decreased and urine specific gravity is increased, dehydration results
Urine (specific gravity)	1.015–1.045	1.015–1.060	If urine volume is increased and urine specific gravity is decreased (isosthenuric), renal disease results
Blood (hematocrit)	37%–55%	22%–45%	An increased hematocrit may indicate dehydration
Blood (serum protein)	6.0–7.8 g/dl	6.0–7.5 g/dl	An increase in serum protein may indicate dehydration

At The Animal Medical Center, a 19-gauge catheter[a] (30.5 centimeters in length, 17-gauge needle) is used for most cats and dogs. Because catheter placement is sometimes very stressful to cats, they are usually tranquilized with a combination of ketamine and diazepam. The dose commonly used at The Animal Medical Center is 0.25 milligrams of diazepam (0.05 ml at 5 mg/ml) and 5 milligrams of ketamine (0.05 ml at 100 mg/ml) intravenously. This usually calms the patient enough to allow for easy catheter placement. For small patients, such as neonates or ferrets, 20-gauge catheters (20 centimeters in length, 13-gauge breakaway needle) may be used.

Proper management of the catheter is extremely important. Fluid volumes are discussed later. Complications include intravenous overload (which causes hypertension), catheter sepsis, phlebitis, and perivascular administration of nonisotonic fluids. The success of this method largely depends on the skill of the health care team and the availability of venous access.

Intraosseous. The intraosseous (IO) route is an excellent alternative method of fluid administration when venous access is not available. Two exemplary situations in which intraosseous administration should be used are when a patient is in hypovolemic crisis and has collapsed veins or when the patient is a small neonate. Intraosseous fluid administration into a nonpneumatic bone, such as the head of the ulna, may also be used in avian patients.[5] Because bone marrow allows excellent uptake of fluids and medications, intraosseous fluid administration may be used to treat hypovolemic shock.

The four preferred sites of injection are the proximal tibial tuberosity, distal tibial tuberosity, proximal medial tibia, and trochanteric fossa of the femur.[4] All four sites allow easy catheterization of the bone marrow and are convenient to bandage. Alternative sites include the wing of the ilium or ischium and the greater tubercle of the humerus. The chosen area is surgically prepared, and a small nick is made in the skin. An 18- to 20-gauge needle, spinal needle with stylet, catheter with stylet, or bone marrow biopsy needle is then introduced into the bone marrow cavity.[4] Next, an administration set is attached and the system is bandaged into place. Fluid volumes are similar to those used for intravenous fluid administration.

Intraosseous fluid administration is contraindicated in the presence of skeletal abnormalities, skin infections over the placement site, and recent fractures to the selected bone.[6] In animals with septic shock, the risk of introducing osteomyelitis must be considered.[6] Possible complications include catheter sepsis and volume overload. Intraosseous fluid administration may be difficult to perform in medium- to large-breed dogs, and success depends largely on the skill of the health care team. Methods of administration and management have been described elsewhere.[6]

DETERMINING THE AMOUNT OF FLUID TO BE ADMINISTERED

After selecting a method of fluid administration, the amount of fluid to be delivered must be determined. This process can be broken down into three parts: rehydration, maintenance, and continuing losses.

Rehydration. Rehydration is the amount of fluid needed to correct the dehydration deficit.[1]

[a]Intracath®, Deseret Medical Inc., Becton-Dickinson & Co., Sandy, Utah 84070.

Volume (ml) of fluid needed for rehydration =
% dehydration × body weight (kg) × 1000

or

Volume (ml) of fluid needed for rehydration =
% dehydration × body weight (lb) × 500

Example: 20-kg (44-lb) dog that is 5% dehydrated
Volume = 5% × 20 kg × 1000 = 1000 ml or 1 L
= 5% × 44 lb × 500 = 1100 ml or 1.1 L

Maintenance. Maintenance is the amount of fluid normally required during a 24-hour period in a hydrated patient. Maintenance fluids include insensible losses, such as those that result from sweating and panting.[1]

Volume = 50 to 60 ml/kg/24 hr (25 to 30 ml/lb/24 hr)

Example: 20-kg (44-lb) dog
Volume = 20 kg × 50 ml/kg/24 hr = 1000 ml or
1 L/24 hr
= 44 lb × 25 ml/lb/24 hr = 1100 ml or
1.1 L/24 hr

Continuing Losses. In addition to rehydration and maintenance fluids, compensation for continuing losses, such as those that result from vomiting and diarrhea, must be added to the fluid plan.[1]

Estimated losses (in milliliters) are added to the fluid plan.

Example: A cat vomits approximately 30 ml of fluid daily and excretes approximately 40 ml of extremely watery diarrhea daily.

70 ml of fluid must be added to the 24-hour fluid plan

Example Problem. A 40-kg dog is 8% dehydrated. The dog is vomiting approximately 400 milliliters of frothy fluid each day. What is the fluid requirement for the first 24 hours in the hospital?

1. Rehydration volume = 40 kg × 8% × 1000 = 3200 ml or 3.2 L
2. Maintenance volume = 40 kg × 50 ml/kg/24 hr = 2000 ml or 2 L
3. Continuing losses = 400 ml/24 hr or 0.4 L

Total fluid plan for 24 hours = (1) + (2) + (3) = 3.2 L + 2 L
+ 0.4 L = 5.6 L

DELIVERING FLUIDS

For the mildly to moderately dehydrated patient that is not in shock, a routine fluid plan can be followed. The fluid volume is best divided into several allotments over a 24-hour period. A reasonably good plan is to take the total fluid volume, divide it by three, and give the fluid three times daily. For example, a 40-kilogram dog that is 8% dehydrated would receive 5.6 liters every 24 hours or 1.8 liters three times daily. The patient must be carefully monitored throughout the fluid plan.

After the first 24 hours of fluid administration, another physical examination is done and a new fluid plan can be determined for the next 24-hour period. Fluid administration is a very dynamic treatment. Because the requirements of the patient may continually change, the fluid plan must be flexible.

FLUID VOLUMES FOR HYPOVOLEMIC PATIENTS

For patients in acute hypovolemic shock, the treatment is intravenous or intraosseous fluid administration of a crystalloid fluid, such as lactated Ringer's solution, or blood products if the hypovolemic shock is the result of acute blood loss. The goal is to expand the blood vasculature, enabling the circulatory system to return to a properly functioning state. Secondary problems can be dealt with after the hypovolemic shock is corrected. To expand the vasculature, one blood volume equivalent of fluid must be administered. The blood volume in an adult patient is 90 ml/kg. The fluid should be given at a rate of 60 to 80 ml/kg/hr for one hour[1] under direct supervision and constant monitoring. In general, the rate of administration should not exceed 80 ml/kg/hr. It is extremely important to monitor the patient in shock while fluid therapy is being administered and to reassess the patient after one hour. If the patient is no longer in a crisis state, dehydration and fluid status can be redetermined and a reasonable plan can be established.

If a patient has a combination of mild volume contraction and dehydration, an alternative fluid plan may be required. A reasonable approach is to administer one quarter to one half of a blood volume equivalent of fluid over one to two hours and then to administer the remainder of the calculated 24-hour dose evenly over the remaining 22 hours. This approach restores vascular volume more quickly without causing volume overload and starts correction of the dehydration deficit.[4]

DETERMINING THE FLUID RATE

After the fluid plan has been devised, it is important to determine the rate at which fluids must be administered.

Fluids are generally delivered through an intravenous administration set attached to a fluid bag or bottle. Administration sets are available in a variety of sizes and shapes. At The Animal Medical Center, an adult administration set (10 drops/ml) and a pediatric set (60 drops/ml) are used. In addition to the administration sets, a special fluid chamber is available for administering fluid volumes less than 150 milliliters. Adult administration sets usually are used on patients that weigh more than 10 kilograms, and pediatric administration sets are used on patients that weigh less than 10 kilograms. Pediatric sets are also used to administer small amounts of fluid.

To determine the rate of fluid administration, several calculations must be performed. First, the so-called drop factor (which is a specific number) must be calculated. The drop factor is used in a second formula that determines the rate of fluid administration in drops per minute.

$$\text{drop factor}^1 = \frac{60}{\text{drops/ml}} \quad \text{(each commercially available administration set provides a different number of drops/ml)}$$

$$\text{rate of fluid administration in drops/min} = \frac{\text{desired ml/hr}}{\text{drop factor}}$$

Example Problem. A 15-kilogram dog needs to receive 750 milliliters over 24 hours (or 250 milliliters three times daily). At what rate should the fluid be administered for an 8-hour period if an administration set that delivers 10 drops/ml is used?

1. Determine the fluid requirement in ml/hr
   250 ml/8 hr = ~ 31 ml/hr

2. Determine the drop factor
   $$\text{drop factor} = \frac{60}{10 \text{ drops/ml}} = 6$$

3. Determine the drip rate in drops/min
   $$\text{drops/min} = \frac{31 \text{ ml/hr}}{6} = \sim 5$$

In summary, the fluids should be set at a rate of 5 drops/min to deliver 250 ml of fluid over an 8-hour period.

For critical patients, use of a constant rate infusion (CRI) pump should be considered. These pumps are effective for delivering very small volumes of fluid (including blood) and certain intravenous medications, such as lidocaine or dopamine. Constant rate infusion pumps are mechanical devices that allow precise, timed delivery of fluids. The drip rate is set in milliliters per hour. There are two basic kinds of constant rate infusion pumps. The most commonly used pump is used in conjunction with a specialized administration set. Using a motorized wheel, fluid is pumped through the lines rather than being administered by gravity. Another type of constant rate infusion pump is a syringe infusion pump, which can be used for volumes of fluids less than 35 milliliters. This is a special pump into which a 35-ml syringe is loaded. An extension set is attached to the syringe, and again the drip rate is set in the pump (in ml/hr). A springlike device pushes the plunger of the syringe at the appropriate rate.

MONITORING THE PATIENT RECEIVING FLUIDS

Improperly administered fluids can result in death. Several parameters must be monitored while fluids are being administered: color and moistness of the mucous membranes, capillary refill time, skin tugor, heart rate, pulse rate and quality, respiratory rate and quality, body weight, urine output, central venous pressure, and overall demeanor of the patient. In addition, the lungs must be auscultated and the results of various laboratory tests (packed cell volume and serum protein) must be continually evaluated.

A potential life-threatening problem associated with fluid administration is volume overload caused by too rapid a rate of administration or too great a volume of fluid infused. Two excellent methods of monitoring the patient to prevent volume overload leading to hypertension are to measure central venous pressure and to auscultate the lungs. The normal range for central venous pressure is from 0 to 10 centimeters of water. A higher value may indicate venous overload. Auscultation of the lungs can detect harsh lung sounds, which may indicate pulmonary edema caused by fluid overbalance. The possibility of pulmonary edema may be confirmed by radiographic examination of the thorax.

A good method of monitoring the patient is to have charts designed to simplify recordkeeping. Charts can be designed for routine fluid administration as well as for intensive care units. The charts used in intensive care units should allow the veterinarian or technician to easily recognize alarming trends in the patient data.

TAPERING THE FLUID PLAN

After the patient has been rehydrated and seems to be recovering, the fluid plan is usually reduced to maintenance requirements only. If the patient has been receiving fluids for more than two days, the fluid plan must be gradually reduced as opposed to being abruptly stopped. During fluid therapy, the kidneys may produce an increased amount of urine because of the increased amount of fluid being administered. If the fluids are suddenly stopped, the kidneys might still produce a large amount of urine, thus leading to patient dehydration. A reasonable plan would be to use the dose being given three times daily on a twice daily basis, thereby reducing the total fluid plan by one third. For a cat receiving 100 milliliters three times daily (a total of 300 ml/day), for example, the regimen should be changed to 100 milliliters twice daily (a total of 200 ml/day). If the patient continues to recover on this amount of fluid, the regimen can be reduced by another one third and administered either at a rate of 100 milliliters once daily or 50 milliliters twice daily (a total of 100 ml/day).

The patient must be monitored closely for any signs of deterioration throughout the duration of therapy. If the patient continues to do well, the fluid plan can be stopped completely. It is important to supply fresh water at all times while tapering the fluids so that the patient can supplement its own needs by drinking water.

KINDS OF SOLUTIONS TO USE FOR FLUID THERAPY

Numerous types of solutions are commercially available for use in fluid therapy. The solutions can be classified into various categories. One way of classifying a fluid solution is by tonicity. Normal osmolality of blood and extracellular fluid is 290 to 310 mOsm/kg.[1] The osmolality of isotonic solutions is the same as that of blood and extracellular water. When infused intravenously, isotonic solutions produce no significant changes in the blood. The osmolality of hypotonic solutions is lower than that of blood; hypotonic solutions can cause red blood cells to swell. The osmolality

(continues on page 556)

HELPFUL HINTS ON FLUID ADMINISTRATION

1. All fluid bags should be labeled with tape; the information on the tape should include the date of opening and the supplements that were added.

2. To predetermine where the fluid volume should stop in a bag or bottle, place the labeling tape horizontally across the bag or bottle.

   Example: 800 ml of fluid must be administered from a 1000-ml bag.

   Place the tape horizontally around the bag at the 800-ml mark so that anyone who walks by knows to stop the fluids at that level.

3. If a whole bag or bottle is to be administered to a patient, place the tape vertically so that anyone who walks by will know that the patient is to receive the entire bag or bottle.

4. When using a pediatric administration set with a 150-ml chamber, the chamber should be filled only with the amount of fluid required for that treatment. Doing so will enable anyone to know that the patient is to receive the entire volume of fluid.

5. For critical patients, make sure to record the time when fluid therapy is started.

6. When the fluid administration is finished, an intravenous catheter should be flushed with a heparin and saline solution to prevent blood clots from forming in the catheter. A mixture of 1000 units of heparin per 250 milliliters of saline is effective.

TABLE III
Composition of Common Crystalloid Fluid Solutions[7]

Solution	Na^+ (mEq/L)	K^+ (mEq/L)	Cl^- (mEq/L)	Ca^{++} (mEq/L)	Mg^{++} (mEq/L)	HCO_3 (mEq/L)	Dextrose (g/dl)	Osmolality (mOsm/kg)
Lactated Ringer's solution	130	4	109	3	0	28 lactate	0	274
Acetated Ringer's solution (Plasmalyte®)	140	5	98	0	3	27 acetate	0	296
0.9% Saline	154	0	154	0	0	0	0	308
5% Dextrose in water	0	0	0	0	0	0	5	278
One-half strength lactated Ringer's solution + 2½% dextrose	65.5	2	55	1.5	0	14 lactate	2.5	263

of hypertonic solutions is greater than that of blood; hypertonic solutions cause red blood cells to shrink.

Another way to classify a fluid solution is to determine whether the solution is composed of a crystalloid or colloid base solution.

Crystalloid Solutions

Crystalloids are sodium-based electrolyte solutions that are commonly used for fluid therapy. The composition of these solutions is similar to that of plasma water; thus, they can be given rapidly and in large volumes without drastically changing the constituents of the intravascular fluid. The composition of common crystalloid fluid solutions is given in Table III.[7]

Isotonic Saline (0.9% Sodium Chloride). Saline is mainly used to expand plasma volume and to correct hyponatremia or metabolic alkalosis.[1] All of the intravenously administered fluid stays in the extracellular fluid, with two thirds being distributed to the interstitial fluid and one third being distributed to the intravascular fluid space.[1] Saline should not be used in patients with suspected or known heart failure or in patients that have a sodium restriction.

One-Half Strength (0.45%) Sodium Chloride plus 2½% Dextrose plus 5 mEq Potassium/250 ml of Fluid. A modified saline solution (½ strength NaCl + 2½% dextrose + 5 mEq K/250 ml of fluid) can be used to treat patients with sodium restrictions. It can be used as a maintenance solution for cats with lower urinary tract disease to avoid iatrogenic hypernatremia.[1]

5% Dextrose in Water. When 5% dextrose in water (D5W) is administered intravenously, the patient's normal hormone mechanism maintains normal glycemia and utilizes the dextrose in the solution; essentially, then, free water is being administered. Five percent dextrose in water divides between the intracellular and extracellular fluid compartments, with two thirds going to intracellular fluid and one third going to extracellular fluid. In the extracellular fluid compartment, three quarters is interstitial and one quarter is intravascular.[1] Because a relatively small amount of fluid (8%) is distributed to the intravascular space,[1] 5% dextrose in water is not a good choice for a fluid solution when the objective is to replenish fluid in the intravascular space (e.g., in patients with hypovolemic shock).

The indications for 5% dextrose in water are as treatment for hypernatremia, as a carbohydrate source administered in addition to other fluids, and as a fluid supplement for patients that cannot tolerate sodium. Five percent dextrose in water should not be used as the sole maintenance fluid therapy because hyponatremia, hypochloremia, hypokalemia, and hypomagnesemia may occur.[1] It should not be given subcutaneously because extracellular fluid already in the body will migrate to the pool of 5% dextrose in water, thereby increasing the volume depletion and possibly leading to shock.

Lactated Ringer's Solution. Lactated Ringer's solution is the fluid of choice in many disease states. It is one of the most versatile fluids available because it can be administered intravenously, subcutaneously, intraperitoneally, and intraosseously. Lactated Ringer's solution is a saline and lactate solution with electrolytes added. It has a reduced sodium content compared with 0.9% sodium chloride.[1] The lactate is broken down by the liver to bicarbonate; thus, it is helpful in the treatment of metabolic acidosis syndromes. In addition, lactated Ringer's solution can be useful as a maintenance solution.

One-Half Strength Lactated Ringer's Solution plus 2½% Dextrose. A modified lactated Ringer's solution (½ strength lactated Ringer's solution + $2\frac{1}{2}\%$ dextrose) has a reduced sodium content that may be helpful in the treatment of hypernatremic patients.

Acetated Ringer's Solution. Plasmalyte® (Baxter HealthCare) is an acetated Ringer's solution in contrast to lactated Ringer's solution. Compared with lactated Ringer's solution, Plasmalyte® has less chloride, more magnesium (lactated Ringer's solution has none), and no calcium (lactated Ringer's solution has some). Plasmalyte® uses acetate as a base that is broken down by the skeletal muscle into bicarbonate. Some researchers believe that acetate should be used instead of lactate when liver disease is present, but there is no definite evidence to support this theory. At The Animal Medical Center, lactated Ringer's solution and Plasmalyte® are used interchangeably; however, Plasmalyte® should not be administered subcutaneously because it causes irritation.

Colloid Solutions

Colloid solutions contain large particles that do not leave the vascular space easily and therefore expand the vascular volume. Colloid solutions are indicated most commonly for patients with hypovolemia and hypoproteinemia (when plasma albumin is lower than 1.5 g/dl).[4] Trauma patients in hypovolemic shock may have capillary damage in many organ systems. Capillary damage increases the likelihood of excessive fluid entry into tissue when crystalloid solutions are given.[4] Excessive fluid entry can cause severe problems with cranial or pulmonary trauma because cerebral or pulmonary edema may occur and lead to death. Thus, it may be beneficial to use a colloid solution to treat shock patients.

Dextran. Dextran is an artificial colloid derived from sugar beets. It is not commonly used in veterinary medicine because serious side effects, such as decreased coagulation and platelet function, renal failure, anaphylactic shock, and decreased immune function, have been reported in humans.[4]

Hetastarch. Hetastarch is a synthetic colloid plasma volume expander that lasts longer and has fewer side effects than dextran. The hetastarch solution is a combination of hydroxyethyl starch and normal saline and is used to treat hypovolemic shock and hypoproteinemia. New particles of the starch are continually formed as α-amylase in the bloodstream breaks down large particles into smaller particles.[4] The small particles are then excreted.

In human studies, a 500-ml infusion of hetastarch raised plasma volume by 9%.[4] Plasma volume returns to baseline in 48 hours. Because hydroxyethyl starch is a starch

molecule, it may cause an increase of serum amylase (unassociated with pancreatitis) for three to five days. Hetastarch is a hypertonic solution and must be administered by slow infusion at a rate of 10 to 20 ml/kg/24 hr.[4] This dose may be given over an eight-hour period in addition to regular fluid therapy. In cases of severe hypovolemic shock that is not responsive to crystalloid therapy, hetastarch may be given in a shock dose rate of 20 ml/kg/hr for one hour under direct supervision. The patient should then be reevaluated. Side effects may include allergic reactions and coagulopathies, although neither has been reported in humans when the rate is less than 20 ml/kg/24 hr.[4] One disadvantage of hetastarch is the significant cost of the product.

Hetastarch should not be used as a maintenance fluid therapy. The solution is designed to be used as a one-time treatment to correct hypovolemia. Normal maintenance fluids should also be administered. If the hypovolemia has not been corrected in 24 hours, another dose of hetastarch may be administered. The patient needs to be reassessed after each treatment.

Common Fluid Additives

In addition to the crystalloid and colloid solutions described, special additives to the fluid plan may help improve support to the patient. The veterinary technician should be familiar with some of the more common additives, such as 50% dextrose, potassium, and vitamins.

50% Dextrose. When a patient is debilitated, anorectic, or prone to hypoglycemia, a dextrose supplement may be required. Short-term anorexia alone in an adult animal does not produce hypoglycemia. A problem may occur, however, in anorectic patients with increased metabolic requirements (associated with fever, sepsis, or hyperthyroidism) or with gluconeogenic disorders (associated with end-stage liver disease, renal failure, or hypoadrenocorticism).[4] The goal of adding dextrose is not to provide adequate calories but to serve as an energy source for the brain. Patients become lethargic, dull, and weak and may have a seizure if hypoglycemia occurs. Enteral or parenteral nutrition may also need to be supplemented in the anorectic patient.

When a patient has a blood glucose value lower than or equal to 80 mg/dl, dextrose should be added to the fluids to make a $2\frac{1}{2}\%$ solution. If the blood glucose continues to remain at or below 80 mg/dl, the solution may be increased to 5% dextrose. In patients with unregulated insulinoma or severe sepsis, it may be necessary to increase the solution to $7\frac{1}{2}\%$ or greater dextrose. If, however, a dextrose drip is increased to greater than 5%, the solution will become hyper-

TABLE IV
Amount of 50% Dextrose
to Add to a Fluid Bag or Bottle

Size of Fluid Bag or Bottle	Amount (in ml) of 50% Dextrose to Add	
	2½% Solution	5% Solution
250 ml	12.5	25
500 ml	25	50
1000 ml	50	100

TABLE V
Potassium Supplementation[3]

Serum Potassium (mEq/L)	Supplemental Potassium per 250 ml of Fluid
3.5–5.5 (Normal)	5 mEq
3.0–3.4	7 mEq
2.5–2.9	10 mEq
2.0–2.4	15 mEq
<2.0	20 mEq

osmotic and may cause phlebitis in small veins. Therefore, dextrose solutions greater than 5% should be administered through a large, central bore vein.

Table IV helps to determine the amount of 50% dextrose to add to a fluid bag. Before adding the dextrose, fluid should be withdrawn (and discarded) in an amount equal to the amount of fluid to be added; if this is not done, the dilution will be incorrect.

Potassium. Potassium supplementation is required in anorectic patients. Potassium is usually available in food and is lost easily in urine. Patients on fluid diuresis are prone to hypokalemia. Normal serum potassium is 3.5 to 5.5 mEq/L.[4] Table V helps to determine the correct dose of supplemental potassium.

Failure to correct hypokalemia can result in muscle weakness, lethargy, anorexia, vomiting, and inability to concentrate urine. Potassium must be given intravenously in a slow drip. If given too fast, potassium can cause adverse cardiac effects and hyperkalemia.

Vitamins. Many water-soluble vitamins, especially B-complex vitamins, are lost rapidly in the polyuric and/or anorectic patient. Any patient on fluid diuresis must be supplemented with B vitamins. In general, 0.5 milliliters of B-complex per 250 milliliters of fluid should be added. If the diuresis or debilitation is severe, this dose can be doubled to 1 millililter of B-complex per 250 ml of fluid.

CONCLUSION

For a number of disease states, including dehydration and shock, the treatment of choice is intravenous fluid administration via an indwelling jugular catheter. Depending on the patient's status, a crystalloid fluid solution with or without fluid supplements should be the primary fluid administered. Careful monitoring and assessment of the patient are critical to successful fluid administration.

ACKNOWLEDGMENTS

I would like to extend my thanks to Dr. Kathy Salmeri and Dr. Michael Garvey of The Animal Medical Center for their assistance.

REFERENCES

1. Schaer M: General principles of fluid therapy in small animal medicine. *Vet Clin North Am* 19:203–212, 1989.
2. Kirk RW, Bistner SI: Simplified fluid therapy, in Kirk RW, Bistner SI (ed): *Handbook of Veterinary Procedures and Emergency Treatment*, ed 4. Philadelphia, WB Saunders Co, 1985, pp 591–617.
3. Zenger E, Willard MD, et al: Oral rehydration therapy in companion animals. *Compan Anim Pract* 19:6–10, 1989.
4. Garvey MS: Fluid and electrolyte balance in critical patients. *Vet Clin North Am* 19:1021–1054, 1989.
5. Crowe DT: Performing life-saving cardiovascular surgery. *Vet Med* 84:77–83, 1989.
6. Otto CM, McCall-Kaufman G, Crowe DT, et al: Intraosseous infusion of fluids and therapeutics. *Compend Contin Educ Pract Vet* 11(4):421–430, 1989.
7. Garvey MS, Fox PR: *The Animal Medical Center Formulary*, ed 2. New York, The Animal Medical Center, 1990.

BIBLIOGRAPHY

Bell FW, Osborne CA: Maintenance fluid therapy, in Kirk RW (ed): *Current Veterinary Therapy*, ed 10. Philadelphia, WB Saunders Co, 1989, pp 37–43.
Kirby R: Critical care—The overview. *Vet Clin North Am* 19:1007–1019, 1989.

Technique in Intravenous Catheterization in Dogs and Cats—Part I

Lorraine M. Crachy, AHT
Athens, Georgia

Perfecting the art of intravenous catheterization is mandatory in providing good patient care. When the technician performs intravenous catheterization and maintenance with a high degree of competency, the procedure saves the veterinarian time, money, and worry. This article describes the three types of intravenous catheters currently used in veterinary practice, as well as placement techniques. Part II will describe bandaging techniques, catheter management, and handling complications associated with intravenous catheters.

Before 1940, intravenous medications were administered to human patients through syringe and needle with a new venipuncture performed for each treatment. During the early 1940s, a new technique was developed in which plastic tubing was passed through the hub of a 17-gauge steel needle that had been inserted into a vein. When the needle was withdrawn from the vein, an adapter was placed on the tubing.[1] This made continuous fluid therapy available and allowed continued access to the vein. The intravenous catheter has been improved over the past 40 years by advances in catheter materials, designs, and placement techniques.

There are three catheter systems currently used in veterinary practice (Figure 1). Winged catheters (Butterfly®—CEVA Laboratories) and injection needles used as catheters will be discussed together. The winged catheter has plastic wings at the needle hub and intravenous tubing extending 8 to 12 in. from the hub. This makes securing the needle easier and allows greater mobility of the needle hub. The over-the-needle catheter[2] (Surflo®—Terumo, Sovereign Indwelling Catheter®—Sherwood Medical) consists of a needle/stylet with a bevel that extends beyond the length of the catheter. The needle bevel is introduced into the vein and is followed by the catheter. When the catheter is completely within the vein, the stylet is removed. This system allows free movement of the limb once the catheter is secured to

the leg. The through-the-needle catheter (Bard®, I-Cath®—C. R. Bard) encloses the catheter within the lumen of the needle; the catheter is threaded through the needle once the needle has been introduced into the vein. The needle is then withdrawn from the vein, and the system is secured to the patient's neck or a limb.

Several criteria must be considered when selecting an intravenous catheter. The advantages and disadvantages of each system are weighed, as are the patient's needs and the veins available.

The use of winged catheters is often criticized, but the winged type catheter has advantages that should be recognized. Winged catheters have the lowest incidence of local infection.[3,4] Technically, winged catheters are the simplest system to insert. In addition, these catheters are often useful in the anesthetized patient where access to the lingual vein, femoral vein, auricular vein, or even the tail vein may be life saving. Winged catheters are beneficial in both very small patients and patients that need numerous venipunctures but not long-term fluid therapy (i.e., thiacetarsamide sodium [Carparsolate®—CEVA Laboratories] during heartworm treatment). However, the disadvantages of winged catheters, although few, often outweigh the advantages. Two drawbacks are that the catheter requires constant supervision because it is sharp and easily punctures or lacerates the vessel wall, and stabilization of the catheter is difficult.

Originally published in Volume 4, Number 6, November/December 1983

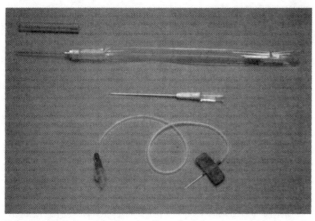

Figure 1—The through-the-needle catheter (*top*), over-the-needle catheter (*center*), and the winged catheter (*bottom*) are displayed.

The over-the-needle catheter has many advantages, especially when therapy is expected to continue for less than 24 hours. It is relatively inexpensive and is much easier to stabilize than the winged catheter, and because of its increased stability, constant supervision is not essential. The over-the-needle catheter is available in a wide variety of gauges and lengths. Minimal perivascular bleeding occurs when over-the-needle catheters are used, since the needle makes the correct size hole for the catheter. A disadvantage of the over-the-needle catheter is that it is easy to contaminate the exposed catheter accidentally. Other disadvantages are that this type of catheter is a problem to maintain for extended periods (over 48 hours) because it is difficult to stabilize in the large bore veins (i.e., jugular veins), and it often compromises venous return in smaller veins. Whenever venous return is compromised, the vessel is subject to phlebitis because of static blood flow around the catheter.[5,6] A catheter intended for long-term use should not compromise venous return; therefore, a long-term catheter should be inserted into a large bore vein. Generally, leg veins are not acceptable for long-term intravenous catheterization, except in very large dogs.

The primary advantage of the through-the-needle type of catheter is that it is the easiest catheter to maintain for extended periods if inserted by sterile technique.[4-6] The through-the-needle catheter is usually placed in a jugular vein. The catheter lengths range from 20 to 90 cm, therefore preventing placement of the catheter in leg veins without passing an area of flexion. There are four major disadvantages of the through-the-needle catheter. First, it is the most expensive of the three catheter systems. Second, some perivascular bleeding occurs because the needle, which is removed from the vein after catheter insertion, is a larger gauge than the catheter maintained in the vein. Third, placement of the through-the-needle catheter is technically more difficult than placement of the other two systems. Fourth, complications from incorrect placement can be life threatening.[5,7]

Several accessible veins can accept one system or all three catheter systems. A vein may be ruled out due to scarring, edema, open wounds, fractures under it, signs of phlebitis, or venous anatomy that would force the catheter through an area of flexion. Each patient and each vein must be evaluated individually, and catheter gauge and length must be chosen to meet a patient's specific needs.

Gauges of catheters and needles are measured by the outside diameters. In determining flow rate, the bore, or inside diameter, becomes the determining factor. By doubling the height of the fluids administered, flow rate is also doubled; but, according to Poiseuille's law, to double the internal diameter of the catheter increases flow rate 16 times.[8] Smaller gauge catheters do not compromise venous return, but flow rate decreases significantly.

Catheter length is chosen by considering patient size and needs and the type of catheter being placed. The longer the catheter, the more stable it becomes, thereby decreasing the mechanical irritation that predisposes the vein to phlebitis.[5] A catheter placed in a limb vein must end before the bend at a joint; otherwise the catheter may kink or be subject to embolus.

When the need for long-term therapy is anticipated, the through-the-needle catheter is the system of choice.[4,6] Veterinary patients usually tolerate through-the-needle catheters better than limb catheters, and through-the-needle catheters are less prone to soiling or mutilation by the patient. Through-the-needle catheters can also be used to measure central venous pressure by extension just into the right atrium. The heart is located between the third and sixth ribs,[9] and the right atrium lies in the cranial aspect of the heart. Therefore, the catheter should extend to the third intercostal space but no farther. If central venous pressure is not to be monitored, a shorter catheter may be chosen. Since the jugular vein is the largest bore peripheral vein, the through-the-needle catheter is the catheter of choice when treating the patient in hypovolemic shock. The through-the-needle is the longest system, making it the most stable. When placed in a large bore vein, there is a reduced risk of early mechanical and or chemical irritation. Irritating drugs should be administered only into large bore veins, which allow dilution of the irritant to prevent chemically caused phlebitis.

Restraint Techniques

Adequate patient restraint is important whenever intravenous catheterization is performed (Figure 2). Before restraining the patient, time should be taken to become familiar with the animal and to evaluate its temperament. During restraint, eye contact accompanied by a soothing or firm voice speaking to an upset patient is often more effective than physical control. The patient must be encouraged to lie still willingly to prevent traumatic catheterization. This is accomplished only through gentle animal handling.

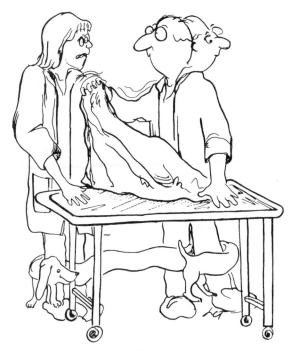

Figure 2—A patient restraint is shown.

Patient Preparation

The main objective in preparing the vein for catheter introduction is to avoid sepsis. To avoid iatrogenic infection, strict adherence to aseptic technique is recommended during each introduction of a catheter. Steps of aseptic technique are:

1. Clip the hair approximately the width of a clipper blade on each side of the vein.
2. Scrub the vein with a surgical soap (Betadine®— Purdue Frederick, Nolvasan®—Fort Dodge Laboratories).
3. Rinse off the scrub with sterile 3×3-in. gauze sponges soaked in isopropyl alcohol or sterile saline.
4. Repeat the scrub and rinse cycle three times over five minutes.
5. Spray the area with povidone-iodine or poloxamer-iodine solution (Prepodyn®—West Chemical Products). A study of surgical hand-washing agents has shown that poloxamer-iodine spray gives a high degree of bacteriostatic effectiveness over time when sprayed on and left to air dry.[10]
6. Allow the area to air dry.

Placement of the Catheter

In the presence of blood, artificial materials such as plastic and steel catheters incite a rapid adsorption of protein, which forms a surface protein layer on the artificial material. Diseases associated with an increase in various serum proteins may result in greater frequency of thrombus formation.[5] To reduce thrombosis, a smooth and atraumatic catheterization procedure must be performed to minimize activation of the clotting mechanisms.

Winged Catheter

To prepare for catheterization, tape should be cut in lengths long enough to go around the limb two to three times. Removal of the tape after catheter placement, is easier if tabs are made by bending sticky side to sticky side on the ends of tape pieces. The fluid and administration set is assembled. To eliminate dead space, the tubing and needle are flushed with sterile saline or fluid from the fluid bottle. Hands must be washed, and the skin should be prepared as described above. A restrainer occludes the vein.

With the left hand, the vein is immobilized by stretching the skin between two points of traction (usually the restrainer's occlusion is one point) to prevent lateral rolling of the vein as well as longitudinal wrinkling. It is important not to immobilize the vein by putting the thumb lateral to it as to do so may cause the vein to collapse. The winged catheter is held with the right forefinger and thumb on the wings. The bevel of the needle is up.

A venipuncture site is selected where the vein is very straight and long enough to accept the length of a catheter. If a site is chosen too close to a point of flexion, the needle will lacerate the vessel wall. Venipuncture is made, and the needle is threaded completely into a vein up to the wings of the catheter (Figure 3). Venipuncture can be accomplished in one of two ways.[2]

Indirect Venipuncture—The needle is pointed in the direction of blood flow and held at a 45° angle, slightly to one side and about ½ in. below the site of entry into the vein. Once into the skin, the angle of the needle is decreased to almost parallel with the skin and the needle is directed completely into the vein.

Direct Venipuncture—The needle is held at a 30° angle over the vein. Carefully, but with a quick motion, the skin is punctured and the needle is advanced completely into the vein in a single motion.

If the catheter hub is not yet attached to the fluid administration set, then blood should be flowing back through the catheter tubing. If the catheter is attached to the fluid administration set, then confirmation of

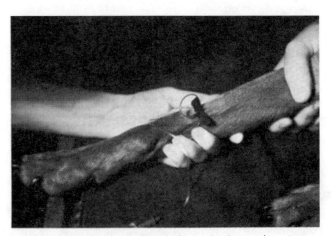

Figure 3—Winged catheter threaded completely into the vein.

intravenous catheterization can be made by lowering the fluid bottle to a level below that of the patient and observing blood flow into the intravenous tubing. Aspiration from an injection port in the fluid administration line is not recommended in winged catheters as it often collapses the vein. The most difficult aspect of using a winged catheter is stabilization of the system. The animal's handler and the operator must act as a team. The vein must remain motionless until the catheter is stabilized. One-half-in. porous tape (Zonas®— Johnson & Johnson Products) is applied directly to the wings of the catheter, wrapped around the limb once, and then wrapped around the limb a second time incorporating the catheter intravenous tubing. To prevent laceration of the vein, this wrapping must be done without moving the needle. If needle movement occurs, needle placement must be reconfirmed. If the catheterization team feels that this stabilization is inadequate, a support wrap or coaptation splint may be carefully applied for added stabilization.[11] The patient must remain under immediate supervision during the entire period of catheterization.

Over-the-Needle Catheter

Preparation for over-the-needle catheters is the same as for winged catheters. If the system is to be bandaged, the necessary bandage material should be assembled. The venipuncture site must include a straight length of vein that can accept the length of the catheter. With leg veins, this site is generally a distal part.

For a patient that is dehydrated, in shock, or thick-skinned, a peephole may be made with a 20-gauge needle before catheterization to visualize the vein more clearly

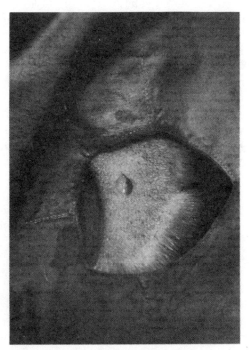

Figure 4—The peephole lies just above the vein.

and to avoid dulling the needle by skin puncture. The skin is pulled laterally or medially away from the vein; the needle is inserted bevel side up through the skin, which normally lies just above the planned venipuncture site. A quick pull up of the needle is made, which will cut a skin-deep, ⅛- to ¼-in. hole. When the skin is allowed to return to its normal position, the hole will lie just above the vein (Figure 4). This peephole is then used for needle insertion, enabling the needle/stylet to puncture the vein. The catheter is held in the right hand at the needle/stylet hub, not at the catheter hub. It is important to keep the bevel of the needle/stylet up. The bevel distance of the needle must be examined to determine how far the needle must be introduced to assure catheter introduction into the vein.

With over-the-needle catheters, venipuncture is easier by the indirect method described above. When blood is flowing into the stylet hub, the catheter is advanced another ⅛ to ¼ in. depending on the bevel-to-catheter distance. A second check must be made to verify that blood continues to flow into the stylet hub. The stylet hub is then held still with the left hand while the catheter is advanced with the right hand. When the catheter is in place, the stylet is removed from it, the intravenous drip set is attached to the catheter hub, and the intravenous infusion drip is started.

The catheter must be held in place with a forefinger and thumb until taping is completed. During the taping, the left hand encircles the patient's limb. The restrainer continues to hold the joint above the catheter in extension until the catheter is secured. When the catheter is secure, the right hand of the restrainer is free to clean blood from the patient. A sterile gauze dressing and antimicrobial ointment[6] must be used at the catheter site.

A length of precut tape, with its sticky side toward the patient, is slipped under the catheter just distal to the venipuncture point. The tape is applied around the limb; the second wrap around the limb secures the catheter hub to the first taping. Tape cannot be placed directly over the venipuncture site as tape is not sterile. The tape-to-tape method prevents the catheter from slipping out when the skin is damp. Taping must begin immediately distal to the point of catheter insertion, since the catheter will pull out to the point where the tape starts.

If the catheter is not to be bandaged in place, a loop is made in the intravenous tubing near the connection to the catheter and taped in place just distal to the first taping. This taping should not be above the catheter taping or it will occlude the vein. In addition, this second taping should not be on or below the next distal joint where any joint movement will pull at the catheter.

Through-the-Needle Catheter

Preparation for catheterization with a through-the-needle catheter is the same as the steps described for placement of the over-the-needle catheter, except that

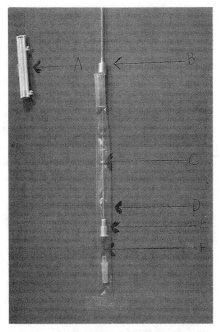

Figure 5—The parts composing the through-the-needle catheter. (*A*) catheter guard, (*B*) needle, (*C*) catheter within the envelope, (*D*) envelope, (*E*) catheter hub, (*F*) stylet.

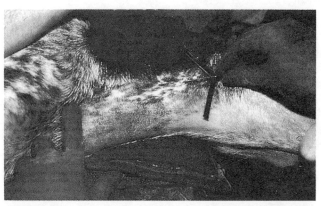

Figure 6—The through-the-needle catheter is directed toward the heart.

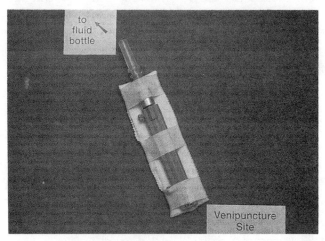

Figure 7—Catheter guard secured to the tongue depressor. Tape wings are then applied to the tongue depressor as close to the venipuncture site as possible.

the through-the-needle catheter is not flushed before placement. A tongue depressor splint is prepared by breaking a tongue depressor in half. Three to four pieces of 1-in. tape are wrapped around it to dull the broken end. This piece of tongue depressor should be longer than the catheter guard by ¾ to 1 in.

Because this catheter is large gauge, can be sutured in place, and is more easily placed when a peephole is made, local infiltration of 2% lidocaine is recommended after skin preparation.

The system should be examined. Different companies add features to their catheters to make it easier to place, secure, or maintain the catheters. Examining and thoroughly understanding the system is imperative before venipuncture is made. The basic through-the-needle catheter consists of a catheter guard, needle, catheter, envelope, catheter hub, and stylet (Figure 5). The catheter is held in the right hand, like a pencil between forefinger and thumb, with the catheter resting on the third finger and on the second joint in the forefinger. Venipuncture is made by the indirect method described earlier for winged catheter placement, but a peephole must be made.[a] The catheter needle is directed toward the heart (Figure 6).

After venipuncture, blood flows into the catheter inside the envelope. The needle is advanced its full distance to make sure it is completely within the vein; the catheter is rechecked for continued blood flow. With the left hand holding the needle in place, the catheter is advanced through the envelope into the vein and the

needle guard is placed. The stylet is removed from the vein, and the intravenous setup is attached and the drip started.

With ½-in. tape, the catheter guard is secured to the tongue depressor splint by attaching the intravenous set adapter to the tongue depressor and securing the needle bevel end of the catheter guard to the tongue depressor (Figure 7). The additional stabilization helps prevent catheter failure due to kinking at the needle tip and pulling apart at the adapter point. The stabilization also incorporates the catheter and administration tubing into one unit.

With ½-in. tape, wings are made at the needle tip end of the tongue depressor system, and the tongue depressor system is angled slightly so that it points behind or toward the patient's ear. The system is sutured in place by making one suture on either side of it. The sutures must be very close to the depressor and to the venipuncture site.

Povidone-iodine antiseptic ointment is applied to the skin puncture site, since it has been shown that antibacterial ointments alone support fungal growth.[5] An ointment should be used because the environment at

---

[a]*Editor's Note:* When using catheters with sharp needles, a peephole may not be necessary.

the catheter site has been so altered that it is susceptible to infection by common skin organisms.[6]

A sterile gauze sponge should be placed over the venipuncture site and partly over the tongue depressor system, and tape should go around the patient's neck. The system must first be wrapped into place with several layers of cast padding (Specialist®—Johnson & Johnson Products), then with gauze roll (Kling®—Johnson & Johnson Products), and finally with an elastic bandage (Elastikon®—Johnson & Johnson Products). This bandaging is important to protect the venipuncture site from environmental contamination and to prevent catheter movement at the venipuncture site, which would cause a mechanically induced phlebitis. Looping the administration tubing at the end of the tongue depressor system and incorporating it into the bandage prevents tension from being placed on the catheter itself.

By taping the administration adapter to the catheter as explained above, the fluid administration system has been closed; there is no way for organisms to enter the system. The system remains sterile as long as it remains a closed system. The administration set should be equipped with an injection port (FluVen 0150®— Venusa Ltd, Venoset,® Venoset® Microdrip—CEVA Laboratories) so that additional intravenous medications may be administered without opening the system. (i.e., without disconnecting the fluid administration set from the catheter). Fluid bottles may be changed during the day using the same administration set.

REFERENCES

1. Myers L: Intravenous catheterization. *Am J Nurs* 45:930-931, 1945.
2. Spencer KR: Intravenous catheters. *Vet Clin North Am* 12(3):533-543, 1982.
3. Crossley K: The scalp-vein needle—A prospective study of complications. *JAMA* 220:985-987, 1972.
4. Burrows CF: Techniques & complications of intravenous and intra-arterial catheterization in dogs and cats. *JAVMA* 163:1357, 1973.
5. Haskins SC: Standards and techniques of equipment utilization, in Sattler FP, Knowles RP, Whittick WG (eds): *Veterinary Critical Care.* Philadelphia, Lea & Febiger, 1981, pp 60-67.
6. Wilmore DW, Dudrick SJ: Safe longterm venous catheterization. *Arch Surg* 98:256-258, 1969.
7. Doering RB, Stemmer EA, Connally JE: Complications of indwelling venous catheters with particular reference to catheter embolization. *Am J Surg* 114:259, 1967.
8. Sawyer DC: *The Practice of Small Animal Anesthesia,* vol 1. Philadelphia, WB Saunders Co, 1982, p 172.
9. Miller ME: *Anatomy of the Dog.* Philadelphia, WB Saunders Co, 1964, pp 131-388.
10. Eitzen HE, Ritter MA, French MLV, Gioe TJ: A microbiological in-use comparison of surgical hand-washing agents. *J Bone Joint Surg [Am]* 61A(3):403-406, 1979.
11. Knecht CD, Allen AR, Williams DJ, Johnson JH: *Fundamental Techniques in Veterinary Surgery,* ed 2. Philadelphia, WB Saunders Co, 1981, pp 205-223, 250-260.

UPDATE

In the discussion on through-the-needle catheters on p. 35 the assumption is that they are being inserted into the jugular vein. This may not be clear from the wording in the text. Through-the-needle catheters should only be placed in large bore veins such as the jugular vein to avoid compromising venous return. Likewise, the catheter of choice for the jugular vein is the through-the-needle variety, which is relatively long and can be easily stabilized in the jugular vein.

Technique in Intravenous Catheterization in Dogs and Cats—Part II

Lorraine M. Crachy, AHT
Athens, Georgia

The discussion in Part I included catheter types and placement techniques. Proper nursing care is required to maintain a well-placed catheter. Bandaging, management, and coping with complications are discussed in the conclusion of this two-part article.

Bandaging

Short-term catheter maintenance does not require bandaging, only stabilization. Examples of uses of short-term catheterization are: delivery of intravenous medications (e.g., placement of a winged catheter for thiacetarsamide sodium therapy during heartworm treatment), fluid therapy given on an outpatient basis, and fluid therapy given during surgery and immediately after surgery.

Time is not the main factor when deciding whether or not to secure a catheter with a bandage. The main factors are (1) the probability of the patient soiling the catheter site, (2) the probability of the patient attempting to remove the catheter, and (3) the patient's medical status. Seriously ill patients have a decreased ability to fight off infections. To stabilize a catheter adequately and because of the large venipuncture site, bandaging is required for all jugular catheters. Bandaging is also required for any patient that is going to be left in a cage for even a few minutes without immediate supervision. A coaptation splint, made of a tongue depressor, metal shoe, or plywood, or a Schroeder-Thomas splint[1] can be used if the catheter will be kinked when the animal moves a joint. Proper choice of the catheter system as well as proper catheter placement can prevent the necessity of splinting.

A support wrap is usually the only requirement when bandaging a catheter site on a leg. Povidone-iodine ointment (Betadine® Ointment—Purdue Frederick) is first applied to the skin puncture site. A sterile gauze sponge is taped over the ointment. Two to three layers of cast padding (Specialist Cast Padding—Johnson & Johnson Products) are wrapped around the leg, starting at the toes but not covering them and continuing up to the joint proximal to the catheter. Two or three layers of gauze roll (Kling—Johnson & Johnson) are then wrapped in the same manner as the cast padding. The support wrap is covered in elastic bandage (Elastikon—Johnson & Johnson) again starting at the toes. The intravenous administration tubing is incorporated into the bandage. This prevents contamination via the injection port, because the administration set is not changed. Fluid bottles can be changed using the same administration set.

Catheter Management

The objectives of catheter nursing care are to maintain a patent catheter and to prevent sepsis (Figure 1). Septic complications are more likely to occur the longer the catheter is in place,[2] or when proper nursing care is not given.[3] Conscientious nursing care can eliminate septic complications. The following is an outline for catheter management.

1. *Introduce catheters by strict aseptic technique.* Unplanned events may force the short-term catheter to remain functional longer than was anticipated. The incidence of septic complications decreases in direct proportion to the time the catheter is left indwelling.[2] Therefore, aseptic technique must not be violated when catheter placement is anticipated to be short-term.

2. *Place long-term (more than 24 hours) catheters into large-bore veins.* The risk of compromising venous

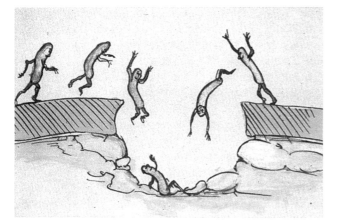

Figure 1—The objectives of catheter nursing care are to maintain a patent catheter and to prevent sepsis.

return is decreased when the catheter is placed in large bore veins. There will be less stasis of blood around the catheter, less catheter-to-wall interaction (less mechanical irritation), and greater dilution of irritating solutions (less chemical irritation).

3. *Affix the catheter to the skin puncture site to prevent catheter movement in the vessel.* This may be accomplished simply with tape or more securely with suture.

4. *Use strict aseptic technique during injection and sampling procedures.* The injection cap should be swabbed with povidone-iodine solution (Betadine® Solution—Purdue Frederick, Prepodyn® Solution— West Chemical Products) prior to needle introduction.

5. *Keep the fluid administration system closed.* When selecting a fluid administration set, it is important that it is fitted with an injection port (FluVen 0150®— Venusa, Venoset® Microdrip®—Abbott Laboratories).

6. *Flush catheter two to four times daily with an anticoagulant solution.* Heparinized saline may be made by adding 2000 U heparin per liter of saline.[4] Bacterial contamination of heparinized saline is a potential hazard.

7. *Maintain a clean, dry, protected puncture site.* This is accomplished by inspection. Routinely change the bandage once daily. Each time the bandage is soiled or wet, the bandage must be removed, the system examined for any signs of failure, the catheter site recleaned as described in prepping the patient prior to catheterization (Part I of this article, Volume 4, Number 6), the skin air dried, povidone-iodine ointment and sterile gauze reapplied, and the system rebandaged.

8. *Rejustify daily the continued use of the catheter.*

9. *Monitor core body temperature three times daily to detect early signs of sepsis.*

10. *Remove the catheter at the first signs of phlebitis, thrombosis, patient discomfort, local inflammation, fever, or catheter malfunction.*

11. *When the catheterized vein is being properly cared for and none of the criteria for catheter removal (No. 10 above) is present, there is much controversy on the maximum length of time a catheter should be left in a vein.*[4-6] In acute disease processes, the patient may respond to therapy within 24 to 72 hours, making continued catheterization unjustified. If the vein has been adequately cared for, the same catheter can remain indwelling for the duration of therapy.[7] The debate lies in whether catheterization should be continued for more than 72 hours if there is no anticipation of patient response to therapy.

If the catheter is removed from an adequately cared for vein, and the vein is not damaged after removal of the catheter (i.e., a pressure bandage is applied to the puncture site for two to three hours after removal of the catheter), then the vein can be reused in 48 to 72 hours, assuming normal healing processes have not been disturbed by the patient's illness. This routine 48-hour vein rotation ideally would allow for intravenous therapy to continue indefinitely. When the decision has been made to rotate venipuncture sites for an animal that already has a patent, aseptic catheter site, the new catheter should be placed before removing the old, but functional, catheter. Some patients, illnesses, clinical situations, and available veins do not permit indiscriminate removal of such a vital part of the patient's therapy. Sometimes patient care requires ultralong-term (more than 72 hours) catheter maintenance without rotating veins or catheters.

Even as early as 1969, when long-term catheters were still placed in external jugular veins, critical-care human patients were being maintained with single catheterizations for 24 days or longer.[7] The protocol for catheter management in these cases was strict aseptic technique and proper nursing care. Catheters in animal patients can also be maintained for extended periods of time, although 24 days and longer may be a real nursing challenge.

Complications

Complications associated with intravenous catheterization can be broken down into three groups: complications directly associated with the patient, complications directly associated with the catheter, and complications after catheter placement.

Complications directly associated with the patient are generally a result of the patient's disease process, the exception being body conformation. Some conformations, such as that of a dachshund, basset hound, puppy, or kitten, by nature render intravenous catheterization difficult. With patience and practice, however, accessible veins can be found and catheterized in these patients.

Disease processes can bring about a variety of complicating factors. Clotting deficiencies may not allow a patient to clot at the venipuncture site. In such cases a small bore catheter should be used, assuming large volumes of fluid will not be needed over a short period of time. A through-the-needle catheter would be less desirable than a bore catheter for these patients because of perivascular bleeding at the venipuncture site. Dyspnea may not allow jugular catheterization. Severely anemic patients are unable to tolerate stress; for them, the cephalic vein may be the site of choice, and they require patience, gentle handling, and a quiet room to minimize stress. Disease processes causing low blood pressure can result in vessel wall spasm.[3] In these cases, the vein should be occluded during the whole prepping period to raise the blood pressure as much as possible, and a peephole should be made to allow for better visualization of the vein. Certain heart or kidney diseases can lead to edema in the extremities making cephalic and saphenous catheterizations nearly impossible, as well as undesirable due to more static blood flow to these areas.

Complications directly associated with the over-the-needle catheter are numerous. Flaring (Figure 2),[3] a common catheter failure, occurs when a piece of the catheter tip peels back, usually at the time of skin puncture. Flaring can be caused by severely dehydrated skin, thick skin (e.g., tomcat neck or forearm skin), or inadequate catheter material. A peephole helps to alleviate this problem. If flaring occurs often during routine catheterizations, the catheter material is a possible cause. The distance from the bevel of the needle to the catheter should be short, and the catheter should not begin abruptly or be made of a thick material. "Accordioning" (Figure 3) occurs when, upon threading the over-the-needle catheter, the catheter material folds (or pleats) between the skin puncture site and the catheter hub.

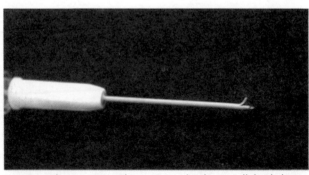

Figure 2—Flaring occurs when a piece of catheter pulls back during skin puncture.

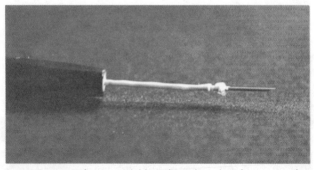

Figure 3—Accordioning is folding that takes place between a skin puncture site and the catheter hub when an over-the-needle catheter is threaded.

The distance from the bevel of the needle/stylet to the start of the actual catheter should be short, assuring that the needle/stylet as well as the catheter is within the vessel lumen when blood is seen in the hub of the stylet. If this distance is too long, the vein may be punctured and blood will appear in the stylet, but when the attempt is made to thread the catheter, it travels alongside the vein because the catheter has never entered the vein. The needle/stylet must be very sharp so that the needle is not dulled by the skin before venipuncture is made. The catheter material must be thin enough so as not to occlude the vessel when using a small-gauge catheter, yet must be thick enough to prevent accordioning of the catheter material when the attempt is made to thread the catheter.

One catheter complication due to technical error is spearing (Figure 4).[3,8] Spearing the catheter is done after removing the stylet (or backing it out even a short distance), deciding the catheter is not properly placed, and reinserting the stylet with the catheter all or partially lodged under the skin of the patient. The stylet must never be reinserted after even partially pulling it back through the catheter. Catheter embolus may result.[3,8]

When purchasing an over-the-needle or a through-the-needle catheter, look for qualities that enhance the ease of catheterization, such as:

1. A sharp needle on the stylet
2. A short bevel-to-catheter distance
3. A one-unit catheter and hub
4. A catheter made of a radiopaque material (in case of catheter embolus)
5. A catheter hub that attaches directly to the administration set
6. A catheter that allows visualization of blood in the stylet
7. A catheter material thin enough not to flare, yet strong enough to advance without "accordioning."

The buyer should not assume that intravenous devices are without defects. A list of complaints is filed with the Freedom of Information staff of the Food and Drug Administration. Complaints about intravenous catheters include leakage from the hub, flaring, contamination

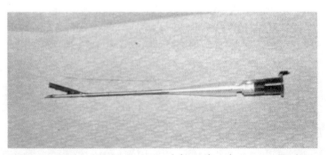

Figure 4—Spearing is reinsertion of the stylet after removing it or backing it partially out of the puncture site because of improper placement.

of sterile catheters, and needle separation from wings.[5] If a catheter defect is encountered, it should be brought to the manufacturer's attention (via the sales representative) and to the attention of the Food and Drug Administration (via a letter to its Freedom of Information staff).

Some of the complications seen in over-the-needle catheters are also seen in through-the-needle catheters. Flaring and spearing cannot occur in the through-the-needle catheter due to its design, but accordioning has been seen by the author. Again, the sharpness of the needle and the material of which the catheter is made are determining factors in catheter quality. Correct placement of the through-the-needle catheter is of primary concern during its insertion. If inserted too far, cardiac perforation can occur. Results of incorrect placement include pneumothorax, hemothorax, chylothorax, cardiac arrhythmias, or pericardial tamponade.[3,8]

The most frustrating complications are those that occur after catheter placement. Proper nursing care can alleviate most postplacement complications or allow their discovery before harm is done to the animal.

Sepsis is the most serious postplacement complication. Local sepsis, phlebitis (Figure 5), occurs when the vessel is involved in an inflammatory process. Signs include redness, heat, swelling, pain, or tenderness at the catheterization site. Phlebitis is most commonly caused by chemical or mechanical irritants or septic technique during catheter placement. Hypertonic solutions or irritating drugs should be given only in large bore veins, where rapid dilution is possible. If an irritating drug must be given in a small bore vein, follow with a large volume (20 to 30 ml) of a buffered, isotonic solution, such as lactated Ringer's. If phlebitis occurs, the catheter should be removed and cultured. To culture, prepare the skin at the puncture site as described in the section Patient Preparation in Part I. The skin should

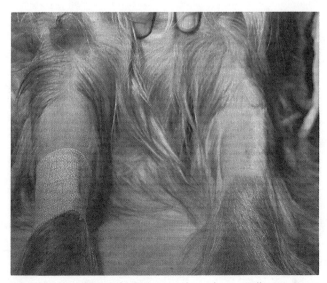

Figure 5—The signs of phlebitis are redness, heat, swelling, pain, or tenderness at the catheterization site.

be allowed to air dry. The catheter is then withdrawn with sterile forceps. The distal 2 to 3 cm of catheter should be cut with sterile scissors and dropped into a tube of thioglycolate broth.[9] Mechanical phlebitis is due to traumatic catheter introduction or movement of the catheter in situ. To minimize traumatic catheterization, all necessary materials should be within an arm's distance before catheter placement and tape should be precut and flushing solutions predrawn before introducing the catheter into the vein. When maintaining a catheter more than 24 hours, be sure to suture it in place and apply an adequate support wrap to minimize catheter movement.

Septic side effects of indwelling venous catheters in human patients have been well documented.[2,8-10] Septicemia and bacterial endocarditis are examples of generalized sepsis. Signs of these side effects include fever, leukocytosis, and cardiac arrhythmias.[11] Catheter-tip culture and serial blood cultures aid in determining the proper antibiotic therapy. Prevention is much more desirable than treating a septic patient. It is important to use aseptic technique when inserting the catheter, as well as during sampling and injection procedures.

Catheter embolus can be caused by spearing, by cutting the catheter upon removal, or by the patient attempting to remove the catheter. If a catheter embolus occurs, a tourniquet is applied to the joint above the catheter and radiographs are taken using soft-tissue technique to locate the embolus. It is necessary to radiograph the chest if the embolus is not found locally. Surgical removal may be necessary. Human literature has reported fatalities due to catheter embolus.[8] Cause of death is most often from sepsis, endocarditis, thrombosis, or perforation of the heart with tamponade. Preventive steps include the following: (1) Always use radiopaque catheters; (2) measure the catheter length before placement and immediately postremoval of the catheter; (3) never risk spearing the catheter; (4) never place a catheter where it will be forced to bend at an area of flexion; (5) securely fix the catheter hub to skin at the site of venipuncture; and (6) never use scissors when removing a catheter. Scissors can be used to remove the elastic bandage material from the support bandage, but the rest of the bandage should be removed by unraveling. Tabs placed on tape ends ease removal of the tape.

Air embolus occurs when a bolus of air is injected into a vein or when venous pressure becomes negative and a vein is open, drawing room air or air from an empty fluid bottle into the vein. Consequences of air embolus may be fatal if large volumes embolize.[12]

Thrombosis can result from mechanical irritants, chemical irritants, or phlebitis.[4] Thromboembolism may be the result of thrombosis and can be diagnosed by physical examination. Signs of arterial occlusion include paralysis, pain, hypothermia of the affected limb, cyanosis, and an absence of pulse.[13] Clinical signs of venous obstruction depend on the anatomic location of the vein and the length of vein involvement. Normal body mechanisms are geared to dissolve the thrombus, making use of collateral vessels for venous return.[13] Only when critical segments of the deep venous system are occluded are clinical signs, such as edema distal to the obstruction, cyanosis, or dilated vessels, seen.[13]

If the fluids for administration have stopped dripping, the cause of thrombosis must be determined as soon as possible. The first step in determining the cause is to straighten the vein by extending the joint above the catheter or extending the neck. The second step is to flush the system with heparinized saline. If the flush cannot be injected nor blood withdrawn, then a clot is present in the lumen of the catheter. The use of high-pressure flush to move the clot out of the catheter lumen is controversial. The University of Pennsylvania veterinary hospital reports no observed clinical problems of thromboembolism with the use of high-pressure flushes.[4] The alternative to flushing a catheter lumen clot is to remove the catheter. In a recent human report, Kaminiski and Pluta have given a detailed description on a safe method of irrigating catheter lumen clots in humans.[14] They encourage the use of a tuberculin syringe either at the injection port or directly at the catheter hub and flushing with heparinized saline. The best treatment is prevention with the heparinized flush. The system should be flushed with heparinized saline at least twice daily and more frequently if there are periods of time when the administration of therapeutic fluids is intentionally stopped (i.e., turn off the fluids, then flush with enough heparinized saline to fill the catheter [heparin lock]).

There are several reasons that fluids can be injected but not withdrawn.[3,4] The catheter may be bent or kinked. If this situation is possible, a measurement can be made with a ruler or another catheter of equal length at the site where the catheter is lying in the patient. If the catheter is being forced around an area of flexion or if palpation of the vein reveals a kinked or bent catheter, then the catheter must be removed to prevent catheter embolus. The catheter might be extravascular; and if it is, it must be removed. Fluids will drip as long as there is loose extravascular space. The catheter tip may be occluded by the vessel wall. In that case, the catheter can be withdrawn slightly, turned, and reinserted. The vessel wall may have collapsed due to hypovolemia, vessel thrombosis, or vessel spasm. If the vessel wall is collapsed due to hypovolemia or vessel spasm, then fluid therapy should improve the condition. If the wall is collapsed due to thrombosis, then the catheter should be removed and placed in another vein. A "flapping" clot may reside at the catheter tip. Aspiration may accomplish clot removal.[14] Lastly, in the case of low blood pressure,

especially when a long catheter has been placed or when the catheter extends past a point of vein occlusion (such as a jugular catheter), withdrawing blood from the catheter can be difficult or even impossible. Blood samples for laboratory analysis should be acquired by a separate venipuncture, not via the indwelling catheter, because withdrawing blood from the catheter may result in blood sample dilution by the therapeutic fluids and possible trauma to the vessel wall.

Acknowledgments

The author thanks Dr. Gary Thayer, Dr. Joan Wheeler, and Dr. Dennis Aron for their editorial assistance, Robert Newcomb for his photography, and Jane Teichner for her illustration. The author's deepest appreciation is extended to Dr. Dennis Aron, whose moral support and encouragement made this article possible.

REFERENCES

1. Knecht CD, Allen AR, Williams DJ, Johnson JH: *Fundamental Techniques in Veterinary Surgery*, ed 2. Philadelphia, WB Saunders Co, 1981, pp 205-223, 250-260.
2. Bolasmy BL, Shepard GH, Scott HW: The hazards of intravenous polyethylene catheters in surgical patients. *Surg Gynecol Obstet* 130:342, 1970.
3. Haskins SC: Standards and techniques of equipment utilization, in Sattler FP, Knowles RP, Whittick WG (eds): *Veterinary Critical Care*. Philadelphia, Lea & Febiger, 1981, pp 60-67.
4. Burrows CF: Techniques and complications of intravenous and intra-arterial catheterization in dogs and cats. *JAVMA* 163:1357, 1973.
5. Spencer KR: Intravenous catheters. *Vet Clin North Am* 12(3): 533-543, 1982.
6. Buxton AE, Highsmith AK, Garner JS, et al: Contamination of intravenous infusion fluid: Effects of changing administration sets. *Ann Intern Med* 90:764, 1979.
7. Wilmore DW, Dudrick SJ: Safe longterm venous catheterization. *Arch Surg* 98:256-258, 1969.
8. Doering RB, Stemmer EA, Connally JE: Complications of indwelling venous catheters with particular reference to catheter embolization. *Am J Surg* 114:259, 1967.
9. Corso JA, Agostinelli R, Brandiss MW: Maintenance of venous polyethylene catheters to reduce risk of infection. *JAMA* 210:2075, 1969.
10. Maki DG, Goldman PA, Rhames FS: Infection control in intravenous therapy. *Ann Intern Med* 79:867, 1973.
11. Cornelius L: Fluid, electrolyte, acid-base and nutritional management, in Bojrab MJ (ed): *Pathophysiology in Small Animal Surgery*. Philadelphia, Lea & Febiger, 1981, pp 12-32.
12. Adornato DC, Gildenberg PL, Ferrane CM, et al: Pathophysiology of intravenous air embolism in dogs. *Anesthesiology* 49:120, 1978.
13. Wingfield WE, Bradley RL: Systemic vascular disease, in Bojrab MJ (ed): *Pathophysiology in Small Animal Surgery*. Philadelphia, Lea & Febiger, 1981, pp 201, 208-209.
14. Kaminiski MV, Pluta J: Irrigation of catheter lumen clots: A safe and effective technique. *Am J Intravenous Ther* 5(4):6, 1978.

A Practical Technique for Catheterization of the Dorsal Pedal Artery in Dogs

Ken Crump, AHT
Veterinary Specialist I

Deb Buhrman-Haferman, AHT
Veterinary Technician B

Anesthesia Department
Veterinary Teaching Hospital
College of Veterinary Medicine
  and Biomedical Sciences
Colorado State University
Fort Collins, Colorado

Arterial catheterization is a procedure not commonly counted among the skills of a veterinary technician. A catheterized peripheral artery, however, can be invaluable during procedures that require constant direct blood pressure monitoring and/or multiple arterial blood samples drawn for blood gas analysis. The dorsal pedal artery in the dog is ideally suited for such catheterization. It is palpable and easily located as it passes over the metatarsal bones of the foot. In this article, a practical technique for peripheral artery catheterization is presented that, with practice, can be easily mastered.

Any time an animal is required to be on mechanically assisted ventilation, an important parameter for monitoring the animal's condition is lost: depth and rate of respiration. A ventilator can be set to meet an animal's ideal requirements. Tidal volume and respiratory rate can be mathematically calculated according to the animal's weight.[1] Conditions may exist in an individual patient, however, that would render such calculations inaccurate. A parameter to adjust these calculations to each patient's needs must be established. Arterial blood samples drawn at intervals for blood gas analysis provide a reliable indicator of balanced respiration. Information obtained from arterial blood gas analysis, such as blood concentrations of O_2 and CO_2 and blood pH, is essential to properly adjust a ventilator.[2]

To avoid unnecessary trauma to the peripheral arteries caused by repeated blood collection, an indwelling catheter can be easily placed and secured in the dorsal pedal artery. In addition to providing access to an artery for blood collection, a dorsal pedal arterial catheter also provides a necessary port to establish continuous direct blood pressure monitoring.[3] Arterial blood gas values and direct blood pressure trends are invaluable tools for establishing and maintaining balanced respiration.

Equipment

To establish a dorsal pedal arterial catheter, the following equipment must be available:

- 2-inch over-the-needle catheter (20-gauge catheter with 22-gauge needle)
- injection cap
- 6 ml flush
- 1-inch-wide tape
- clippers
- surgical scrub
- cotton ball
- germicidal ointment.

It is important that the flush be heparinized. Because of the arterial blood pressure, blood backflowing into the catheter can form a clot, occluding the catheter. One rec-

Originally published in Volume 8, Number 8, September 1987

ommended formula for heparinized flush calls for 1 ml of heparin (1000 units/ml) added to 500 ml of sterile normal saline.[4] The catheter should be filled with flush before an attempt at placement is made. Preflushing the catheter allows immediate visualization of blood flashback.

The strips of tape to secure the catheter must be prepared before the procedure is begun. Once the catheter is in place, it is essential that it be secured immediately. Three strips of tape are required to secure the catheter. Each strip should be 8 to 10 inches long. One strip of tape should be 1/2 inch wide, while the other two strips should each be 1 inch wide. All three strips should be put in a convenient place so that they will be readily available once the catheter is in place.

Anatomy

The technician is presented with an unusual task in locating the dorsal pedal artery. Unlike the peripheral veins that technicians commonly catheterize, the dorsal pedal artery is not readily seen. Consequently, the technician must rely on anatomic landmarks. To find the dorsal pedal artery, the technician should follow the course of the femoral artery.

The femoral artery progresses down the medial aspect of the hindlimbs. As it passes the condyle of the tibia, the femoral artery tapers to form the cranial tibial artery. The cranial tibial artery tapers further to form the dorsal pedal artery. The dorsal pedal artery passes over the cranial aspect of the tarsus, across the metatarsus, and branches and tapers to carry oxygenated blood to the foot and toes (Figure 1).

Palpation

As is common in veterinary medicine, that which cannot be seen must be visualized by careful palpation. Because the dorsal pedal artery cannot be seen, the technician must become proficient in palpation. The technician can gain proficiency by practicing on any cooperative dog. The practice animal can be in virtually any position for palpation, but for the purpose of catheterization, it is necessary that the patient be in lateral recumbency.

When positioning the patient for dorsal pedal arterial catheterization, the anesthetized dog is placed in left lateral recumbency. The right hindleg is flexed against the body and secured up and out of the way with 1-inch tape. The left hindleg is extended and secured to the table (Figure 2). The extended leg is clipped and surgically prepped over the medial and cranial aspects of the metatarsus. The technician can then isolate the dorsal pedal artery by palpating with the left hand (Figure 3). The room should be quiet and free of distraction so the technician can concentrate on mentally visualizing that which is being isolated by the fingertips. The mental image of the artery must have definition. The technician should be able to see, in his or her mind, the artery as it courses just below the skin. The catheterization attempt is successful only after a successful "blind stick" into the artery. With the supplies ready, the dog properly positioned, and the artery isolated, the technician is ready to place the catheter.

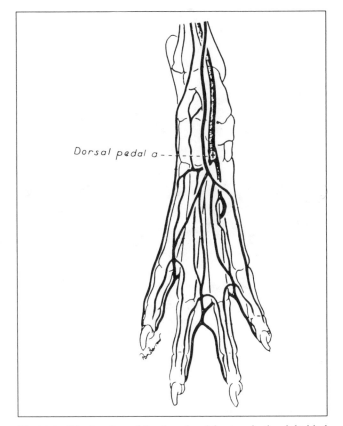

Figure 1—The location of the dorsal pedal artery in the right hind paw. (From Evans HE, deLahunta A: *Miller's Guide to Dissection of the Dog,* ed 2. Philadelphia, WB Saunders Co, 1980, p 220. Reprinted with permission.)

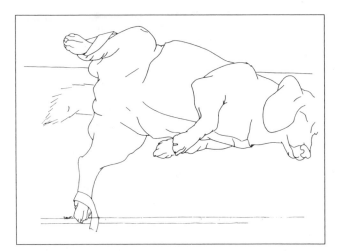

Figure 2—The anesthetized dog is positioned in left lateral recumbency.

Placement

Placing a dorsal pedal arterial catheter requires patience and concentration. The technician should not expect to be immediately proficient at this technique. Many early attempts will be met with frustration. Unlike venipuncture, in which the vessel is easily seen by applying pressure at strategic points, the dorsal pedal artery must be isolated by palpation and defined by mental image. With practice,

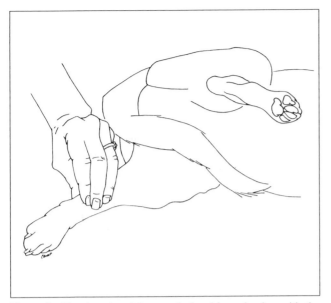

Figure 3—The dorsal pedal artery isolated by palpating with the left hand.

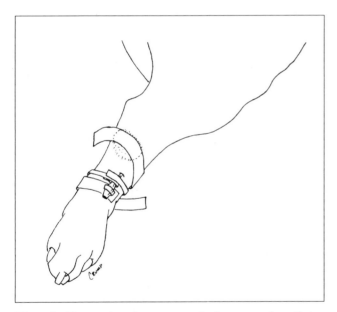

Figure 4—Three strips of tape are required to secure the catheter.

however, the technician can expect to consistently cannulate the dorsal pedal artery.

The catheter should be filled with flush before the placement attempt is made. Preflushing the catheter allows immediate visualization of blood flashback. As with venipuncture, blood flashback into the hub of the needle indicates a successful "stick."

With the dorsal pedal artery clearly defined and isolated by the left hand, the technician positions the catheter in his or her right hand between the thumb and forefinger. The hub is held in a manner that allows it to be clearly seen. The bevel of the needle should face up. The needle should enter the skin just distal and parallel to the artery. It should

be kept in mind that the artery is very superficial. It is easy to make the initial entry at too steep an angle and consequently enter too deeply. Once through the skin, slowly advance the needle and catheter toward the endmost point of the artery as isolated by the left index finger. Because the only indication of a successful "stick" is blood flashback, the technician's eyes should never leave the hub of the needle. The first sign of blood flashback indicates that the bevel of the needle has entered the artery. The needle should then be advanced 1 mm into the artery to push the tip of the catheter through the artery wall. Then the hub of the needle should be held firmly in place and the catheter advanced down the needle and into the artery. The needle is then withdrawn while the catheter is held in place. Blood will immediately pulse out of the catheter if the catheter has been successfully seated. Place the injection cap into the catheter and flush immediately. The catheter is ready to be taped securely in place.

Securing the Catheter

Once the catheter is in place and flushed, it must be secured immediately (Figure 4). The arterial blood pressure, unlike venous pressure, is often sufficient to push the catheter out of the artery. Three strips of tape are required to secure the catheter. Each strip should be 8 to 10 inches long. One strip of tape should be 1/2 inch wide. The other two strips are to be 1 inch wide.

The 1/2-inch-wide strip of tape is used to secure the catheter to the dog's foot. This strip should be placed, sticky side up, beneath the exposed portion of the catheter. The catheter should lay on top of the tape about 1 inch from one end of the strip. Wrap the long portion of the strip of tape over the top of the catheter and around the foot. This will adhere the catheter to the tape as well as secure the catheter to the foot. Flush the catheter after it has been secured; this will confirm proper placement of the catheter in the artery even after manipulation.

The first strip of 1-inch-wide tape is used to secure the injection cap to the catheter and isolate it from the hair and skin of the foot. Slide this strip, with its sticky side down, under the injection cap. Wrap the tape around the foot and over the top of the injection cap. This method not only provides a tape barrier between the injection cap and the exposed skin and hair, but also provides easy access to the injection cap. By lifting the tape from the top of the injection cap, the cap can be adjusted or removed as needed. After the necessary adjustments to the cap are made, the tape can then be replaced over the top of it. Once the injection cap is secured, flush the catheter again.

The second strip of 1-inch-wide tape is used to make a bandage for the site where the catheter enters the skin. Apply germicidal ointment to the puncture site and place a cotton ball over it. Wrap the second strip of 1-inch-wide tape around the cotton ball and the foot to hold the cotton in place. It is important to remember, when placing all three strips of tape, not to wrap them too tightly. Each strip only needs to be tight enough to perform the function for which it is intended. Wrapping the tape too tightly may impair venous return from the foot and cause swelling or more serious damage.

Maintenance and Removal

After an arterial catheter is secured in place, it differs from a venous catheter in only one significant way. It must be flushed repeatedly or kept patent by constant infusion of flush. Arterial blood pressure is constantly trying to force blood into the catheter. Clots forming in a catheter or at the very tip of a catheter can turn a successful cannulation into a useless exercise in frustration. Arterial pressure also makes it necessary to develop a different technique for intermittent flushing. The tiny pressure release that occurs as the bevel of the needle passes out of the injection cap allows a volume of arterial blood to rush back into the catheter. It is necessary, therefore, to continue to deliver flush as the needle on the flush syringe is withdrawn from the injection cap of the catheter. The constant delivery of flush in this manner eliminates the pressure release, and consequently prevents arterial blood flow into the catheter. To keep the catheter patent, it is necessary to flush it every five to ten minutes or maintain a constant infusion of flush for as long as the catheter is in place.

Removing a dorsal pedal arterial catheter is very similar to removing a cephalic vein catheter. The 1-inch-wide tape is removed from the injection cap and the 1/2-inch-wide tape securing the catheter to the leg is snipped with bandage scissors. The catheter is then withdrawn from the skin while pressure is applied to the cotton ball at the puncture site. Under normal circumstances, pressure is applied for several minutes and the bandage is then left in place for at least 12 minutes to prevent a hematoma and/or frank bleeding. This differs only slightly from the procedure for removing a venous catheter, during which pressure is applied to a venous puncture site for one minute or less.

Troubleshooting

This technique is not without its difficulties. In the following section, some of the common problems and ways to overcome them are discussed.

Decreased Arterial Blood Flow

Dogs that have been confined in a cage for several days before a dorsal pedal arterial catheterization attempt is made present a particular problem. Our experience indicates that exercise increases the blood flow through the peripheral arteries. Therefore, being confined in a small area for several days may decrease the blood flow through the dorsal pedal artery, making it difficult to palpate and almost impossible to catheterize. If the need for a dorsal pedal arterial catheter is anticipated, try to confine the patient in a run before the procedure. If a run is unavailable or impractical, exercise the dog frequently before the anticipated procedure.

Loss of Body Heat During Anesthesia

It is most common for a dog to lose body heat during anesthesia. Even the most diligent attempts to maintain normal temperature during anesthesia can result in a dog with cold feet. It is difficult to palpate and catheterize the dorsal pedal artery in a cold foot. This problem can be remedied by taping warm socks on the dog's feet before administering anesthesia. When it is time to catheterize the dorsal pedal artery, simply remove the socks.

Difficulty in Seating the Catheter

Problems often occur when seating the catheter once the needle has penetrated the artery wall. The most common mistake is to pull the needle out of the artery as the catheter is advanced down the needle and into the artery. The technician must take special care not to move the needle while advancing the catheter.

Fraying of the Catheter Tip

The dorsal pedal artery lies on the metatarsal bones with no underlying cushion of muscle or fat. This facilitates catheterization by providing a rigid backstop to trap the artery against while piercing it with the needle. When a placement attempt is made too deeply, however, the needle can easily strike a metatarsal bone. This contact can cause the end of the catheter to fray. A frayed catheter tip will almost certainly traumatize an artery beyond practical use. If the technician feels the needle or catheter tip deflect off of bone during a catheterization attempt, the needle and catheter should be withdrawn at once and a new attempt with a fresh catheter should be made.

Occlusion of the Artery

It is possible to occlude the artery while trying to palpate and isolate it. As the technician concentrates on defining the artery in his or her mind, it is possible that the pressure applied to the artery during palpation might occlude blood flow through it. The arterial pulse could still be felt, but the technician would not know when the bevel of the needle had entered the artery—the pressure-occluded artery would not allow blood to flash back into the hub.

Patients that Cannot be Anesthetized

It may be necessary to collect arterial blood samples from a patient that cannot be anesthetized. Information derived from arterial blood gas analysis may be crucial to evaluate the condition of an animal suffering from severe trauma or pneumothorax. In a situation in which it is contraindicated to anesthetize the patient, a dorsal pedal arterial catheter can be placed by manually or chemically restraining the patient and administering a local anesthetic around the intended puncture site.

Conclusion

The dorsal pedal artery in the dog is ideally suited for catheterization. It is a superficial vessel backed by bone and is relatively easy to palpate. Catheterizing the dorsal pedal artery requires concentration, careful palpation, skill with a needle, and practice. A veterinary technician can readily develop the skills required for catheterization and add a new dimension to patient monitoring.

Acknowledgment

The authors wish to acknowledge Dr. E. L. Gillette, Oncology Unit, Colorado State University, whose high expectations motivate us toward greater technical competence.

REFERENCES

1. Lumb WV, Jones EW: Oxygen administration and artificial respiration, in *Veterinary Anesthesia*. Philadelphia, Lea & Febiger, 1984, pp 133–163.
2. Haskins SC: Blood gases and acid–base balance. Clinical interpretation and therapeutic implications, in Kirk RW (ed): *Current Veterinary Therapy III*. Philadelphia, WB Saunders Co, 1983, pp 201–215.
3. Kittleson MD, Olivier NB: Measurement of systemic arterial blood pressure. *Vet Clin North Am [Small Anim Pract]* 13(2):321–336, 1983.
4. Forney SD, Allen RC: *Formulary of the Colorado State University Veterinary Teaching Hospital*. Fort Collins, CO, College of Veterinary Medicine and Biomedical Sciences, Colorado State University, 1985, p 28.
5. Evans HE, deLahunta A: *Miller's Guide to the Dissection of the Dog*, ed 2. Philadelphia, WB Saunders Co, 1980, pp 202–223.

Intraosseous Infusion of Fluids in Small Animals

Intraosseous cannulation should be used when rapid administration of fluids or drugs is necessary and a central or peripheral vein is not readily available.

Melani Poundstone, DVM
TenderCare Veterinary Medical Center
Greenwood Village, Colorado

Intraosseous infusion was first used in the 1940s in children when medical conditions made intravenous catheter placement difficult. Intraosseous placement provides immediate vascular access to systemic circulation when intravenous catheter placement is impossible. Although its use in veterinary medicine has increased over the years, intraosseous infusion still is not being used to its full potential. The purpose of this article is to encourage use of intraosseous fluid infusion and to make it less intimidating for the technician.

ANATOMY

Sinusoids in the bone marrow drain into medullary venous channels, which then drain into nutrient and emissary veins.[1,2] The emissary veins subsequently drain into the systemic venous system.[1,2] The rigid nature of the marrow cavity maintains open access to systemic venous circulation even in cases of hypovolemia. Intraosseous infusion provides a direct line to systemic circulation and is not subject to vascular collapse in shock states, as is the venous system.[1-4]

Emergency Drugs and Fluids That Can Be Administered by the Intraosseous Route

Drugs

Atropine

Calcium

Dexamethasone

Diazepam

Digitalis

Dobutamine and dopamine
  hydrochloride

Epinephrine

Gluconate

Lidocaine

Sodium bicarbonate

Fluids

Colloids (dextrans and plasma)

Crystalloids (lactated Ringer's
  solution, Ringer's solution, normal
  saline, dextrose solutions)

Whole blood

INDICATIONS AND CONTRAINDICATIONS

Intraosseous cannulation should be used when rapid administration of fluids or drugs is necessary and a central or peripheral vein is not readily available. In cases of shock, placement of a peripheral intravenous catheter is difficult because of peripheral circulatory collapse. The marrow cavity, however, remains unaffected and thus provides a better alternative for fluid and drug administration. Intraosseous lines also can be placed in neonates or small dogs and cats where peripheral catheterization is difficult because of the size of the vein.

Intraosseous infusion is contraindicated in cases of septic shock (the infusion may cause osteomyelitis), in pneumatic bones of birds, in bones that are or have been fractured, and if an abscess is present over the catheterization site.[2,5]

FLUIDS AND DRUGS ADMINISTERED BY INTRAOSSEOUS INFUSION

One advantage of intraosseous infusion is that large volumes of fluids can be administered. Crystalloid solutions as well as colloids and whole blood can be given by this route. Widely varied drugs, including many of the emergency drugs (such as sodium bicarbonate, which cannot be administered by the endotracheal route) can be given via this method[2-6] (see Emergency Drugs and Fluids That Can Be Administered by the Intraosseous Route). Bone marrow suppressive agents (such as chemotherapeutic drugs) should never be given by this route.

TECHNIQUE

Figures 1 through 8 demonstrate the intraosseous technique step by step. The preferred sites for intraosseous administration are the tibial crest and the trochanteric fossa of the femur. The wing of the ilium or greater tubercle of the humerus also can be used. First, the site chosen is clipped and surgically prepared. A 1% lidocaine solution is then infiltrated into the skin, surrounding tissue, and periosteum over the site. A spinal needle or a 16- to 18-gauge hypodermic needle may be used in neonates or smaller-sized animals. A small stab incision is made to prevent blunting of the needle. The needle is then directed into the bone. This article only discusses placement in the tibial crest because placement in this anatomic location is much easier than in the trochanteric fossa of the femur. In addition, accidental trauma to the sciatic nerve is avoided by tibial crest placement.

The tibia is grasped on each side of the crest with a thumb and forefinger. Then, after insertion of the needle through the stab incision, pressure is applied to the needle and, with a twisting motion, the needle is inserted through the cortex of the bone. The needle is directed away from the growth plate in a distal direction while being kept centered between the two fingers. As soon as it is advanced through the first cortex, the needle should slide down the marrow cavity. The needle is then advanced to the hub, and placement of the catheter is verified. Watching for simultaneous movement of the catheter when the limb is moved is the most commonly used method for verification of catheter placement.[2,3] Aspiration of bone marrow and radiography also can be used to assess proper placement (Figure 9). The catheter should then be flushed with several milliliters of a heparinized saline solution to assess patency of the catheter and to check for extravasation. During placement, it is important not to penetrate both cortices with the needle. Extravasation of drugs and fluids can occur if the second cortex is perforated with the needle. Even

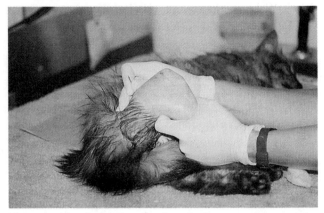

Figure 1—The site is clipped and surgically prepared for cannulation.

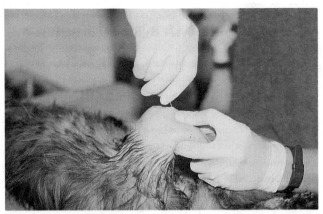

Figure 2—The tibia is grasped on each side of the tibial crest with a thumb and forefinger. With the stifle bent, the needle is introduced into the cortex and directed away from the growth plate in a distal direction.

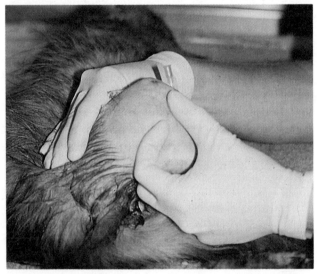

Figure 3—The needle is advanced to the hub, and placement of the catheter is verified.

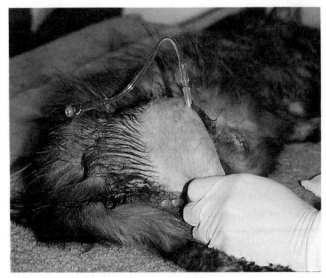

Figure 4—A fluid administration set is attached to the hub of the needle.

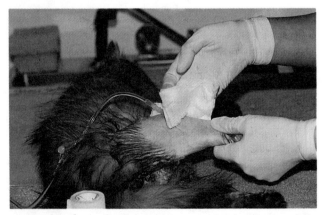

Figure 5—A triple antibiotic ointment is placed around the catheter site and covered with a gauze pad.

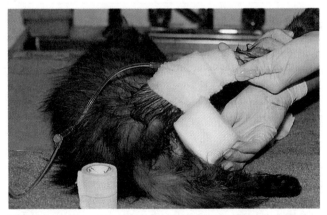

Figure 6—A layer of cotton wrap is placed over the gauze pad.

with proper placement, bone plugs can make administration of fluids and drugs difficult. Bone plugs can be avoided by any of the following methods: (1) A stylet can be used with the spinal needle during placement. The stylet is withdrawn after the needle has been placed in the proper location in the medullary cavity. (2) A 22-gauge needle

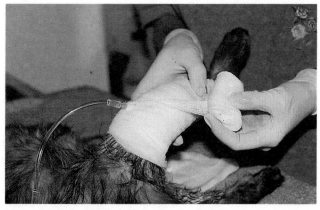

Figure 7—A layer of elastic gauze is placed over the cotton to hold it firmly in place.

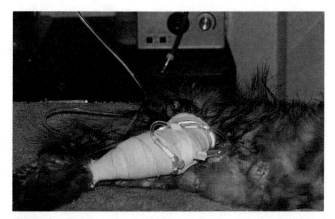

Figure 8—Finally, a layer of elastic adhesive tape is placed and the drip set is taped to the bandage.

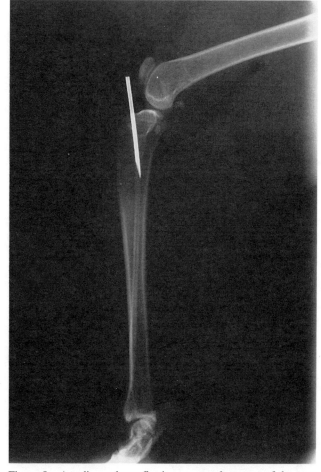

Figure 9—A radiograph confirming proper placement of the needle in the tibial crest.

can be placed inside a 16- or 18-gauge hypodermic needle to act as a stylet. (3) Another needle, inserted into the same hole as the needle that became plugged, may be used as a replacement.

An administration set can now be attached to the hub of the needle. After fluid therapy, the hub can be capped. The needle is then secured by placing a tape butterfly around the hub of the needle. The hub should be affixed to the skin by suturing or by use of a small amount of super-bonding glue. A triple antibiotic ointment is then placed around the site, which is covered with a gauze pad. To prevent bending of the needle as well as contamination of the site, the needle is wrapped using cast padding, elastic gauze, and elastic adhesive tape.

MAINTENANCE

Care for an intraosseous catheter is the same as that for a central or peripheral venous catheter. When not in use, the catheter should be flushed every six hours with heparinized saline solution and replaced every 72 hours; the site also should be changed at this time.[2,4,5] Aseptic technique should always be used when the catheter is being handled. Because of the potential of initiating osteomyelitis, an intravenous route should be used after the patient has stabilized.

CONCLUSION

Special training or equipment is not necessary for placement of an intraosseous catheter. Intraosseous infusion is a reliable method to infuse fluids and drugs to a hypovolemic patient when intravenous infusion is impossible. Shock doses of fluids, whole blood, plasma, and emergency drugs can rapidly be administered using this route.

REFERENCES

1. Fiser DH: Intraosseous infusion. *N Engl J Med* 322:1579-1581, 1990.
2. Otto CM, Kaufman GM, Crowe DT: Intraosseous infusion of fluids and therapeutics. *Comp Clin Educ [Small Anim Pract]* 11:421–431, 1989.
3. Crowe DT: Symposium on critical care: Performing life-saving cardiovascular surgery. *Vet Med* 84(1):83–84, 1989.
4. Wingfield WE, Henik RA: Cardiopulmonary arrest and resuscitation,

in Ettinger SJ (ed): *Textbook of Veterinary Internal Medicine*. Philadelphia, WB Saunders Co, 1989, p 177.

5. Lamberski N, Daniel G: The efficacy of intraosseous catheters in birds. *Proc Assoc Avian Vet*:17–19, 1991.

6. Crowe DT: Cardiopulmonary resuscitation in the dog: A review and proposed new guidelines—Part II. *Semin Vet Med Surg [Small Anim Pract]* 3(4):344–346, 1988.

Management of Shock. Part I. Recognition and Therapy

R. J. Kolata, DVM, MS
Diplomate, ACVS
Experimental Surgery Laboratory
School of Medicine
St. Louis University Medical Center
St. Louis, Missouri

Patients develop shock through a variety of mechanisms. Although each mechanism initiates a particular chain of events that can be categorized (e.g., vasculogenic shock, cardiogenic shock), the central defect producing shock is deficient oxygen transport to the majority of body tissues.[1]

This primary issue is the focus of this two-part series on the management of shock. Three key facets must be considered when discussing the management of shock: recognition and therapeutics (Part I) and patient monitoring (Part II).

Shock Recognition

Vital to the early recognition of shock is an awareness of the clinically encountered circumstances in which a patient may develop shock. In this regard, it is helpful to classify insults that can precipitate into shock and to describe the conditions with which these insults are associated:

1. **Reduction of blood volume**. This may result from external or internal hemorrhage accompanying trauma or surgery or with a hemorrhagic crisis, such as rupture of a tumor or ingestion of dicumarin. Blood volume can also be reduced by loss of plasma through exudation from large burns or inflammation of body cavities (specifically, peritonitis). Loss of fluid and electrolytes can also reduce blood volume; this occurs with dehydration, vomiting, diarrhea, diuresis, and sequestration of fluid with intestinal obstruction. Loss of blood volume can arise through these three mechanisms simultaneously, as occurs in animals presented with fractures and/or soft tissue trauma accompanied by hemorrhage into tissue planes and transudation of plasma and fluids into bruised or wounded soft tissue (Figure 1).

2. **Changes in blood and fluid distribution**. This circumstance occurs with anaphylaxis; endotoxemia associated with invasive infection; and vasomotor paralysis from central nervous system depression caused by drug intoxication, gastric dilatation-torsion, and (rarely) central nervous system injury.

3. **Inadequate cardiac pumping**. This condition is seen in animals with advanced heart failure, heartworm disease, some cardiac dysrhythmias, and such myocardial injuries as contusion or ruptured chordae tendineae. Inadequate cardiac pumping may also accompany drug- or toxin-induced myocardial depression.

Although mechanisms responsible for shock can be defined separately, in a clinical setting they often work simultaneously. For example, septic shock attributed to invasive peritonitis from a ruptured colon begins with changes in blood distribution. Subsequently, inadequate cardiac pumping develops because of reduced venous return, which is caused by loss of fluids into the peritoneal cavity as well as toxin-induced vasodilation.

Originally published in Volume 7, Number 8, September 1986

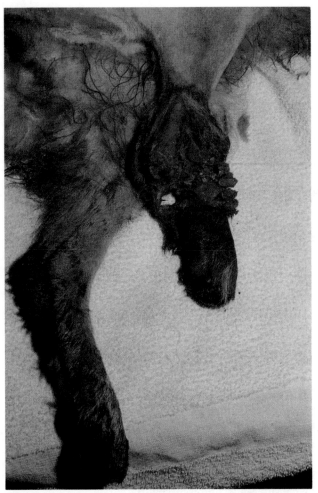

Figure 1—Severe trauma involving soft tissue and bone can cause shock without significant hemorrhage.

Recognition of the clinical signs of shock is vital to successful management. It is axiomatic that the longer shock exists in a patient, the more difficult treatment is. Therefore, early awareness of the signs associated with shock is vital. Some of the signs that alert the practitioner or technician to the presence of shock are associated with the cause (e.g., external hemorrhage with trauma or profuse vomiting and diarrhea with parvovirus infection). Other signs are more specific to shock and reflect compensatory change or changes signaling failure to compensate for inadequate tissue perfusion and oxygenation. These signs can be attributed to activity of the sympathetic nervous system. Tachycardia, diminished pulse strength and heart sounds, pale dry mucous membranes, prolonged capillary refill time, cool extremities, tachypnea, depressed sensorium, and weakness are usually apparent. In postoperative patients, abnormally slow recovery from anesthesia may be an early signal of shock.

Summary of Signs

Tachycardia, tachypnea, slow capillary refill time (Figure 2), and cold extremities reflect sympathetic activity di-

rected toward compensation for reduced blood flow and oxygen delivery and may also reflect pain. Reduced pulse strength and heart sounds reflect reduced cardiac filling and stroke volume. Weakness and depression reflect reduced oxygen availability, reduced nutrient availability, and other possible changes (such as acidosis and hyperkalemia).

Therapeutics

The goal of treatment of shock must be to ensure adequate oxygen delivery to tissues. To reach this goal, three activities are necessary: (1) the cause of shock must be eliminated or controlled, (2) adequate circulatory volume must be reestablished, and (3) the detrimental effects of tissue hypoxia must be reversed. *Most important* to remember during this discussion of therapeutics is that treatment must be titrated to match the needs of the patient; therefore monitoring (which will be discussed in Part II) is as critical to successful management as proper selection and use of therapeutic agents.

arrhythmogenic	the capacity to induce arrhythmias or irregularities of rhythm
capacitance vessel	a vein capable of dilating and holding blood with little change in internal pressure but a large increase in volume
chordae tendineae	the tendinous cords that connect each cusp of the two atrioventricular valves
chronotropic	changes in rate, that is, an increase or a decrease in the heart rate
colloids	large molecules that are dispersed in physiologic liquid and tend to hold water molecules to the same degree as blood proteins
hemodynamic	pertaining to movements involved in the circulation of the blood
hyperkalemia	abnormally high potassium concentration in the blood, usually because of defective renal excretion
hypoxia	decreased oxygen supply to tissue (below physiologic levels despite adequate perfusion of the tissue by blood)
inotropic	influencing muscular contraction
sensorium	term often used to designate the condition of a patient relative to consciousness or mental alertness

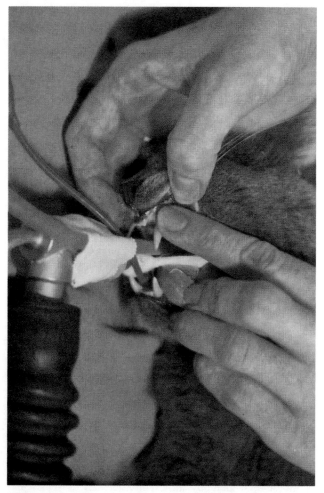

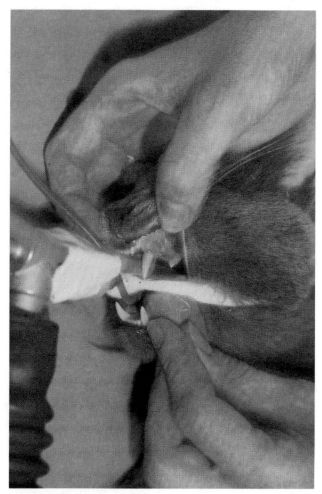

Figure 2A   **Figure 2B**

Figure 2—Capillary refill time is determined by firmly pressing against the attached maxillary gingiva (**A**) and counting the seconds required for the color to return (**B**).

Fluids

Ensuring an adequate circulating volume is a cornerstone in the treatment of shock (Figure 3). Three types of fluids are used for volume replacement: (1) blood; (2) colloids, such as dextran, hydroxyethyl starch, and plasma; and (3) electrolyte solutions. Each type of fluid has advantages and disadvantages. Blood restores both red cells and plasma (Figure 4) but has problems associated with compatibility, availability, and storage. In addition, blood is inappropriate for cases in which the volume deficit involves plasma or water and electrolytes.

Colloids have a longer storage life than blood does and have fewer compatibility problems. These solutions restore colloidal osmotic pressure when plasma proteins are lost and help to expand and maintain circulatory volume while reducing tissue edema; however, they are expensive and have no oxygen-carrying capacity. More specifically, dextran can interfere with normal blood-clotting mechanisms.

Electrolyte solutions are the most commonly used volume replacements. They are inexpensive, have long storage lives, and cause few reactions; however, these solutions have no oxygen-carrying capacity or colloidal osmotic activity. Their lack of oncotic activity allows them to leak rapidly from the vascular space into the interstitial space, thus promoting tissue edema.

Although none of these solutions is the ideal volume replacement, research and clinical experience show that electrolyte solutions are advantageous for initial management of shock and that blood and colloids can be reserved for situations in which their specific advantages are necessary.[2]

In the early stage of shock, patients usually respond rapidly to the control or elimination of initiating causes and to volume replacement, thus allowing hemodynamic stability to be restored. When shock is prolonged either because the initiating factors cannot be or are not adequately controlled or because treatment is not initiated until some time after the onset of hypotension, additional therapeutic agents are required to resolve shock.

Sodium Bicarbonate

Animals in shock accumulate a metabolic acid load from anaerobic glycolysis. In early shock, this acidosis can be resolved by restoring adequate circulation because hepatic metabolism eliminates lactic acid. Prolonged shock with

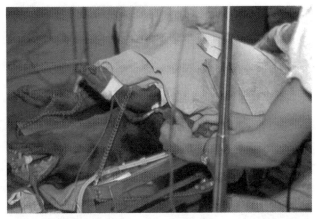

Figure 3—In extreme cases of shock, it may be necessary to administer fluids rapidly by direct infusion.

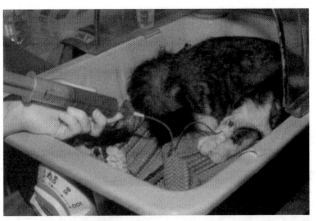

Figure 4—A technique for administering whole blood to a cat in hemorrhagic shock.

accompanying acidosis, however, results in myocardial depression and vasodilation, which inhibit prompt response to volume replacement. Under these circumstances, administration of sodium bicarbonate can be beneficial. Ideally, blood pH should be measured and sodium bicarbonate requirements calculated. When this is not possible, sodium bicarbonate can be given empirically at a rate of 2 to 4 mEq/kg, with one half of the dose administered as a bolus and one half given in fluids during the next four hours. Because blood pH needs to be returned only to a level above 7.20, overalkalization should be avoided, as it can decrease serum-ionized calcium and potassium concentrations and lead to adverse effects on the heart.

Glucocorticoids

The use of glucocorticoids, such as hydrocortisone, methylprednisolone, or dexamethasone, has been advocated in the treatment of shock. These drugs stabilize cell and lysosomal membranes and prevent release of proteolytic enzymes, which generate vasoactive peptides that in turn cause negative hemodynamic effects. Glucocorticoids also allow glycolysis to proceed during hypoxia by increasing the efficiency of glycolytic enzymes. This glycolytic action provides energy needed for maintenance of cell membranes and organelles.

The benefits of glucocorticoids have been most evident in animals presented with septic or endotoxic shock. Studies have found that glucocorticoids protect the body against liver gluconeogenesis and tissue glycolysis and thereby prevent the hypoglycemia associated with the terminal stage of endotoxic shock. Glucocorticoids have also been shown to reduce the activation of complement, which is believed to be an important cause of tissue damage in septic shock. The mortality associated with experimental septic shock in dogs has been dramatically reduced by administration of an appropriate antibiotic and methylprednisolone in high doses and at frequent intervals.[3] The effects of glucocorticoids have been found to be dose dependent, with low doses having little or no effect and extremely high doses being toxic.[4] The most effective dose

ranges are from 50 to 100 mg/kg of hydrocortisone, 15 to 30 mg/kg of methylprednisolone, and 4 to 8 mg/kg of dexamethasone. These doses should be given intravenously and repeated every four to six hours until the animal is stabilized. Also important is that these drugs be given early in shock; in experimental animals, pretreatment provided a greater effect than did administration of one of these drugs after shock had advanced to a more detrimental stage.[4]

Antiprostaglandins

Antiprostaglandin drugs, such as indomethacin, ibuprofen, and flunixin meglumine, moderate and reverse some of the adverse hemodynamic consequences of sepsis and endotoxemia. Like glucocorticoids, these drugs have been shown to be most useful for treating animals in septic and endotoxic shock. Although antiprostaglandins apparently do not increase chances of survival, they do enhance the effectiveness of other forms of treatment.[5]

Vasoactive Drugs

Vasoactive drugs can be useful in the treatment of volume-resistant shock, that is, shock that does not respond or responds only transiently to volume expansion. This circumstance occurs often with animals in septic shock, in the late stages of hemorrhagic and traumatic shock, or in cardiogenic shock. To improve overall blood flow by relaxing arteriolar constriction and to protect the viscera from progressive ischemia, a number of drugs are recommended.[6] Catecholamines (particularly dopamine, dobutamine, and isoproterenol) and α-receptor blocking agents (such as phentolamine and chlorpromazine) are frequently used to provide vasodilation and improve organ blood flow.

Dopamine, a precursor of norepinephrine, has mild alpha, stronger beta, and specific dopaminergic vasodilating action in the mesenteric, cerebral, renal, and coronary vessels. In low doses (1 to 10 μg/kg/min), dopamine increases blood flow in these vascular beds and exerts a positive inotropic action on the heart (increases the force of contraction) with little change in blood pressure. When treating an animal in shock, dopamine infusion should be initiated at

5 µg/kg/min and the dose rate increased as necessary to normalize urine output and peripheral perfusion.

Isoproterenol is a synthetic catecholamine and a selective β-receptor stimulator that has inotropic and chronotropic actions that strengthen and speed contractions of the heart. Isoproterenol causes vasodilation of arterioles in the skeletal and mesenteric vascular beds while reducing blood volume in the large venous beds. These effects increase cardiac output and peripheral blood flow. Disadvantages of isoproterenol are its cardioaccelerating and arrhythmogenic effects and its tendency to increase metabolic demand for oxygen. The dose range for isoproterenol is 0.2 to 0.8 µg/kg/min. The infusion rate can be adjusted to improve peripheral blood flow without elevating the animal's heart rate beyond 160 to 200 beats/min, depending on the size of the animal.

A newer drug, dobutamine, is being used to augment cardiac output after volume loading. Like dopamine, it is a catecholamine; but, unlike dopamine, it acts directly on the heart only, producing inotropic and mild chronotropic effects with little peripheral vascular effect. Dobutamine has no direct renal or mesenteric effect, but reflex vasodilation is evident as cardiac output increases. Compared with isoproterenol, dobutamine is less arrhythmogenic; however, like isoproterenol, it increases myocardial demand for oxygen. Dobutamine is indicated in cases where cardiac output and tissue perfusion do not increase despite volume loading. The drug is given by intravenous infusion at a rate of 2 to 15 µg/kg/min. The heart rate and parameters of peripheral perfusion should be monitored to guide dosing. Enough of the drug should be given to improve and stabilize tissue perfusion without accelerating the heart rate over 160 to 200 beats/min, depending on the size of the animal.

In contrast to catecholamines, phentolamine and chlorpromazine are α-receptor blocking agents. Phentolamine reduces arteriolar resistance, thereby increasing capillary flow. It increases the rate and strength of myocardial contraction and increases cardiac output if the venous return is maintained. Phentolamine is given as a bolus at a dose of

0.5 µg/kg, followed by infusion of 5 µg/kg/min to maintain peripheral blood flow.

Chlorpromazine, like phentolamine, is an α-blocker but also has central nervous system effects. Unlike phentolamine, it has few and weak cardiac effects. Overall effects are reduced arteriolar resistance, increased venous capacities, and increased peripheral blood flow. Cardiac output must be maintained by volume infusion. The recommended dose is 0.1 to 0.3 µg/kg given as repeated boluses until the desired vasodilation is achieved and then at 30-minute intervals.

The animal should be weaned from vasoactive drugs slowly and in stages decreasing the infusion rate when hemodynamic variables are stabilized. The period of treatment may be as short as 8 hours or as long as 48 hours.

Oxygen

For animals with pulmonary injury associated with shock or with pneumonia or pulmonary edema, oxygen is often beneficial. In conscious, spontaneously breathing animals, oxygen can be provided by oxygen cage or by nasal or transtracheal catheter. The oxygen cage has the advantages of ease of administration and ability to control oxygen concentration. The catheter methods allow access to the animal for monitoring procedures and administering other treatments without disrupting oxygen delivery but require nursing care and attention.

Intranasal oxygen can be provided by inserting into the nasopharynx a soft plastic or rubber catheter lubricated with topical anesthetic gel. The catheter should be sutured to the animal's head, secured with a cervical bandage, and connected to an oxygen source with a flow of 1 to 5 L/min delivered. Transtracheal oxygen can be provided in the same fashion except that a 14- to 16-gauge Intramedicut® Catheter (Sherwood Medical) is inserted percutaneously into the lumen of the midcervical trachea (Figure 5). The catheter should be bandaged in place and connected to an oxygen source with a flow of 1 to 3 L/min delivered.

If spontaneous breathing is ineffective, mechanical ventilation must be instituted. This requires tracheal intubation either orally or by tracheostomy. The animal then is connected to a ventilator, and breathing is mechanically controlled or assisted. In this case, it is advisable to monitor the animal's blood gases to ensure proper adjustment of the ventilator.

Glucose

Provision of metabolic substrates in the form of glucose has been beneficial for some patients in shock. In studies of dogs in experimental septic shock, a combination infusion of glucose, insulin, and potassium has been shown to increase chances of survival.[7] The author has found this combination to be beneficial in some clinical patients.

A mixture containing 3 grams of glucose, 1 unit of insulin, and 0.5 mEq of potassium per kilogram of body weight should be given in a total volume of 250 ml of saline. One third of this solution is administered rapidly over 15 minutes and the rest at a rate that delivers 1 gram of glucose

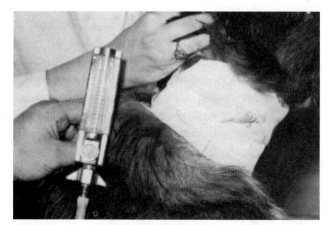

Figure 5—Oxygen may be administered directly into the trachea through a sterile intravenous catheter.

per kilogram of body weight per hour. If no favorable response is evident after the first hour, the infusion can be discontinued. If a favorable response is evident, the rate of infusion should be titrated to achieve the maximum response at the minimum rate of infusion. Administration of this glucose-insulin-potassium mixture can be discontinued when hemodynamic stability is sustained for at least 15 minutes after infusion has stopped.

Summary

Selection and delivery of appropriate drug therapy are essential to restoring and stabilizing circulation volume and oxygen delivery. The appropriate therapeutic protocol is based on accurate assessment of the patient's condition and recognition of the underlying causes of shock. Also essential to patient recovery are proper monitoring and evaluation of the restorative process, which will be the focus of discussion in Part II of this two-part presentation.

REFERENCES

1. Shoemaker WC: Pathophysiologic basis of therapy for shock and trauma syndromes: Use of sequential cardiorespiratory measurements to describe natural histories and evaluate possible mechanisms. *Semin Drug Treat* 3:211-229, 1973.
2. Moss GS, Proctor HJ, Homer LD, et al: A comparison of asanguineous fluids and whole blood in the treatment of hemorrhagic shock. *Surg Gynecol Obstet* 129:1247-1257, 1969.
3. Hinshaw LB, Bellen BK, Archen LT, et al: Recovery from lethal *Escherichia coli* shock in dogs. *Surg Gynecol Obstet* 149:545-553, 1979.
4. Weil MH, Shubin H, Nishijima H: Corticosteroid therapy in circulating shock. *Int Surg* 59:589-592, 1974.
5. Hardie EM, Kolata RJ, Rawlings CA: Canine septic peritonitis: Treatment with flunixin meglumine. *Circ Shock* 2:159-173, 1983.
6. Lewis CM, Weil MH: Hemodynamic spectrum of vasopressor and vasodilator drugs. *JAMA* 208:1391-1398, 1969.
7. Manny J, Ratinovici N, Manny N, et al: Effect of glucose-insulin-potassium on survival in experimental endotoxic shock. *Surg Gynecol Obstet* 147:405-409, 1978.

Management of Shock. Part II. Patient Monitoring*

R. J. Kolata, DVM, MS
Diplomate, ACVS
Experimental Surgery Laboratory
School of Medicine
St. Louis University Medical Center
St. Louis, Missouri

Three facets must be considered when managing a patient in shock: recognition, therapeutics, and patient monitoring. The first two were discussed in Part I (Vol. 7, No. 8), while Part II focuses on patient monitoring. This activity is vital to restoring and stabilizing circulatory volume and oxygen delivery and to selecting and delivering appropriate drug therapy.

As a result of technologic advances, many physiologic variables can be monitored. Combined, they can be used to calculate indexes and parameters that give detailed pictures of a patient's cardiopulmonary status. Unfortunately, most of the instruments required to make these measurements are too costly for use in small animal practices. Diligent monitoring of some easily measured variables, however, along with knowledgeable consideration of their interrelationships, will provide useful information on which to base rational and timely treatment of shock patients. This discussion includes easily obtained variables most likely to be used in clinical practices.

Body Temperature

Body temperature is controlled by the hypothalamus. Heat is produced by metabolism, and heat conservation or dissipation is carried out through the ventilatory and cardiovascular systems. The body temperature of warm-blooded animals must be controlled within a narrow range so that tissues and organs can function optimally.

In addition to core temperature, measurement of skin temperature can be useful in monitoring a shock patient (Figure 1). Because heat is carried to the extremities by blood flow and because skin vessels are controlled by the sympathetic nervous system, measurement of the skin temperature between the third and fourth digits of the hindlimb can be used to obtain information on peripheral perfusion. In an ambient temperature of 20° to 23°C (68° to 74°F), the temperature taken at the toe-web is from 2° to 5°C (3° to 8°F) less than the rectal temperature in a dog with nor-

mal sympathetic tone, cardiac output, and local blood flow. A difference greater than 6°C (10°F) between the rectal and toe-web temperatures indicates that peripheral perfusion is reduced by vasoconstriction or obstruction of flow. Temperature differences greater than 20°C (35°F) indicate extreme vasoconstriction and are associated with severe shock. This measurement has been found to be of value in monitoring postoperative patients and is an accurate indicator of low cardiac output.[1]

Monitoring Procedure

Body temperature monitoring is most conveniently done using a thermistor probe and an electronic thermometer. Skin temperature monitoring requires a thermometer with a range of 20° to 40°C (68° to 103°F).

*Part I of this two-part series appeared in the September 1986 issue (Vol. 7, No. 8) of *Veterinary Technician*.

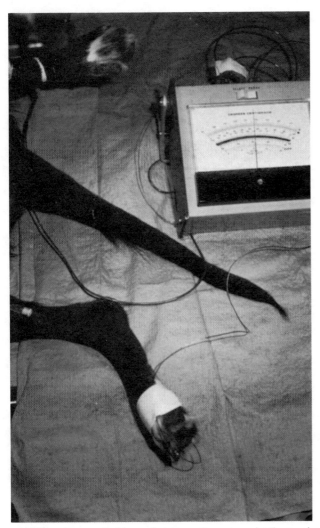

Figure 1—Core and skin temperatures are conveniently monitored using an electronic thermometer.

Breathing Pattern

The function of breathing is to exchange gas between the atmosphere and the blood. Breathing rate and character are influenced by pathologic conditions and by a wide range of reflexes; however, they are not directly correlatable with oxygen demand or the efficiency of ventilation. Nonetheless, breathing rate, character, volume, and sounds are important indicators of changes in oxygen demand and effectiveness of breathing.

Many conditions induce changes in the rate of breathing. Tachypnea in a patient in shock can signal hemorrhage, pneumothorax, pulmonary edema, pneumonia, pain, or increased body temperature.

Changes in the pattern of breathing are signs of intrathoracic or intrapulmonary abnormalities. Breathing will be deep and show signs of increased effort (i.e., retraction of the thoracic inlet and intercostal muscles) if there is restriction of lung expansion by partial airway obstruction or effusion of fluid or blood into the pleural space. When restriction of expansion of the lungs or chest causes inspiration to become difficult and low in volume, expira-

tion becomes active in order to force air from the lungs rapidly so that another breath can be taken. During this sort of breathing, ventilatory effort will be obvious and an expiratory grunt may be heard. These abnormal patterns of breathing, although indicators of problems within the ventilatory system, do not indicate inadequate blood oxygenation. Despite decreased tidal volume, an increased rate may provide a great enough minute volume for adequate oxygenation.

Areas of diminished breathing sounds indicating congestion, atelectasis, or effusion as well as wheezing and crackles indicating fluid or secretions in the airways and alveoli may be heard on auscultation. As with the patterns of breathing, abnormal breathing sounds may not be associated with insufficient ventilation but are important in monitoring the course of the abnormality causing them.

Monitoring Procedures

Assessing and monitoring of ventilatory efficiency is done by careful observation, use of a stethoscope, spirometry, and (when indicated) radiography. Changes in the rate, character, and sounds of breathing do not correlate directly with changes in blood gas values and are only presumptive evidence of impaired ventilation. These changes are important signs, however, and should be monitored routinely.

Tidal volume can be estimated by observing the chest wall. Placing an ear near the patient's mouth and nose to feel and hear the puff of expired air is also a means, although crude, of estimating tidal volume. The most objective way of assessing tidal volume is the use of a spirometer attached by a short ridged tube to a tight-fitting face mask.

Radiography shows pleural accumulation of gas or fluid as well as such pulmonary changes as edema, pulmonary hemorrhage, or atelectasis.

Blood Gases

Arterial blood gas measurements are used to assess the efficiency and adequacy of breathing and, along with mixed venous blood gases, to assess tissue oxygenation.

Arterial carbon dioxide partial pressure (P_{CO_2}) is used to characterize ventilatory status. Elevated P_{CO_2} indicates hypoventilation, and decreased P_{CO_2} indicates hyperventilation. Blood carbon dioxide in conjunction with blood pH are used to determine a patient's acid-base status.

Arterial oxygen partial pressure (P_{O_2}) is used to assess the efficiency of ventilation. It is only slightly influenced by the rate and depth of breathing and is more strongly influenced by the balance between pulmonary blood flow and alveolar ventilation. Problems that reduce the ratio of ventilated–perfused alveoli (e.g., pneumonia, pulmonary contusion, and atelectasis) cause a decrease in oxygen tension despite hyperventilation.

Monitoring Procedures

Blood gas analysis is done using a machine with electrodes for measuring oxygen and carbon dioxide tensions and blood pH.

Blood samples for analysis are obtained from an artery. They are drawn under anaerobic conditions in heparinized syringes. If only the acid-base status is required, venous blood is suitable. The sample should be analyzed immediately, although samples can be stored on ice for up to three hours without clinically important changes taking place.

Packed Cell Volume

Packed cell volume (PCV) is an important variable because of its association with the transport of oxygen. Changes in the packed cell volume are common in shock patients and are usually associated with blood loss or dehydration.

Optimum packed cell volume is considered to be in the range of 30% to 40%.[2] A packed cell volume above 45% is associated with decreased oxygen transport caused by decreased capillary flow. A low packed cell volume is tolerable if it develops slowly so that physiologic compensation can become effective. Patients with abnormally low PCVs, however, do not tolerate stress as well as those with normal PCVs.

The oxygen demand of a shock patient may increase from 20% to 50% above baseline. If the packed cell volume of this same patient is reduced by one half, the cardiac output must double to meet tissue requirements and must triple to meet maximum demand.[3] Such increases may not be possible in a very ill or hypovolemic patient. In addition, myocardial oxygenation is inadequate if the packed cell volume is acutely lowered to 20% (hemoglobin of 7% to 8%) or less.[4] If myocardial oxygenation is inadequate, left ventricular failure may develop, particularly when the cardiac output must be elevated to meet the oxygen demands induced by trauma or sepsis.

In critically ill patients, packed cell volumes in the range of 27% to 33% have been found to be most compatible with survival.[5] Optimum packed cell volume corresponds to a hemoglobin concentration of 10% to 12%.

Monitoring Procedures

Assessing the color of the patient's mucous membrane is used as a crude estimate of the packed cell volume and hemoglobin content. Packed cell volume is conveniently monitored by using capillary tubes and a microhematocrit centrifuge. Colorimetric methods are available to measure hemoglobin.

Heart Rate

The heart is a pump that outputs according to its rate of pumping and its stroke volume. Although it is an important determinant of cardiac output, the heart rate does not correlate directly with output. Nonetheless, rates outside the normal range, both high and low, are associated with reduced cardiac output. Although the number of beats per minute alone does not describe cardiac function, trends in rate do reflect some changes in function. Pain and excitement cause transient elevations. A continuously high resting rate or a rate that is gradually increasing with time indicates hypoxemia, deteriorating myocardial function, or

inadequate intravascular volume. Bradycardia, which is caused by vagal stimulation and hypothermia, can reduce the oxygen transport and allow development of dysrhythmias that may further reduce output.

Heart rhythm is also important with regard to output. Ventricular dysrhythmias can elevate heart rate while decreasing cardiac output caused by inadequate filling. Because optimum cardiac output is necessary for adequate oxygen delivery and because rate and rhythm influence output and cardiac work, monitoring of these variables is important with shock patients.

Monitoring Procedures

Heart rate can be measured by palpation of the apex impulse on the chest wall; palpation of the arterial pulse; auscultation; use of a Doppler flow detector; recording of arterial pulse waves using a catheter, strain gauge, and recorder; or electrocardiograms (which are discussed in the section on Cardiac Electrical Activity).

Each method has its advantages and disadvantages. Palpation of the apex impulse detects cardiac activity but can be unreliable in obese patients and those in shock. Palpation of the arterial pulse has the same advantage and disadvantage plus may be inaccurately low in patients with some dysrhythmias. Auscultation provides accurate assessment of rate as well as some indication of the strength of cardiac activity because the audible volume of the heart sounds roughly correlates with the strength of contraction and ejection volume. Amplifiers that connect to stethoscopes can be purchased to assist auscultation and make such monitoring more convenient.

An informative technique for continuous monitoring of the heart rate is to place an ultrasonic Doppler flow probe detector over a suitable artery and connect it to a signal amplifier (Figure 2). The audible signal of each pulse wave can be heard and can be used to monitor heart rate and blood flow. A disadvantage of this method is the probe's sensitivity to position and movement.

Electronic heart rate meters that trigger at the R wave can be used for continuous heart rate monitoring. Their

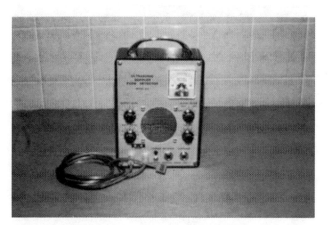

Figure 2—A Doppler flow probe and signal amplifier can be used to monitor heart rate and arterial pressure.

usefulness is limited, however, because no information about the mechanical activity of the heart is obtained.

Cardiac Electrical Activity

Depolarization and repolarization of cardiac muscle fibers is normally an orderly process and one that is coupled to mechanical activity. Factors influencing development of cardiac dysrhythmias include local myocardial injury, hypothermia, hypoxemia, hypercapnia, acidosis, changes in potassium concentration, and the effects of drugs and anesthetics. In many instances, a synergy exists between the inciting factor and the patient's sympathetic nervous system; an example is the depressant effect of halothane on the myocardium lowering the threshold for the arrhythmogenic effects of catecholamines. Shock patients with problems known to be associated with dysrhythmias (e.g., gastric dilatation-torsion or myocardial contusion) require electrocardiographic monitoring throughout the recovery period.

Monitoring Procedures

Electrocardiographic monitoring is ideally done using an instrument with an oscilloscope and a paper recorder. Because diagnostic-quality recordings are not necessary, a three-lead system placed in an appropriate configuration on the chest wall and using modified alligator clips or needle electrodes can be used to obtain leads II or III. Proper grounding of the patient is important because satisfactory grounding will reduce interference from other electrical equipment.

Arterial Pulse

The arterial pulse is a product of left ventricular contraction. Its character depends on stroke volume, rate and force of ejection, and vascular tone. Evaluation of the pulse is an acceptable way to make a subjective evaluation of cardiovascular function quickly and easily.

Variations in stroke volume, force of ejection, and vascular tone change the pulse character in definable ways. A small stroke volume ejected rapidly into a vascular tree having increasing tone, as occurs in patients in early shock, produces a sharp, high-amplitude, short-duration pulse in the femoral artery and an imperceptible pulse in the distal artery. Conversely, a normal volume ejected with less than normal vigor into a dilated vascular tree, as may exist during anesthesia, produces a soft, low-amplitude, long-duration pulse in the femoral artery and a weak distal pulse.

Palpation of proximal and distal artery pulses can give a crude estimation of blood pressure. The weaker the proximal pulse and the more difficult it is to palpate the distal pulse, the lower the blood pressure is likely to be.

Palpating the arterial pulse can also help detect and monitor some dysrhythmias, as rhythm and pulse strength vary irregularly.

Monitoring Procedures

Arterial pulse is most readily monitored by palpating a peripheral artery. The femoral artery is most commonly used; but the lingual, labial, brachial, distal ulnar, cranial tibial, plantar, and median coccygeal arteries can also be used.

To obtain the most complete information when palpating arterial pulses, familiarity with the character of the pulses of normal animals is necessary. Variations from the expected character or rate should initiate more objective investigation and assessment of the cardiovascular system.

Arterial Pressure

Arterial pressure depends on cardiac output and vascular tone. A range of arterial pressures can be found in normal animals, and the pressure can vary from minute to minute in each patient. The variation is within a relatively narrow range because pressure must be maintained to allow autoregulation of blood flow within organs. If arterial pressure is below the critical pressure of about 60 mm Hg, blood flow within organs becomes pressure dependent and perfusion will be inadequate and organ function begin to fail.

Monitoring Procedures

Arterial pressure can be estimated by palpating the pulse or can be measured directly or indirectly. Direct measurement of arterial pressure is best done using an arterial cath-

Figure 3—A Doppler flow probe along with an inflatable cuff and an aneroid manometer are used together to measure arterial pressure.

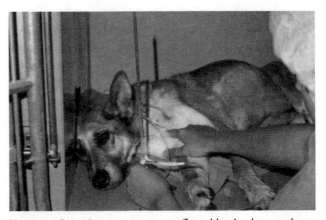

Figure 4—Central venous pressure reflects blood volume and cardiac filling. It is monitored using a central venous catheter and a saline manometer.

eter, a transducer, a signal processor, and a recorder, although an aneroid manometer can be used. Direct measurement of arterial pressure is accurate and has the advantage of allowing access to arterial blood for blood gas analysis; however, this procedure has the disadvantage of being invasive; that is, such complications as thrombosis, embolisms, hemorrhage, and infection can occur and frequently nursing care is required. In addition, the electronic equipment is expensive and requires maintenance.

Indirect blood pressure measurements are most conveniently made using one of two types of ultrasonic detectors: (1) a flow detector that detects the movement of red cells or (2) a flow detector that detects movement of the arterial wall during the pulse wave. Both detectors are used with a pneumatic cuff to occlude flow and an aneroid manometer to measure pressure (Figure 3). Both of these methods are accurate and correlate well with direct measurements if a cuff of proper width is used. Two disadvantages of indirect measurement are (1) at low pressure it may be difficult to find a peripheral artery over which to place the sensor and (2) both methods are least accurate at low pressures, which represent the pressure range of greatest interest. A third disadvantage is that sensor location is critical and easily disturbed by patient movements. Nonetheless, both indirect methods have the advantage of being relatively inexpensive, easy, noninvasive, and safe; and (as mentioned previously) the Doppler flow detector can be used to monitor heart rate and blood flow as well as pressure. Aneroid manometers used for either direct or indirect measurement of pressure should be calibrated periodically to ensure accuracy.

Central Venous Pressure

Central venous pressure (CVP) is used clinically to monitor fluid volume infusion because of its relationship to blood volume, although this relationship is indirect. Blood pressure in the cranial vena cava depends on intrathoracic pressure, tone of capacitance vessels, blood volume, rate of venous return, and right ventricular function. When right ventricular function is adequate, the central venous pressure is controlled by the tone of the capacitance vessels and intrathoracic pressure. Pneumothorax will raise intrapleural pressure and tend to elevate central venous pressure. When blood volume or venous return exceeds the upper or lower limits of possible venous compensation, the central venous pressure will be outside the normal range. The ability of changes in venous tone to compensate for changes in volume makes continuous monitoring a more reliable guide than simply taking isolated measurements.

Central venous pressure does not reflect pulmonary venous or left atrial pressure and therefore cannot reliably identify conditions predisposing the patient to pulmonary edema. In patients without pulmonary vascular disease or left ventricular failure, however, this inability does not interfere with its value as a guide for fluid volume replacement. The disadvantages are the same as those for arterial

pressure monitoring, that is, invasive, expensive, and requiring nursing care and maintenance.

Monitoring Procedures

Central venous pressure is measured using a large-bore catheter with its tip in the cranial vena cava near the right atrium. The catheter is usually connected to a saline-filled manometer, and the pressure is read in centimeters of saline (Figure 4). Because of the low pressures measured, the technical aspects of CVP monitoring are crucial if accuracy and reliability are to be achieved. Catheter position is important and should be verified before measurements are made. Radiographs are the most accurate way of determining catheter position, but it is more convenient to assume accurate placement by seeing pressure fluctuations of about 5 mm of saline corresponding to inspiration and expiration. The reference point of measurement must be at right atrial level. The system should be flushed to remove all air bubbles, and the reference point must be verified before each measurement. Pressure readings should be taken during several breathing cycles to ensure accurate measurement.

Even when every effort is made to follow proper technique, values obtained by a saline manometer can be falsely high by as much as 2 to 4 cm of saline because of the slow-frequency response of the system.[6] Accurate CVP values are obtained by using a transducer and electronic recorder.

Capillary Refill Time

Capillary refill time (CRT) is a measurement of tissue perfusion. When arterial pressure is reduced or, more important, when arterial and arteriolar vasoconstriction are present, perfusion of a capillary bed is diminished and slower than normal. Consequently, mucous membranes are pale; and, if an area of membrane is blanched by applying fingertip pressure, when that pressure is released, blood flow and hence return of color into the area are slower than normal. It must be pointed out that capillary refill time reflects vasomotor tone and not blood pressure. Low pressure with vasodilation, which occurs with a dead or deeply anesthetized patient, can result in a normal capillary refill time; while an apprehensive patient, and one therefore with peripheral vasoconstriction but normal blood pressure, may have a prolonged refill time.

Monitoring Procedures

Capillary refill time can be assessed by applying digital pressure to the oral mucous membranes for a short time (one to two seconds) and rapidly releasing that pressure. The time for the blanched area to return to the color of the surrounding membrane is the capillary refill time. Using a stopwatch to time the return of color allows consistency in evaluation; however, the time is generally judged as normal or abnormal by simple observation. Because a patient's packed cell volume as well as available light affect recognition of the return of color, changes in either should be considered when judging changes in the capillary refill time. Normal is considered to be less than two seconds.

Urine Output

The kidneys regulate the volume, tonicity, and chemical composition of extracellular fluid; in doing so, they receive about 20% of the cardiac output.

Intravascular volume is an extremely important stimulus for changes in urine output. Decreases in intravascular volume cause an increase in antidiuretic hormone (ADH) secretion, with a decrease in urine volume. As volume is further decreased, glomerular filtration pressure is decreased and further reduction in urine volume occurs. If arterial pressure decreases to about 60 mm Hg, renal autoregulation fails, glomerular filtration stops, and urine production ceases. Because of these renal responses to intravascular volume and pressure changes, measuring urine output provides (by inference) information about blood volume, intravascular pressure, and tissue and organ perfusion.

Monitoring Procedures

Measurement of urine output requires collecting and measuring urine produced during a preselected interval. The most effective method of collecting urine is by using an indwelling urethral catheter that continuously empties into a closed sterile container (Figure 5). Intermittent drainage using an indwelling catheter can be done by occluding the catheter between collections. This method is subject to error because of urine loss around the catheter when the bladder distends between collections. Aseptic insertion and management of the catheter must be done to avoid urinary tract infection. Measurement of the specific gravity of the urine as well as the volume collected provides additional information about intravascular volume and fluid balance. High specific gravity (>1.030) low-volume urine is associated with dehydration, and the converse (specific gravity <1.015) is associated with overhydration or renal failure.

Serum Proteins

Serum proteins are important components of the internal environment. They have several vital functions. Globulins produced by lymphocytes are active in specific immunity, and α-globulins produced by the liver are important in nonspecific immune response. This nonspecific response has been shown to be significant after trauma or surgery. The albumin component of serum proteins is the single most important. Albumin is important for maintenance of plasma volume and proper hydration of tissue through its colloidal osmotic effect. It is an important binding and transport system for drugs, metabolic products, and hormones and is a reserve of protein for catabolism and repair. These functions are so important that patients with hypoproteinemia, particularly hypoalbuminemia, have higher complication and mortality rates than those with normal protein concentrations. Plasma protein and albumin concentrations at one half of normal values can be tolerated by an otherwise healthy shock patient. It is advisable to keep these values as close to normal as possible, however, particularly in patients expected to have a prolonged recovery.

Shock patients lose proteins because of preexisting dis-

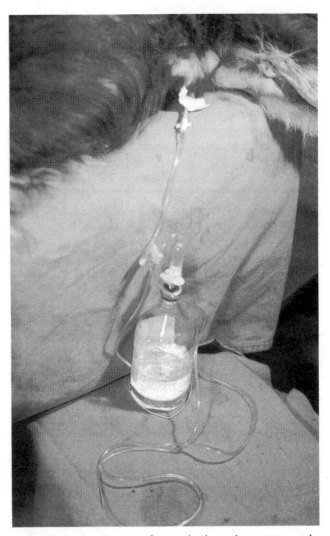

Figure 5—A closed system for monitoring urine output can be readily assembled using an intravenous administration set and an empty sterile fluid bottle.

ease, hemorrhage, tissue injury, and inflamed and traumatized mesothelial membranes and tissue surfaces. Plasma protein concentration is inversely related to intravascular water concentration, with high protein concentration suggesting dehydration and low protein concentration suggesting overhydration and the need for plasma transfusion.

Monitoring Procedures

Total protein and albumin can be measured by colorimetric methods. Total protein can also be measured by a refractometer, using the plasma from the blood taken for the hematocrit (i.e., to determine the packed cell volume).

Acid-Base Balance

Acid-base abnormalities are common in shock patients. Of the four classically described acid-base states, perhaps the most commonly encountered are metabolic acidosis and metabolic acidosis with respiratory compensation. Metabolic acidosis is found in patients with poor tissue perfusion, which occurs during shock or during prolonged anesthesia. Respiratory compensation occurs by increased breathing and by eliminating carbon dioxide.

Perhaps the most important effects of acid-base changes are those occurring to the heart and oxygen transport systems. Acidosis depresses ventricular function when severe (pH <7.2), and alkalosis (pH >7.5) inhibits oxygen delivery to tissues. Acid-base changes also influence the distribution of electrolytes, with acidosis causing elevation of plasma potassium and alkalosis decreasing plasma-ionized calcium.[7]

Monitoring Procedures

Acid-base balance is most rapidly and accurately assessed by measuring blood pH and P_{CO_2} with a blood gas analyzer. After these variables are known, acid-base status can be determined by using a nomogram.

Another method of assessing acid-base status is to titrate an anaerobically obtained blood sample with acid to estimate the bicarbonate content. If the pH is unknown, errors in interpretation of the results of titration will occur because the effects of metabolic alkalosis and of compensation for respiratory acidosis are to raise plasma bicarbonate levels and the effects of metabolic acidosis and of compensation for respiratory alkalosis are to decrease plasma bicarbonate levels.

Electrolytes

Electrolyte abnormalities are linked to fluid balance and acid-base abnormalities.[7] Loss of blood and plasma results in a proportionate loss of extracellular electrolytes. Acidosis tends to cause an increase in plasma potassium and alkalosis a decrease in serum-ionized calcium. Losses of fluid and electrolytes take place in patients with such conditions as vomiting, diarrhea, gastrointestinal obstruction, and peritonitis. Each of these problems causes loss of a particular combination of electrolytes. Vomiting causes hypochloremia and alkalosis from losses of hydrogen and chloride. Diarrhea tends to result in losses of sodium, potassium, and magnesium plus water, resulting in dehydration and acidosis.

In most cases of trauma with shock, there is loss of potassium, which can lead to hypokalemia after resuscitation.

Monitoring Procedures

Physical signs of major electrolyte abnormalities are nonspecific and apparent only at extremes in concentration. The most accurate and reliable method of determining sodium, potassium, and chloride concentrations are flame photometry or ion-selective electrodes. Photometric and titration methods are also available for determining chloride levels.

Clinically important changes in potassium can be detected and monitored by interpreting electrocardiograms.[8] Hyperkalemia tends to impair conduction from the sinoatrial node to the atrioventricular node. At potassium concentrations of 6.0 to 6.5 mEq/L, peaked T waves are seen. Wide QRS complexes and flattened P waves are associated with potassium concentrations of 6.5 to 7.0 mEq/L. Atrial

standstill, depressed S–T segments, and wide QRS complexes are seen when potassium reaches 7.0 to 9.0 mEq/L; and cardiac arrest can occur at concentrations greater than 9.0 mEq/L.

Hypokalemia tends to increase the rate of discharge of nodal tissue and decrease conduction through the ventricle. In patients with hypokalemia, electrocardiographic findings are bradycardia, prolonged Q–T intervals, and small biphasic T waves. Hypokalemia is not as accurately detected by electrocardiograms as hyperkalemia is.

Hypoxemia causes changes in electrocardiograms that may be confused with changes in potassium concentration. These can be differentiated, however, because hypoxemia causes peaking of T waves and elevation of the S–T segment without the P wave and QRS changes that occur with potassium abnormalities.

Summary

Management of a patient in shock may be as simple as providing intravenous fluids and a quiet place to recover from the effects of a small self-limiting hemorrhage or as complex as providing fluids, oxygen, blood transfusions, and other supportive therapy for a postoperative patient that suffered blood loss and surgical trauma in addition to the effects of the problem that required surgery.

Regardless of the magnitude and duration of a patient's state of shock, successful treatment requires early recognition of the problem and selection and delivery of appropriate therapy guided by a knowledge of the patient's physiologic needs, all of which are obtained by diligent and timely monitoring.

It is vitally important to be aware that monitoring a shock patient requires surveillance of a number of variables simultaneously to obtain sufficient information to ensure adequate treatment. Because many of these variables are interdependent, particularly those assessing blood volume flow and cardiac function, it is necessary to measure several of them concurrently and evaluate them with regard to one another in order to obtain optimum information about the patient's condition. Without this evaluation, a patient may die unexpectedly because monitoring has been inadequate and timely, appropriate treatment therefore not delivered.

REFERENCES

1. Kolata RJ: Significance of changes in toe web temperature in dogs in circulatory shock. *Proc 28th Gaines Vet Symp*:21–26, 1978.
2. Fan FC, Chen RYZ, Schwessler GB, et al: Effects of hematocrit variations on regional hemodynamics and oxygen transport in the dog. *Am J Physiol* 238:545–551, 1980.
3. Shoemaker WC: Cardiorespiratory patterns of surviving and nonsurviving postoperative patients. *Surg Gynecol Obstet* 134:810–814, 1972.
4. Jaw K-M, Heldman J, Chien S: Coronary hemodynamics and oxygen utilization after hematocrit variations in hemorrhage. *Am J Physiol* 240:326–334, 1980.
5. Czer LSC, Shoemaker WC: Optimal hematocrit value in critically ill postoperative patients. *Surg Gynecol Obstet* 147:363–367, 1978.

6. Mann RL, Graziano CC, Turnball AD: Comparison of electronic and manometric central venous pressures. *Crit Care Med* 9:98–102, 1981.
7. Tasker JB: Fluids, electrolytes, and acid-base balance, in Kaneko JJ (ed): *Clinical Biochemistry of Domestic Animals*, ed 3. New York, Academic Press, 1980.
8. Coulter DB, Engen RL: Differentiation of electrocardiographic changes due to asphyxia and to hyperpotassemia in dogs. *JAVMA* 160:1419–1423, 1972.

The Technician's Role in the Management of Dogs with Congestive Heart Failure

David B. Joseph, AHT

Northridge, California

Congestive heart failure is the syndrome that occurs as the result of abnormal sodium and water retention and an accumulation of extracellular fluid in the lungs. Patients and clients benefit when veterinary technicians have a proper understanding of this disease process. With prompt medical treatment and appropriate drug

Originally published in Volume 11, Number 9, October 1990

therapy, affected patients can lead relatively normal lives.

Case Example

A 77-pound, 12-year-old, castrated male golden retriever with dyspnea (labored breathing) was presented to Porter Pet Hospital. Physical examination of the patient demonstrated pink mucous membranes, and auscultation of the thorax demonstrated muffled heart sounds. The heart rate was 102 beats/min. On palpation, the abdomen was normal. The temperature was 101.0°F. Additional diagnostic studies included electrocardiogram, thoracic radiographs, hemogram, serum biochemistry profile, and urinalysis.

Radiographs demonstrated pulmonary congestion, some pleural effusion, and moderate tracheal elevation. The electrocardiogram showed sinus arrhythmia and suggested left atrial enlargement. The patient was given 125 milligrams of intramuscular furosemide. Later that day, the dog was breathing much better and was released to the owner with a prescription of furosemide to be given orally at a dosage of two (50-mg) tablets per day. The owner was asked to return the dog to the hospital the next day for a checkup.

Radiographs taken 24 hours later demonstrated a considerable reduction in pulmonary fluid. The owner was advised to continue the prescription as indicated and to return the patient in one week for reevaluation. On examination, the dog was improving and no congestion was apparent. The dose of oral furosemide was reduced as follows: for three days, 100 milligrams was given twice daily; then 50 milligrams was given twice daily for two days. The patient was maintained on 50 milligrams twice daily.

The dog was stable for approximately nine months and then was returned to the hospital for radiographs and an electrocardiogram. The radiographs demonstrated increased congestion, and the electrocardiogram showed sinus arrhythmia and P-mitral. The prescription was oral captopril (25-mg tablets) given three times a day and a change in diet. The diet was Prescription Diet® Canine h/d® (Hill's Pet Products). The patient was maintained at a dosage of 12.5 milligrams of oral captopril three times a day. Several months later, the dog was presented to a local emergency clinic for collapse and possible atrial fibrillation. Advised of the poor prognosis, the owners decided on euthanasia.

Anatomy of the Heart and the Cardiac Cycle

A review of the heart anatomy and cardiac cycle facilitates understanding of the disease process of congestive heart failure. The heart is a large muscular pump composed of a special type of striated muscle tissue that contains a complex network of veins, arteries, and nerves. The heart is divided into four chambers: the right atrium, right ventricle, left atrium, and left ventricle.

The cardiac cycle begins with the filling of the right atrium with venous blood, which is then pushed through the atrioventricular valve and into the right ventricle. From the right ventricle, venous blood is delivered to the lungs via the pulmonary artery; here the blood is oxygenated and returned to the left atrium via the pulmonary vein. From the left atrium, the oxygenated blood flows through the mitral valve and into the left ventricle; from here, the thick-walled left ventricle pumps blood through the aorta, to the network of arteries, and to the rest of the body.[1]

Cause

There are three categories of congestive heart failure: primary failure of contractility, systolic mechanical ventricular overload, and diastolic mechanical interference. Primary failure of contractility, which occurs if primary myocardial disease is present, is a common cause of congestive heart failure. Systolic mechanical ventricular overload produces a chronic overload of the affected ventricle and thus results in decreased ventricular contractility and subsequent congestion. This syndrome occurs frequently with chronic atrioventricular valve fibrosis and with congenital heart disease, such as patent ductus arteriosus.

Diastolic mechanical interference occurs if a prohibiting factor, such as pericardial effusion, restricts ventricular filling. The interference, which can be caused by pericardial disease, does not necessarily lead to congestion.[2]

The most common cause of left-sided heart failure or congestive heart failure is mitral valve regurgitation. This condition usually occurs in old patients. Evidence suggests that male dogs are affected more frequently than female dogs. In a 1979 study conducted by Buchanan, 62% of patients that were at least 8.5 years of age had mitral valve disease alone.[3]

Proper closure of the mitral valve requires six components working as a unit. The components are the mitral leaflets, chordae tendineae, mitral annulus, papillary muscles, left ventricular wall, and left atrial wall. Failure of one or more of these structures can produce mitral valve disease.

Mitral valve disease can occur if a fibrous formation of tissue prevents one or more of the components from working to ensure proper closure of the mitral valve. A backward flow of blood can reenter the left atrium and can lead to mitral valve regurgitation, which is named for the audible murmur that is detected via stethoscope during auscultation of the chest.

There is no initial problem with congestion because cardiac output compensates to adjust to the new demands of the body. As mitral valve regurgitation progresses, the heart undergoes a loss of contractility and left-side enlargement. Decreased cardiac efficiency and an increased heart rate result.

Role of Fluid Retention

It has been known for years that the cardiovascular system and renal function are codependent. Patients with congestive heart failure and decreased cardiac output also have decreased urinary output. Normal cardiac function allows the proper amount of blood to pass through the kidneys, and the sodium-to-water ratio remains within normal limits.

A failing heart reduces blood flow; poor renal perfusion and renal vasoconstriction result. Renal vasoconstriction causes the redistribution of blood in the kidney such that renal cortical blood flow is reduced while relatively normal medullary flow is maintained.[4] When extracellular levels of sodium drop and potassium levels increase, the kidneys produce renin; this substance acts on angiotensinogen in the plasma. Enzymes convert angiotensin 1 to angiotensin 2, which acts as a potent vasoconstrictor.

This process occurs in the lungs and in the zona glomerulosa (part of the adrenal gland), which in turn releases aldosterone. The secretion of aldosterone further augments the retention of sodium by the kidneys. This process stimulates secretion by the kidneys. Cardiac work load increases as more fluid enters the bloodstream. Ultimately, fluid leaves the vascular compartment. The resulting clinical signs are ascites and/or edema, particularly pulmonary edema.

Clinical Signs

In most patients with mitral valve regurgitation, associated clinical signs usually become evident after seven years of age. Patients usually present with a dry and hacking cough, listlessness, and dyspnea (especially in the early morning or after exercise). Coughing is one of the body's earliest responses to congestion of blood in the lungs.

On physical examination of a patient with possible left-sided heart failure, a systolic heart murmur may be auscultated. Other clinical signs include resting tachycardia (fast heart rate), diminished pulse amplitude, systemic venous engorgement, and moist pulmonary rales.[5] A systolic murmur can produce a "wash-wash" sound instead of the normal "lub-dub" sound. Excess fluid in the lungs (pulmonary edema) can sometimes be heard while listening to the thorax with a stethoscope. In some patients, severe pulmonary congestion leads to respiratory distress and collapse. Immediate medical attention is required.

Diagnosis

When a patient is admitted to the hospital, several diagnostic tests should be performed to accumulate a data base for appropriate diagnosis and treatment. Before diuretics or other medications are given, a venous blood sample should be obtained in order to evaluate the patient's hemogram and serum chemistry. An electrocardiogram should be taken using at least six leads; 10 leads are preferred to assess adequately the electrical activity of the myocardium. The six preferred leads are leads I, II, III, aVR, aVL, and aVF. In patients with left-sided heart failure or mitral valve regurgitation, the electrocardiogram may demonstrate a tall or wide P wave as well as a widening of the QRS complex.

Thoracic radiographs should be taken with the patient in right lateral recumbency. A ventrodorsal view is also useful. If the patient is in respiratory distress, a dorsoventral view should be taken and so labeled. Evaluation of the radiographs by the veterinarian can demonstrate cardiomegaly (on the lateral view), tracheal elevation, and pulmonary edema. The ventrodorsal view confirms left- or right-side enlargement and the extent of pulmonary congestion. The ventrodorsal view helps to rule out or confirm masses in the lungs or heart. The technician must take high-quality radiographs while subjecting the patient to a minimum of stress.

Management
Initial Therapy

The goal of initial therapy is to alleviate pulmonary congestion, restrict sodium intake, correct electrical imbalances, and begin a beneficial course of therapy. Before therapy is instituted, a data base of the patient's laboratory values, electrocardiogram, and radiographs should be evaluated. If there is no evidence of additional systemic disease, therapy is initiated.

If pulmonary congestion is radiographically evident, the most effective method of removing extracellular fluid is to administer a diuretic. The most commonly used diuretic, furosemide, is given orally at a dosage of 1 to 4 mg/kg as often as three times daily.[6] An oral bronchodilator (to dilate or expand the pulmonary bronchi), such as aminophylline, can be given at a dosage of 6 to 9 mg/kg three times daily if the patient is dyspneic.[7]

Another bronchodilator that is available to practitioners, sustained-release theophylline, offers timed-release action to alleviate dyspnea longer. The agent can be given orally at a dosage of 6 to 11 mg/kg three times daily.

Emergency Treatment of Acute Congestive Heart Failure

In a congestive heart failure patient that is undergoing long-term therapy, there can be an acute onset of respiratory signs. Immediate medical attention is required to save the patient's life.

Acute congestive heart failure occurs quickly and without warning as a result of trauma that causes immediate accumulation of pleural fluid in the lungs. Acute congestive heart failure can occur in puppies that chew on electrical cords or in dogs with cardiomyopathy. Chronic congestive heart failure is a long-term problem; after a long period of therapy, treatment is no longer effective. In all cases of congestive heart failure, stress (e.g., from radiographs, blood collection, or oral medication) should be avoided if possible until the patient is stabilized.

Emergency treatment should include the following elements:

- Placing an intravenous catheter
- Administering oxygen for 5 to 10 minutes to increase the blood oxygen content and to give the technician time to follow the veterinarian's orders
- Slowly administering intravenous aminophylline (4 to 8 mg/kg) diluted with 20 milliliters of D5W solution
- Administering intramuscular or intravenous furosemide (2 to 4 mg/kg).

If these steps are followed, the condition of the patient can improve in 30 minutes.

This treatment can be repeated in two hours. If the patient is still failing, intravenous dobutamine (2.5 μg/kg/min) is recommended to increase cardiac contractility. Dobutamine must be diluted before use and given in a slow infusion. One vial (250 mg) can be diluted in one liter of D5W solution; 1 drop/kg/min is administered via a standard microdrip venoset.

Maintenance Therapy

Good maintenance therapy is essential in the management of patients with congestive heart failure. Treatment must be carefully chosen to achieve the effect dictated by the veterinarian's instructions, the patient's needs, and the client's expectations.

Several drugs are available to veterinarians. Technicians should be familiar with the mode of action and results associated with each of these drugs.

The most commonly used cardiovascular drugs in veterinary clinics are digoxin, captopril, and hydralazine hydrochloride. Again, it is essential to have a proper data base (i.e., complete blood count, serum chemistry, radiographs, and electrocardiogram) before long-term drug therapy is instituted. The technician can make the veterinarian aware of reactions to medication and client compliance with a prescribed course of therapy. The technician must be able to inform the client of several complications that can result from cardiorespiratory therapy.

Three major complications can arise from such therapy: untoward generalized systemic effects (e.g., hypotension or organ underperfusion), adverse drug interactions, and direct or indirect toxic effects on target and nontarget organs.[1]

The main objectives of maintenance therapy are to reduce the cardiac work load and to ease sodium retention. The magnitude of work load reduction is determined by the severity of the disease: the more severe the disease, the greater the exercise restrictions imposed on the patient.

Heart failure can be classified in four phases. Phase 1 is clinically inapparent and requires no exercise restriction. In Phase 2, the patient is comfortable at rest but experiences fatigue, dyspnea, or coughing during physical activity. Strenuous exercise should be avoided. In Phase 3, the patient is comfortable at rest but minimal exercise causes coughing, dyspnea, and fatigue. If the patient is lying down, dyspnea may result; only moderate home exercise should be allowed, and stair climbing should be forbidden.

Phase 4 is much more severe. The patient has difficulty breathing while at rest and may be slightly cyanotic. Such signs as cough and fatigue are aggravated by any type of stress or exercise. Total exercise restriction must be imposed.

The first goal of therapy is to minimize clinical signs. Vasodilators, such as captopril, are relatively new on the market. Captopril is administered orally at a dose of 0.5 to 2.0 mg/kg[1] and is available in 12.5- and 25-milligram tablets. The drug is an angiotensin-converting enzyme inhibitor. It acts by blocking the conversion of angiotensin 1 (secreted by the kidneys) to angiotensin 2. Natriuresis (renal excretion of sodium) and increased renal perfusion result.

Captopril causes a moderate degree of arterial and venous vasodilation. It is recommended that serum urea nitrogen and serum creatinine levels be monitored because such complications as acute renal failure and hyperkalemia have been associated with the use of captopril. Other side effects are hypotension and anorexia, even at low doses.

Another vasodilator, hydralazine hydrochloride, is given orally at a dosage of 0.5 to 3.0 mg/kg twice daily. The action of this agent differs from that of captopril. Hydralazine causes a high degree of arterial dilation but is a less-effective venous dilator than captopril. Hydralazine reduces the volume of blood regurgitation in the mitral valve by decreasing the diastolic blood pressure, increasing the stroke volume, and increasing cardiac output; there is a resulting decrease in venous blood pressure.[6] As mitral valve regurgitation lessens and lung congestion subsides, the effectiveness of the cardiac cycle increases. The disadvantages associated with long-term use of vasodilators include varying dosages, hypotension, tachycardia, sodium retention, and gastrointestinal signs.

The use of the cardiac glycoside digoxin in patients with congestive heart failure is intended to improve myocardial contractility and stabilize (decrease) the heart rate. This therapy can be used in conjunction with diuretic therapy (before vasodilators) or alone (after diuretics and vasodilators fail). Digoxin exerts its effects by increasing myocardial contractility and thus permitting greater stroke volume and decreasing congestion.

A disadvantage of digoxin is its narrow therapeutic value; the drug can produce toxicity at relatively low doses. The toxicity level may overlap into the therapeutic dose and lead to early signs of digoxin toxicity. Clinical signs can take as long as 10 days to become evident. The signs usually occur when the patient is on the maximum dose allowed but can occur at any time. Therapy involves discontinuing the drug for 24 to 48 hours or until signs cease; digoxin is then reintroduced at a lower dose.

Most dogs recover from digoxin toxicity rapidly because of the rapid clearance of the drug from the body. A blood test that is available at local laboratories indicates levels of digoxin in the blood; the test may be helpful in determining whether toxicity has occurred or whether therapeutic levels have been reached.

The maintenance dosage of digoxin in dogs is 0.02 mg/kg/day given in one or two doses. The dosage in cats is 0.01 to 0.16 mg/kg/day.[6] Loading doses (above-normal doses during the first few treatments) of digoxin were once administered to achieve therapeutic levels of the drug rapidly. Because there is no therapeutic advantage to loading doses, they are no longer recommended.

Dietary Management

Good nutritional management of patients with congestive heart failure is essential. Technicians can assist clients with the general diets that are available and can explain necessary supplementation. Technicians should be aware of the eight goals of dietary management:

- Reduce sodium intake
- Prevent hypoproteinemia
- Prevent potassium deficiency
- Provide calories from carbohydrates
- Reduce the amount of catabolic waste from protein metabolism, thus decreasing functional renal load
- Provide sufficient nutrition to maintain proper body weight
- Supplement B-complex vitamins
- Provide a high-ash diet to aid in sodium excretion.

Sodium restriction is the primary objective of all diets for patients with congestive heart failure. Dogs and cats reabsorb sodium from the kidneys more effectively than humans do. It is therefore essential to limit sodium intake to approximately 10 mg/kg/day. The ideal food for dogs with advanced or moderate congestive heart failure is Prescription Diet® Canine h/d® (Hill's Pet Products), which contains less than 95 milligrams of sodium per 100 grams of dry matter. The diet also supplies the required potassium (an element usually lost via drug diuresis) as well as other nutrients necessary to proper nutrition of patients with congestive heart failure.

Wherever sodium goes, water follows. Diuretic therapy affects the sodium-to-potassium ratio of the patient. If there is a high level of aldosterone, potassium loss might result in hypokalemia. Signs of hypokalemia include general weakness, changes on the electrocardiogram, azotemia, reduced glucose tolerance, altered blood pressure, and poor urine concentration.[3]

Such diets as Prescription Diet® Canine h/d® provide 150 to 250 mg/kg of potassium with no further supplementation. Too much potassium can lead to hyperkalemia, which in turn can lead to cardiac arrhythmias.

Client Education

When the patient is stable, the proper doses of medication have been established, and the veterinarian has discussed the treatment with the client, it is often the technician who answers common client questions and explains medication techniques. The client must understand that it is essential that medications be given at regular intervals.

Technicians should be prepared to give helpful tips and instruction.

Among the first changes is the diet of the patient. When a diet is to be changed, the client should be instructed to make the transition as gradually as possible. To alleviate concern about how much salt or potassium the patient is getting, the technician should encourage the use of diets that are complete and require slight or no supplementation. A 7- to 14-day transition may be needed to accustom the patient to a new food product. Low-sodium diets are less palatable than diets with higher sodium content.

Instruct clients to mix the new diet into the old diet gradually while decreasing the amount of the old diet. A smooth transition should result. If an immediate diet change is necessary, I recommend that the food be warmed and seasoned with a small amount of garlic powder.

Hypoproteinemia can occur in old dogs and cats as protein uptake is diminished by faulty metabolism. This condition causes extra retention of fluid. Supplemental protein should be avoided because most old patients have some form of renal failure. If the client wishes to use homemade recipes, the diet should contain 14% to 18% protein from dry matter. The protein should be high quality and easily digested.

In old dogs and cats, the gastrointestinal tract can have decreased blood flow as a result of poor arterial circulation. Meals should be fed frequently and in small quantities.

Supplementation is necessary if owners prefer not to use prepared diets. During diuretic therapy, the body excretes large quantities of fluid and B-complex vitamins. The intake of B vitamins should be increased to five times the normal amount. This can be accomplished by adding brewer's yeast (1 g/kg/day) or B-complex preparations to the diet.[3]

Because adequate water intake is critical, free access to water should be available at all times. A lack of water causes electrolyte imbalances and dehydration and can result in acute renal failure. Water that contains no sodium (available at many distributors) may be preferred; water treated by home water-softening systems contains high salt concentrations. If the patient has advanced heart failure, only distilled water should be used.

The client must understand that a pet with chronic congestive heart failure will be on medication for the rest of its life. Clients should be encouraged to contact the doctor or technician if questions or problems arise. Technicians play a key role in explaining the proper method for administering medication in the treatment of patients with congestive heart failure.

It is important to allow the owner to administer the first dose while still in the examination room. This practice enhances the client's self-confidence and trust in the technician. Design a schedule for medication that coincides with the client's work schedule, particularly if medication and/ or feeding must be done three times a day or more.

Summary

Congestive heart failure is a lifelong disease that can be managed well with proper diet and proper therapy. The technician's vital role involves educating clients about giving medications, recognizing the possible side effects of responding to acute exacerbations, and counseling clients about diet management.

Congestive heart failure is usually incurable but manageable. The patient can live an extended, high-quality life. The main goals of cardiac therapy are to reduce sodium and to decrease fluid in the lungs or abdomen. Aggressive, safe therapy can dramatically benefit the patient. The technician must ensure that the client has accurate instructions about the diet and schedule of medication and that these instructions are followed exactly.

Acknowledgments

The author is grateful for the help and support of James Craig, VMD, MS, Porter Pet Hospital; Elizabeth White, AHT, Director, Animal Health Technology Program, Pierce College, Woodland Hills, California; and Vetronics Corporation.

■

REFERENCES

1. Thomas WP: Long-term therapy of chronic congestive heart failure in the dog and cat, in Kirk RW (ed): *Current Veterinary Therapy. IX.* Philadelphia, WB Saunders Co, 1989, pp 368–376.
2. Ralston SL: Dietary considerations in the treatment of heart failure, in Kirk RW (ed): *Current Veterinary Therapy. IX.* Philadelphia, WB Saunders Co, 1989, pp 302–307.
3. Ross JN: Heart failure, in *Small Animal Clinical Nutrition.* Topeka, KS, Mark Morris Associates, 1987, pp 11-1–11-35.
4. Bauer T: Diagnostic approach to cardiopulmonary disorders, in Kirk RW (ed): *Current Veterinary Therapy. IX.* Philadelphia, WB Saunders Co, 1989, pp 188–194.
5. Reed JR: Acquired valvular heart disease in the dog, in Kirk RW (ed): *Current Veterinary Therapy. IX.* Philadelphia, WB Saunders Co, 1989, pp 231–237.
6. Fox PR: Complications of cardiopulmonary drug therapy, in Kirk RW (ed): *Current Veterinary Therapy. IX.* Philadelphia, WB Saunders Co, 1989, pp 308–315.
7. Kirk RW: Cardiac emergencies, in *Handbook of Veterinary Procedures and Emergency Treatment,* ed 4. Philadelphia, WB Saunders Co, 1985, pp 51–56.

Fluid and Electrolyte Therapy in Cardiac Patients

Clifford R. Berry, DVM
Veterinary Technology Program
St. Petersburg Junior College
St. Petersburg, Florida

Christophe W. Lombard, DrMedVet
Department of Medical Sciences

Jennifer Lombard, RANA
Veterinary Teaching Hospital

College of Veterinary Medicine
University of Florida
Gainesville, Florida

The role of fluid therapy for the cardiac patient requires an understanding of the pathogenesis of congestive heart failure. Under conditions of poor circulatory function, certain compensatory mechanisms result in salt and water retention in order to preserve cardiovascular output. Not only are the deleterious effects of loading a cardiac patient with fluids important to recognize but also the rate of fluid administration as well as the effects of acute withdrawal of diuretics, any of which can result in pulmonary edema and death.[1] This article covers the pathogenesis of congestive heart failure, the electrolyte abnormalities commonly seen in heart failure patients, and the role of fluid therapy in the treatment of the small animal cardiac patient.

Pathophysiology of Heart Failure

Congestive heart failure can have many predisposing factors and disease states that can result in a decreased forward ejection or stroke volume of blood to the rest of the body.[2] The most common cause of congestive heart failure in dogs is a disease called *endocardiosis* or *chronic valvular disease*, which leads to insufficiency of the atrioventricular valves.[3] Other causes of cardiac failure include dilated cardiomyopathy, bacterial endocarditis with aortic valvular insufficiency, congenital heart disease, and many of the other acquired heart diseases. The organs that are most sensitive to a decrease in blood perfusion include the brain, the myocardium itself, and the kidneys. Each of these organs has compensatory mechanisms that are stimulated by poor cardiac output. The end result of these compensatory changes is the maintenance of an adequate blood supply not only to the organ itself but to the rest of the body.[4-7]

The kidneys play an important role in the maintenance of normal fluid and electrolyte homeostasis in the body. Once the kidneys start becoming hypoxic and/or detect a decrease in the renal arterial blood flow or renal arterial pressure, a number of reactions are set into motion, with the net result being sodium and water retention. The hormone *renin* is released by the kidney and activates a circulating protein called *angiotensinogen*, which is converted into angiotensin I. Activated angiotensin I is then converted to angiotensin II by an enzyme found primarily in the lungs. Angiotensin II has three primary actions: (1) peripheral vasoconstriction of the arterioles; (2) stimulation of the release of aldosterone from the adrenal cortex; and (3) stimulation of thirst, thereby increasing fluid intake.[3,4] *Aldosterone* is a mineralocorticoid hormone that regulates sodium and potassium levels in the bloodstream. The increase in the aldosterone blood levels results in retention of sodium and water and excretion of potassium by the kidneys.[5,7]

The central nervous system, by way of pressure and volume receptors that are located in the circulatory system, reacts to the decrease in effective plasma volume and pressure by increasing sympathetic discharge from the autonomic nervous system.[3,5] The end result of this reflex is peripheral vasoconstriction as well as an increase in heart rate and myocardial contractility. In addition, antidiuretic hormone (ADH) is secreted by the neurohypophysis (i.e., caudal part of the pituitary gland), resulting in increased water retention by the distal convoluted tubules and collecting ducts of the kidneys. These three basic homeostatic mechanisms, which are initially beneficial to the cardiac patient by improving cardiac output, ultimately result in excessive fluid accumulation[3] and congestive heart failure. The signs of congestive failure have been reviewed.[8] Once cardiac failure occurs, a vicious cycle in which progressive cardiac failure will result in more fluid retention and cause the heart to work harder (increased myocardial oxygen demand and cardiac work) is initiated, which in turn will result in further cardiac failure and further edema formation.[3-5]

Electrolyte and Acid-Base Imbalances
Sodium

Total body sodium is increased by the mechanisms previously discussed, although serum sodium usually is normal in value (140 to 155 mEq/L).[5] Sodium is the major cation responsible for creating the osmotic gradient and drawing water back into the body from the filtrate in the kidney tubules. Sometimes, the serum sodium levels may in fact be slightly low (hyponatremia) because of a dilutional effect. In these cases, the constant release of antidiuretic hormone has resulted in excessive water retention, which is not related to either sodium retention or the osmotic gradients created by excessive sodium.[5,7] When giving fluids to a cardiac patient, the sodium content of the fluids to be given should always be considered. It is best to use fluids that have low sodium content or no sodium at all. Therefore, the intravenous fluid of choice is 5% dextrose in water.[5,6,9] Dilutional hyponatremia can also be caused iatrogenically by overadministration of these fluids to the heart failure patient.

Potassium

Serum potassium levels may be decreased, normal, or increased in heart failure patients. Hyperkalemia can exist predominantly in low cardiac output in which prerenal azotemia (elevated blood urea nitrogen and creatinine levels) are concomitantly present.[5,7,10] Also, the use of potassium-sparing diuretics (e.g., spironolactone), excessive potassium chloride oral supplementation, or concurrent hypoadrenocorticism can predispose the cardiac patient to hyperkalemia. Severe hyperkalemia, especially in the presence of hyponatremia, can lead to some severe and often life-threatening abnormalities in cardiac rhythm.[11] The end result electrocardiographically is atrial standstill and a sinoventricular rhythm (Figure 1). Sustained low cardiac

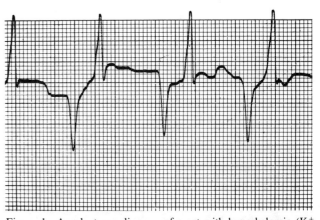

Figure 1—An electrocardiogram of a cat with hyperkalemia (K^+ = 9.5 mEq/L) secondary to urethral obstruction. Notice the bradycardia (heart rate = 75 beats/min), lack of P waves, peaked T waves, and a wide and bizarre QRS pattern. Paper speed: 50 mm/sec. Sensitivity: 2 cm = 1 mV.

output and diminished renal blood flow can lead to concurrent primary renal failure. Evaluating the patient's urine concentration ability before using diuretics is important in determining the patient's renal function. Renal failure patients will tend to have high serum potassium levels; and, in advanced cases in which renal shutdown (acute renal failure) has occurred, hyperkalemia is again a life-threatening problem. A low urine specific gravity will be present in patients with primary renal disease, even before diuresis.

Hypokalemia can be a common sequela in chronic congestive heart failure and may result from prolonged anorexia (decreased potassium intake) or elevated circulating aldosterone levels (increased potassium excretion by the kidneys). Potassium excretion is also enhanced when diuretics that are not potassium sparing (such as furosemide) are used. As with sodium, an iatrogenic dilutional hypokalemia can occur when overzealous fluid administration is followed. In addition, an intravenous dextrose solution used in cardiac patients promotes the uptake of potassium into the cells of the body through the action of the hormone *insulin*. Hypokalemia is particularly life-threatening when concurrent medications, such as digitalis, are given.[5,11] Low potassium levels predispose the animal to digitalis toxicity, the combination of which can potentiate cardiac arrhythmias. Also, when the animal is alkalemic (blood pH greater than 7.42), potassium excretion in the renal tubular epithelial cell is promoted because the kidneys are trying to retain acid (to buffer the alkalemia) in the form of the hydrogen ion. Because this hydrogen ion is reabsorbed from the filtrate by the tubular epithelial cell, potassium is exchanged and excreted.[10]

Acid-Base Status

Acid-base disorders are usually complex in nature in patients with cardiac disease. The severity of the acid-base imbalance depends on many factors, including tissue oxygenation, lactic acid accumulation, and renal excretion of acids.[4,5,10] Respiratory acidosis is usually present in acute, decompensated heart failure in which carbon dioxide is not exchanged adequately at the alveolar-capillary level and builds up in the bloodstream, thus creating acidosis. Acidosis can also result from an inadequate blood volume being pumped to the lungs, causing carbon dioxide (acid) retention. A large pericardial or pleural effusion can cause compression atelectasis of the lungs so that inadequate amounts of air or blood will flow to areas of gaseous exchange and a severe ventilation-perfusion mismatch occurs.[5]

Metabolic alkalosis (blood pH greater than 7.45) can also be found in the heart failure patient. This is usually secondary to chronic use of furosemide and to hypokalemia. In order to compensate, the kidneys will try to retain potassium and excrete the hydrogen ion. The end result is called *contraction alkalosis*.[10] Also, digitalis toxicity can result in excessive vomiting. This loss of hydrochloric acid may result in metabolic alkalosis. Respiratory alkalosis can be a result of increased respiratory rate and excessive loss of carbon dioxide because of congestive heart failure and pulmonary edema.

In the previous two paragraphs, examples of isolated acid-base disorders were described. In the cardiac patient, however, compensatory mechanisms have usually taken place so that the blood pH has normalized. In other words, the metabolic acidosis that commonly occurs in a cardiac patient has been compensated for; and the end result is a blood pH in the normal range (7.38 to 7.42).[4,5]

Fluid Therapy and Management of the Cardiac Patient
Patient Evaluation

Each cardiac patient should be clinically assessed and the status of its condition categorized in one of the New York Heart Association (NYHA) clinical classes (Table I); classification is based on a thorough history, physical examination, and clinical severity of congestive heart failure.[8] This classification provides the veterinarian or veterinary technician with a method for determining the response of the patient to therapy. For example, initial evaluation of an NYHA Class I to III cardiac patient should include an electrocardiogram, chest radiographs, blood work, and urinalysis.

If the patient is placed in NYHA Class IV and is in respiratory distress with cyanosis, a diagnostic workup should be postponed and the animal placed in an oxygen cage.[2,12] Furosemide should be administered subcutaneously or intravenously to help relieve the pulmonary edema. Morphine sulfate can also be given in order to reduce the animal's anxiety.[1,12] Morphine administration, however, should be done with caution and the patient put under constant supervision because this drug is a known respiratory depressant and can cause respiratory acidosis. This therapeutic approach to NYHA Class IV patients should be followed only if they have left-sided cardiac failure.

Recognition and treatment of four basic emergency settings related to the cardiovascular system are necessary for survival of the Class IV cardiac patient that falls into the

TABLE I
Classification of Congestive Heart Failure Patients[a]

Class	Description
I	No exercise intolerance (no dyspnea or coughing with normal activity or exercise); cardiac murmur present; normal electrocardiogram and radiographs
II	Animal comfortable at rest but ordinary activity produces fatigue, dyspnea, or coughing; chamber enlargement patterns recognizable on electrocardiogram and radiographs
III	Animal comfortable at rest but minimal exercise may produce fatigue, dyspnea, and coughing; orthopnea (respiratory distress) may develop when the animal is recumbent for prolonged period of time; arrhythmias may be present on electrocardiogram and pulmonary edema present on thoracic radiographic examination
IV	Congestive heart failure present at rest; signs of dyspnea, cyanosis, and coughing exaggerated with minimal exertion; thoracic radiographs and electrocardiogram reveal severe cardiomegaly or chamber enlargement patterns, respectively

[a]Some information contained herein was obtained from the New York Heart Association and from Ettinger SJ, Suter PF: *Canine Cardiology.* Philadelphia, WB Saunders Co, 1970.

subgroup of a life-threatening cardiovascular emergency that requires immediate attention and appropriate therapy. The four syndromes in this subgroup are (1) cardiogenic shock, (2) acute heart failure, (3) pericardial tamponade, and (4) cardiac arrhythmias.[13] Each of the four settings has different fluid therapy requirements and therefore should be treated as separate conditions. Physical examination findings and fluid therapy requirements are presented in Table II.

After any Class IV patient has been stabilized for at least 24 hours, a complete workup should be performed. This should include a complete blood count, serum chemistries, urinalysis, and chest radiographs. Usually these patients require constant electrocardiographic monitoring. It is imperative to analyze a rhythm strip on an hourly basis during this time to detect subtle changes that may be caused by developing electrolyte imbalances or the appearance of new arrhythmias. An S-T segment depression (which may be caused by hypokalemia or hyperkalemia) and prolongation of the Q-T interval (which may be caused by hypocalcemia, hypokalemia, or hypothermia) are two examples of how electrolyte abnormalities can be detected by the presence of electrocardiographic changes.[11]

Patient Monitoring

All of the basic monitoring procedures needed by the veterinary technician in the critical care setting have been described in the literature.[14] These include weight, body temperature, capillary refill time, mucous membrane color, arterial pulse, indirect blood pressure measurement, electrocardiogram, blood gases, and daily packed cell volume

TABLE II
New York Heart Association Classification of Acute Class IV Patients[a]

	Cardiogenic Shock	*Acute Heart Failure*	*Pericardial Tamponade*	*Cardiac Arrhythmias*
Temperature	Decreased	Normal to decreased	Normal	Normal to decreased
Heart rate	Rapid	Rapid	Normal/increased	Decreased or increased
Heart sounds	Normal	With/without murmur, gallop rhythm	Muffled	Irregular
Membrane color	Pale to white	Pale/cyanotic	Pale pink	Pale/cyanotic
Pulses	Weak, rapid	Weak, rapid	Weak	Irregular with/without pulse deficits
Heart failure signs	Recumbent	Pulmonary edema	Pleural effusion, ascites	Weakness, syncope, edema
Electrocardiographic findings	Sinus tachycardia	Chamber enlargement, tachycardia with/without arrhythmias	Low voltage, electrical alternans[11]	Arrhythmia present[11]
Initial therapy	Fluid therapy,[9,16] oxygen therapy with/without hydrocortisone sodium succinate	Furosemide,[12] vasodilators, cage rest, oxygen therapy	Pericardiocentesis	Appropriate antiarrhythmic therapy[13]

[a]Patients are categorized into four basic syndromes based on the findings at physical examination and electrocardiographic results. The goal of initial therapy is to stabilize the patient and determine the underlying causes of shock.

and total protein. A central venous pressure (CVP) measurement can be set up by using an indwelling jugular venous catheter and a water-filled manometer. The manometer should be placed so that the mark for 0 cm of water is at the same height as the right atrium (mid-thoracic region just caudal to the elbow).[15] The manometer can then be opened to the jugular venous catheter; the fluid line will fall until the central venous pressure is reached (Figure 2). The optimum pressure for a dog in heart failure has been suggested to be 8 to 11 cm of water. Central venous pressures also can be used to monitor diuretic and fluid therapy as well as serve as an accurate measurement of right-sided cardiac filling pressures.[4,14,15] An elevated central venous pressure (greater than 12 cm of water) is usually associated with elevated right-sided filling pressures and edema formation. In animals in acute shock, fluids should be administered at a rapid rate. The concern for loading the patient with fluids and thus creating a "wet" lung situation, however, requires special monitoring of the central venous pressure. These measurements can govern the rate of fluid administration and help prevent against overloading the cardiac patient with fluids. The following guidelines for monitoring central venous pressure can assist the veterinary technician in evaluating fluid administration[16]:

1. Measure the central venous pressure.
2. Infuse the patient for 10 minutes as follows:

CVP	Rate (ml/kg/min)
<8	4
8 to <14	2
>14	1

3. Following infusion, measure the central venous pressure.

Rise in CVP (cm of water)	Decision
>5	Stop
>2 to <5	Wait 10 minutes
<2	Continue infusion

In order to obtain the values of pulmonary venous pressure and left atrial filling pressures, a special balloon-tipped catheter (Swan-Ganz Thermodilution Catheter—Edwards Laboratory) is "floated" into a pulmonary lobar artery. A percutaneous technique for pulmonary arterial catheterization has been described using local anesthesia only.[17] This technique is usually performed under fluoroscopic guidance or pressure-monitored control. This cathe-

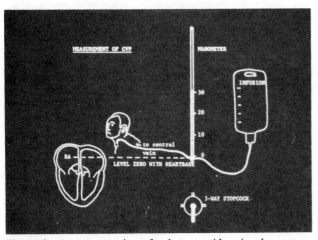

Figure 2—A representation of a human with a jugular venous catheter in place and connected to a fluid-filled manometer for a central venous pressure measurement. Note that the height of the base of the manometer (stopcock) is at the level of the right atrium.

TABLE III
Drip Speeds of Different-Sized Infusion Sets

Calculated Fluid per Hour (ml/hr)	*Amount of Fluids per Minute (ml/min)*	*Number of Drops of Fluid per Minute Based on Infusion Set Size*		
		10 drops/ml	*20 drops/ml*	*60 drops/ml*
10	0.17	2	3	10
20	0.35	3	7	20
30	0.50	5	10	30
40	0.65	7	13	40
50	0.85	8	17	50
60	1.00	10	20	60
70	1.20	12	23	70
80	1.35	13	27	80
90	1.50	15	30	90
100	1.65	17	33	100
120	2.00	20	40	120
140	2.35	23	47	140
160	2.70	27	53	160
180	3.00	30	60	180
200	3.30	33	67	200
250	4.15	42	83	250

ter can also measure cardiac output (liters per minute) by using a previously described thermodilution technique.[5] A capillary wedge pressure greater than 20 mm Hg (determined when the balloon of the catheter tip is inflated and the catheter is wedged into a pulmonary lobar artery) is considered to be elevated and is associated with pulmonary edema formation.[5]

Fluid Therapy

Indications for fluid therapy in cardiac patients would include (1) dehydration, (2) renal failure, (3) administration of intravenous cardiotonic or antiarrhythmic drugs, (4) correction of any electrolyte and/or acid-base imbalance, and (5) cardiogenic shock. Use of previously described central venous pressure guidelines is necessary to ensure that the cardiac patient is not loaded with fluids.[15,16]

Patients in cardiac failure and requiring fluid therapy should be placed on sodium-free isotonic solutions, such as 5% dextrose in water. Daily fluid requirements include submaintenance calculations (20 ml/kg/day), rehydration of the patient (% dehydration × body weight in kg × 1000 ml = ml needed to rehydrate the patient), plus evaluation of other fluid losses (urinary output, vomiting, or diarrhea). Body weight, oral fluid intake, urinary output (using a urine collection system or volume estimates), packed cell volume and total protein, and central venous pressures are all essential methods for monitoring patients when giving intravenous fluids. Total sodium intake should be limited to 12 mg/kg/day or 0.5 mEq/kg/day. If metabolic acidosis is present and warrants therapy, the amount of sodium present in sodium bicarbonate must be included when figuring total daily sodium intake (23 mg of sodium per mEq of sodium

bicarbonate). Potassium administration should be done only if severe hypokalemia (potassium level less than 2.5 mEq/L) has been documented. Doses of 0.5 to 2.0 mEq/kg are used for intravenous administration over a 24-hour period. Anuria, oliguria, hyperkalemia, and the use of potassium-sparing diuretics (spironolactone) are all contraindications for supplementing the cardiac patient with potassium.[5,10]

Intravenous administration of various cardiac drugs to improve cardiac output or suppress arrhythmias must be done as a constant-rate infusion drip because of the short half-lives of these various drugs. These patients must be carefully monitored, and the intravenous setups must be properly placed and accurate drip rates maintained to ensure accurate delivery of the drugs being used.[14]

Because small amounts of fluids are usually given, the intravenous setup requires a pediatric drip set (35 drops/ml); if the animal is receiving fluids for dehydration or maintenance, the two fluid lines must be separated, as the rate of administration of the dehydration or maintenance fluids usually exceeds the rate of drug administration. The following formula can be used for constant-rate infusion drips:

$$\frac{\text{body weight (kg)} \times \text{dose (µg/kg/min)} \times 60 \text{ min/hr}}{\text{concentration (µg/ml)}}$$

$$= \text{ml infused over one hour}$$

Table III provides drip rates (drops/min) for pediatric and adult fluid administration sets; these rates can be used to calculate the amount of fluids that should be administered to the patient over a one-hour time period.

Summary

Many homeostatic mechanisms play a role in the pathogenesis of congestive heart failure and edema formation. The end result is a volume overloading of sodium and extracellular fluids (including blood plasma). Careful monitoring of the hydration and electrolyte status of cardiac patients is mandatory because these animals usually have multiple-system failure. Defining the exact cause of failure and using fluid therapy only when indicated are essential parts of the treatment regimen for congestive heart failure patients.

REFERENCES

1. Cohen JS: A summary of complications of fluid therapy, in Schaer MS (ed): *Fluid and Electrolyte Balance. Veterinary Clinics of North America.* Philadelphia, WB Saunders Co, 1982, pp 545–558.
2. Morgan RV: Cardiac emergencies—Part I. *Compend Contin Educ Pract Vet* 3(7):649–657, 1981.
3. Thomas WP: Long term therapy of chronic congestive heart failure in the dog and cat, in Kirk RW (ed): *Current Veterinary Therapy VII. Small Animal Practice.* Philadelphia, WB Saunders Co, 1980, pp 368–376.
4. Hamlin RL: Fluid and electrolyte balance in congestive heart failure. *JAAHA* 8:224–228, 1972.
5. Bonagura JD: Fluid and electrolyte management in the cardiac patient, in Schaer MS (ed): *Fluid and Electrolyte Balance. Veterinary Clinics of North America.* Philadelphia, WB Saunders Co, 1982, pp 501–513.
6. Chew DJ, Kohn CW, DiBartola SP: Disorders of fluid balance and fluid therapy, in Fenner WR (ed): *Quick Reference to Veterinary Medicine.* Philadelphia, JB Lippincott Co, 1982.
7. Chew DJ: Electrolytes and osmolality, in Fenner WR (ed): *Quick Reference to Veterinary Medicine.* Philadelphia, JB Lippincott Co, 1982.
8. Lombard JC, Lombard CW: The role of the veterinary technician in the outpatient visit of a pet with heart disease. *Vet Tech* 6(9):442–445, 1985.
9. Cornelius LM: Fluid therapy in small animal practice. *JAVMA* 176(2):110–114, 1980.
10. Schaer MS: Disorders of potassium balance and acid-base disorders, in Schaer MS (ed): *Fluid and Electrolyte Balance. Veterinary Clinics of North America.* Philadelphia, WB Saunders Co, 1982, pp 399–410.
11. Tilley LP: *Essentials of Feline and Canine Electrocardiography*, ed 2. Philadelphia, Lea & Febiger, 1985.
12. Kittleson M: Drugs used in the management of heart failure, in Kirk RW (ed): *Current Veterinary Therapy VIII. Small Animal Practice.* Philadelphia, WB Saunders Co, 1983, pp 368–376.
13. Muir W, Bonagura JD: Cardiovascular emergencies, in Sherding RG (ed): *Contemporary Issues in Small Animal Practice: Medical Emergencies.* New York, Churchill Livingstone, 1985, pp 37–94.
14. Lombard JC, Lombard CW: The monitoring of cardiac patients in the intensive care unit by the veterinary technician. *Vet Tech* 6(10):489–494, 1985.
15. Vintinner LP: Central venous pressure monitoring in the dog. *The AHT* 3(4):196–200, 1982.
16. Webb AI: Fluid therapy in hypotensive shock, in Shaer MS (ed): *Fluid and Electrolyte Balance. Veterinary Clinics of North America.* Philadelphia, WB Saunders Co, 1982, pp 515–532.
17. Henderson RA, Dillon AR, Brawner WR, et al: Technique for percutaneous pulmonary arterial catheterization in conscious dogs. *Am J Vet Res* 46(7):1538–1539, 1985.

Central Venous Pressure Monitoring in the Dog

Larry P. Vintinner, BS
Animal Health Instructor
Animal Health Technology
Newbury Junior College
Holliston, Massachusetts

The central venous pressure (CVP) is a blood pressure measurement taken from the anterior vena cava. CVP is used to estimate the fluid requirements of the patient (effective circulating blood volume) and the efficiency of the heart's pumping. Measuring the CVP aids in the clinical evaluation of a patient in shock, an elderly patient undergoing surgery, and a patient in any situation in which blood volume and cardiac function are of concern.

The CVP is a measurement of effective blood volume, cardiac pumping action, and the vascular bed. If the heart is healthy, the CVP is the first parameter to drop when circulation is deficient, and it is the last parameter to return to normal after the animal responds to appropriate therapy.[1] Therefore, the CVP can provide a valuable guide to fluid replacement therapy and to the pumping ability of the heart. Continuous monitoring of the CVP probably provides the best immediate information about the patient regarding the severity of shock and the quality of the animal's response to therapy.[2]

A low or normal CVP indicates that blood replacement can be begun or safely continued. An elevated or rising CVP with falling blood pressure, increased capillary refill time, reduced pulse pressure, and signs of pulmonary edema indicates a fluid volume overload and myocardial failure.[3,4]

Procedure

Following sedation or use of a short-acting general anesthetic, the animal is placed in a lateral or supine (ventrodorsal) position. The hair is clipped over the external jugular vein, and the area is given an aseptic surgical scrub with an iodine-based preparation.[5] A commercial manometer unit[a] is fastened to an intravenous stand at about 2 to 5 inches above the top of the surgical table. Exact positioning of the manometer is explained later in this article.

If a commercial manometer unit is not available, an improvised manometer unit can be constructed using a second intravenous infusion set and a desk ruler. Securing the improvised manometer unit to the intravenous stand may be done in one of two ways. In the first method, the intravenous infusion tubing is fastened vertically to the intravenous stand with adhesive tape. The ruler is placed underneath the tubing as a measurement guide and is also fastened to the intravenous stand with adhesive tape (Figure 1). In the second method, a fabricated CVP device is used, as shown in Figures 2 and 3.[b,c] This device makes attachment and adjustment of the manometer unit to the intravenous stand efficient and easy. Following preparation of the manometer, a 1-L bottle of isotonic infusion fluid and an intravenous infusion set are readied for use.

A percutaneous puncture of the external jugular vein is made with a 14- to 18-gauge, 2-inch needle with a catheter inside.[d] The catheter is advanced into the anterior vena cava until the catheter tip approaches the third intercostal space (the tip of the catheter at the entrance to the right atrium), establishing direct fluid continuity with the right atrium.[6] The catheter is secured with adhesive tape or a gauze bandage around the animal's neck, making sure to incorporate the hub of the catheter. The intravenous infusion tubing and the manometer are then connected to the catheter via a

[a]CVP Manometer #4607, Abbott Laboratories, North Chicago, IL 60064.

[b]Jumbo Holder #1J, Hold-All Manufacturing, Inc., Suffern, NY 10901.
[c]Rubber stopper #R5145-3, American Scientific Products, Bedford, MA 01730.
[d]Venocath-14 #4614, Abbott Laboratories, North Chicago, IL 60064.

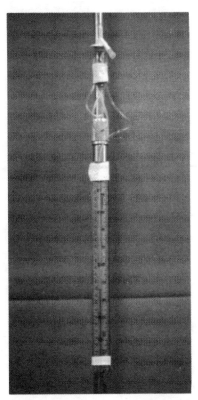

Figure 1—A desk ruler is fastened to an intravenous stand with infusion tubing placed in the center groove. Dye has been added to the fluids to provide color contrast. The fluids are at the 12-cm level.

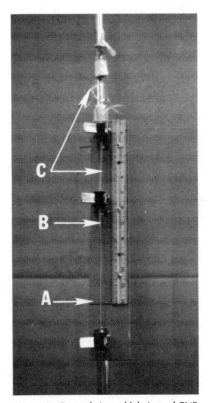

Figure 2—Frontal view of fabricated CVP device, with *A*, the 0-cm reference line; *B*, the fluid level at 12.5 cm; and *C*, the infusion tubing with excess tubing and the drip chamber fastened to the intravenous stand.

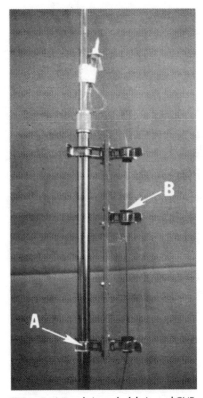

Figure 3—Lateral view of a fabricated CVP device, with *A*, the support clamp; and *B*, the rubber stopper (24-mm diameter, modified with a ¼-inch center hole and a ¼-inch vertical groove for insertion of infusion tubing).

three-way stopcock.[c] The screw clamp on the fluid infusion set is opened, and the stopcock is positioned to allow fluid to flush out the catheter (stopcock closed to the manometer). After catheter patency has been assured, the stopcock is positioned to allow the manometer to fill up to or above the 15-cm mark (stopcock closed to the catheter).

The CVP varies widely, depending on the level at which the zero-reference point of the manometer is positioned in relation to the right atrium of the animal's heart. If the dog is in left or right lateral recumbency, the zero-reference point of the manometer unit is aligned and level with the midline of the trachea at the thoracic inlet[1] (Figure 4). If the dog is in the supine position, the zero-reference point of the manometer is aligned and level with the third intercostal space and halfway between the sternum and spinal cord[1] (Figure 5). A carpenter's level[f] that is fastened to a taut string or cord provides an excellent guide to the proper adjustment of the level of the manometer and anatomical reference points (Figure 4).

[c]Three-way Stopcock, Propper Manufacturing Co., Inc., Long Island City, NY 11101.
[f]Line Level #555, Johnson Level and Tool Manufacturing Co., Inc., Milwaukee, WI 54405.

Interpreting CVP Readings

The stopcock is positioned (closed to the infusion set) so that there is a column of fluid from the anterior vena cava to the manometer. When the column of fluid, which is preset at 15 cm, falls under that level, it represents the pressure in the anterior vena cava. A fluctuation of 2 to 5 mm in the fluid, coinciding with heartbeats and

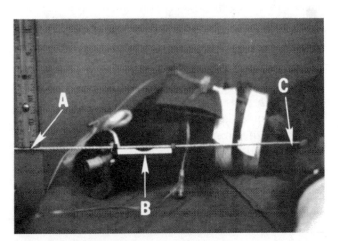

Figure 4—A fabricated CVP device in use. Note *A*, the zero-reference point; *B*, the carpenter's level; and *C*, the black line, designating the lateral anatomical reference point at the midpoint of the trachea at the thoracic inlet.

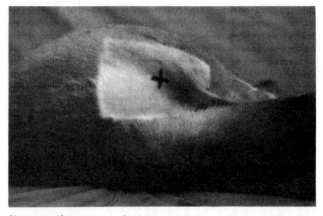

Figure 5—The anatomical reference point, *X*, for ventrodorsal positioning is the third intercostal space, halfway between the sternum and the spinal cord.

respirations, indicates that the catheter tip is correctly placed and accurate readings can be obtained. Positional changes of the animal (lateral to supine) may cause reading fluctuations of 3 cm or more in fluid level.[3]

With the zero-reference point in place, the normal CVP values for dogs and cats vary from 0 to 10 cm.[4] When the CVP reading is below 6 to 8 cm of fluid, blood volume replacement is indicated. A CVP that stabilizes at levels between 8 to 10 cm of fluid usually indicates an expanded blood volume, and fluid administration should be slowed or stopped.[2,3] A CVP measurement rising close to or above 15 cm indicates a fluid overload and impending myocardial insufficiency.[2] With an elevated CVP, all fluid administration must be terminated; blood volume reduction may be necessary and can be performed via the CVP catheter. Because the CVP of dogs and cats normally varies between 0 and 10 cm, administration of intravenous fluids depends on the results of other clinical parameters such as hematocrit, color of mucous membranes, heart rate, respiration rate, and capillary refill time.

Clinical Use

If the purpose of measuring the CVP is to monitor venous pressure, and fluid administration is of secondary importance, periodical positioning of the stopcock to flush out the catheter and to prevent blood clot formation in the catheter is advised. If the primary purpose is to rapidly infuse fluids to restore functional blood volume, then the stopcock should be periodically positioned to measure the CVP level and to evaluate the animal's response to therapy.

While employing this technique, the author has used catheters of varying sizes (14 gauge, 16 gauge, and 18 gauge). The 14-gauge catheter provides excellent manometric fluctuations of approximately 5 mm which correspond with cardiac and respiratory actions. This fluctuation was distinctly visible in the manometer, greatly aiding visual inspection of a patent, operational

system. Fluctuations of approximately 2 mm were observed when the 18-gauge catheter was used. The slight fluctuations were difficult to observe and hindered identification of the fluid level in the manometer. The smaller catheter also tended to become more readily occluded with blood clots and required frequent flushing with infusion fluids.

When the 14-gauge catheter was used, subcutaneous hematomas developed in several animals following catheter removal from the jugular vein. No such complication occurred when the 18-gauge catheter was employed. Application of a pressure bandage at the puncture site during the recovery period aided in controlling the frequency and size of hematomas. Ultimately, the appropriate catheter size is determined by factors such as the animal's size and physical condition, the fluid infusion rate, and personal preference.

Summary

In a small animal veterinary practice, the cost of a commercial manometer and the infrequency of its use may not justify its purchase. However, the availability of a common metric desk ruler and an ample supply of intravenous infusion sets make CVP procedures possible with minimal additional equipment, i.e., a through-the-needle catheter of appropriate size and a three-way stopcock. A CVP device like the one illustrated in Figure 2 is a simple yet efficient device which provides support for the intravenous tubing and a measurement scale (metric ruler). In addition, the manometer can be easily aligned with the animal.

As indicated by the range of CVP values, individual animal fluctuations, and animal-manometer positioning, the CVP is a more valuable guide to overhydration and impending cardiac congestion than it is an indicator of under- or over-administration of fluids. However, the CVP procedure is a valuable asset when it is used in conjunction with other standard evaluation procedures. Understanding the CVP and its application is a useful aid in animal health care for the veterinarian and animal health technician.

REFERENCES

1. Jennings PB, Anderson RW, Martin AM: Central venous pressure monitoring: A guide to blood volume replacement in the dog. *JAVMA* 151:1283-1292, 1967.
2. Soma LR: *Veterinary Anesthesia.* Baltimore, The Williams & Wilkins Co, 1971, pp 551-552.
3. Burrows CF: Shock: Pathophysiology and management, in Kirk RW (ed): *Current Veterinary Therapy VI, Small Animal Practice.* Philadelphia, WB Saunders Co, 1977, pp 42-43.
4. Ross JN Jr: Heart failure and shock, in Ettinger SJ (ed): *Textbook of Veterinary Internal Medicine,* vol 2. Philadelphia, WB Saunders Co, 1975, pp 858-859.
5. Burrows CF: Inadequate skin preparation as a cause of intravenous catheter-related infection in the dog. *JAVMA* 180:747-749, 1982.
6. Kirk RW, Bistner SI: *Handbook of Veterinary Procedures and Emergency Treatment,* ed 2. Philadelphia, WB Saunders Co, 1975, pp 404-406.

A Method for Collecting and Storing Feline Whole Blood*

MEDICAL UPDATE is a regular feature of *Veterinary Technician*®. The Editor in Chief, Richard B. Ford, DVM, MS, can be contacted for further information at 204 Emerywood Drive, Raleigh, NC 27615. This month's MEDICAL UPDATE was written especially for *Veterinary Technician* readers by Louise R. Price, RAMT, of Tufts University School of Veterinary Medicine, North Grafton, Massachusetts.

An increasing number of blood transfusions in cats at Tufts University School of Veterinary Medicine resulted in the need to create an aseptic means of storing feline blood. Many cats become severely anemic and require immediate transfusion. It is inconvenient for technicians to leave their duties in order to draw blood from donor cats, and the time involved in drawing blood from a donor further compromises the condition of the recipient. In addition, significant costs are involved in keeping multiple donors in the hospital.

If blood is stored in an open system, risk of bacterial contamination increases because blood is an ideal medium for bacteria. A blood collection bag is considered a closed system because it is open only at the tip of the needle, which is used for donor venipuncture. Once the administration ports of a blood bag are entered, how-

*Supported in part by Tufts University School of Veterinary Medicine Transfusion Medicine Academic Award NHLBI, K07HL01860.

ever, the unit is considered an open system. Another example of an open system is collection in syringes to be donated immmediately to the recipient or injected into a blood collection bag. The ideal bag for storing feline blood accommodates 50 milliliters of blood to be stored as a closed system (Figure 1). Because no such bag is commercially available, the following technique was created and has been in use at Tufts University School of Veterinary Medicine since 1987.

Preparation of the Blood Bag

A standard double blood bag designed for storing human blood (Fenwal, Division of Travenol Laboratories [Figure 2]) can be used. The primary bag contains 63 milliliters of citrate phosphate dextrose adenine (CPDA) anticoagulant solution—the recommended anticoagulant for 450-milliliter blood collection. At Tufts University School of Veterinary Medicine, standard feline blood collection is 50 milliliters with 7 milliliters of citrate phosphate dextrose adenine.

The additional citrate phosphate dextrose adenine is transferred from the primary bag to the satellite bag by breaking the plasma outflow seal and manually rolling the primary bag in order to remove the anticoagulant (Figure 3). The outflow tube is then clamped with a one-hand sealer clip (Fenwal, Division of Travenol Laboratories [Figure 4]), and the satellite

bag is removed. The remaining blood bag contains approximately eight milliliters of citrate phosphate dextrose adenine in the collection line. Although seven milliliters is the ideal amount, toxicity has not occurred in recipients.

Collection of Blood

All materials must be on hand before the tranquilizing agent is administered to the donor. Speed and organization are important because the following means only provides adequate sedation for approximately five minutes. The donor cat, which should weigh at least 10 pounds, is sedated with an intravenous combination of 0.5 milligrams of midazolam hydrochloric acid (Versed®—Roche Laboratories, Division of Hoffmann-La Roche), 10.3 milligrams of ketamine hydrochloric acid (Ketaset®—Fort Dodge Laboratories), and 0.2 milligrams of atropine. This combination also allows a smooth recovery. An ocular emollient is used to prevent dryness of the corneas. The hair over either jugular vein is clipped, and the skin is washed with a surgical scrub and alcohol rinse. Aseptic preparation is critical in avoiding bacterial contamination of stored blood.

The cat is placed in sternal recumbency with both front legs hanging over the side of the table. A hemostat is placed on the blood tube just proximal to the attached needle. An assis-

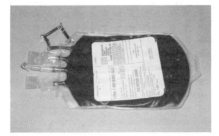

Figure 1—A closed-system blood bag containing 50 milliliters of feline whole blood.

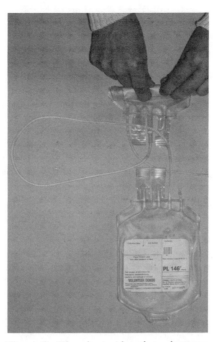

Figure 3—The citrate phosphate dextrose adenine is transferred from the primary bag to the satellite bag by breaking the plasma outflow seal and manually rolling the primary bag.

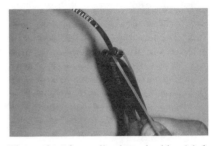

Figure 5—In order to prevent air from entering the line, the collection line is clamped with a hemostat before the needle is removed.

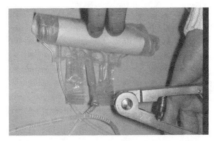

Figure 4—The outflow tube is clamped with a one-hand sealer clip.

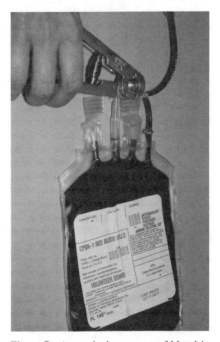

Figure 6—After collection, the blood left in the line is stripped twice with a tube stripper to allow the blood to mix with the anticoagulant in the bag.

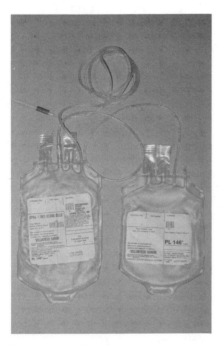

Figure 2—A standard double blood bag for storing human blood.

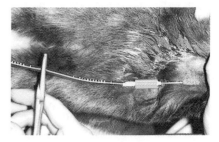

Figure 7—A two-inch segment of blood is left in the line for future cross matching.

tant positions the cat's head to expose the vein. The thumb or forefinger is pressed over the vein slightly cranial to the thoracic inlet. When optimum venous exposure is achieved, the needle is slowly inserted through the skin and into the vein. The hemostat is then released. Blood flows immediately into the collection line and to the primary bag, where it mixes with the anticoagulant. The primary bag is occasionally agitated to facilitate mixing of blood with the anticoagulant. The bag is placed on a scale during collection until the weight increases by 50 grams. The weight of the bag is taken into account as part of the total weight; when collection is complete, therefore, the scale will read 80 grams

(indicating that 50 milliliters of blood has been drawn).

The collection line is clamped with the hemostat *before* the needle is removed from the vein; such clamping prevents air from entering the line (Figure 5). With a gauze square, the assistant applies moderate pressure to the vein for two to three minutes. Immediately after collection, the blood left in the line is stripped twice with a tube stripper (Fenwal, Division of Travenol Laboratories), which forces the blood into the bag to mix with the anticoagulant; the blood then reenters the line (Figure 6). Blood in the line is stripped into the primary bag; a two-inch segment of blood is left in the line and sealed with a sealer clip for

future cross matching (Figure 7). The blood is stored at 39°F (4°C) for a maximum of 30 days.

Fluid Return to the Donor

Donors may occasionally become tachypneic with pale mucous membranes after blood donation. To prevent this, 150 milliliters of previously drawn lactated Ringer's solution is given intravenously to the donor immediately after donation to maintain the circulatory volume. A 20- or 21-gauge butterfly needle in the cephalic vein can be used to deliver fluids before the cat recovers from sedation.

Administration of Blood

Stored blood can be warmed in a 98.6°F (37°C) water bath for 10 minutes before administration. A standard blood component recipient set (Fenwal, Division of Travenol Laboratories) is attached to one entry port of the bag. The blood is administered during a one-hour period. When the transfusion is almost complete, 10 millilters of 0.9% saline can be added to the blood bag via a sampling site coupler (Fenwal, Division of Travenol Laboratories) inserted into the second port. Adding saline helps to ensure that all blood in the line is given to the recipient. Normal saline is the only fluid that should ever come in contact with the blood.

Conclusion

This method is very successful at Tufts University School of Veterinary Medicine because it allows blood to be stored and conveniently administered; the method is also cost effective because donor cats are brought in on a scheduled basis and not housed at the university. The previously used, traditional method of feline blood transfusion involved slow injection of freshly collected blood. This method was time consuming for technicians and increased the risk of citrate toxicity or volume overload for the recipient in the event that the blood was administered too rapidly. The greatest advantage of the current method is that cats are afforded blood transfusions on a timely basis. □

Nutritional Support of Critically Ill Patients—Part I

CLINICAL NUTRITION is a regular feature of *Veterinary Technician®*. This month's feature, which is Part I of a two-part presentation, was adapted from a presentation at the International Veterinary Emergency and Critical Care Symposium in September of 1988. The author, Dennis T. Crowe, Jr., DVM, is a Diplomate of the American College of Veterinary Surgeons and is affiliated with the Department of Small Animal Medicine of the College of Veterinary Medicine, University of Georgia, Athens, Georgia.

"All deaths are hateful to miserable mortals, but the most pitiable death of all is to starve."

Homer, Odyssey XII:341

The recognition, development, and routine use of nutritional support have collectively represented a major advance in the care of critically ill or injured humans and animals. This article examines the effects of poor nutrition in critically ill veterinary patients, discusses the indications for and methods of nutritional support, and provides guidelines for the choice of methods. Patients can be given nutritional support through chemically enhanced oral feeding, forced oral feeding, orogastric tube feeding, and various forms of ostomy tube feeding. Parenteral methods of feeding include use of a central vein for total parenteral nutrition or a peripheral vein for protein-sparing or partial parenteral nutrition. More information about specific methods of delivery has been published.[1-3]

Effects of Poor Nutrition on Critically Ill Patients

Within 8 to 12 hours of the deprivation of energy and protein, glycogen stores in the liver are depleted and body proteins (primarily from muscle, the gut, and the liver) become the main source of glucose through glucogenesis in the liver. After 48 hours of deprivation, decreases in plasma fibronectin, which is an important glycoprotein necessary for the enhancement of macrophage function, can be measured. Decreases in cellular and humoral immune function can be measured in otherwise nonstressed animals after five days of deprivation of energy and protein.

In patients with severe burns, traumatic injuries, or severe sepsis, serious tissue catabolism occurs and the patient loses lean tissue and fat (as much as 1.5 to 2 times the loss observed in otherwise nonstressed undernourished individuals). The loss of muscle mass causes muscular weakness, which is associated with lethargy; affected patients appear tired and lack vitality. Muscular weakness of the smooth muscle of the gastrointestinal tract generally becomes apparent within five days of the onset of poor nutritional intake. The eventual result is ileus and poor digestive capabilities (which are also attributable to decreased production of digestive enzymes and atrophy of gastrointestinal mucosa).

As further muscle mass is lost, weakness of the respiratory muscles (the diaphragm in particular) leads to progressive respiratory compromise. Cardiac muscle also eventually fails.

A decrease in plasma volume occurs as albumin concentrations in the blood decrease. The half-life of albumin in dogs averages eight days. The half-life in cats is five to six days. It is shorter in patients experiencing catabolic states and in small dogs and cats. A decrease in albumin levels may begin to be detectable within one week of the onset of protein–energy deprivation and stress. Lower albumin levels affect oncotic pressure and Starling forces; and animals are less resistant to volume losses caused by bleeding, plasma losses from burns, or peritonitis and are prone to shock. In experiments, hypoproteinemic animals (e.g., with 1.5 grams of protein per 100 ml of blood) reached the same degree of shock after loss of 15% of their blood volume that animals with normal amounts of albumin in the blood (i.e., 3 grams of protein per 100 ml of blood) reached after loss of 30% of their blood volume.

Because of the effect of hypoalbuminemia on Starling forces, intestinal absorption of nutrients is also impaired. Animals that are hypoalbuminemic as a result of nutritional depletion have a high incidence of surgical wound edema and dehiscence, wound infection, delayed healing of fractures and other wounds, prolonged wound edema, and generalized swelling of limbs and dependent areas of the body.

In undernourished animals, the liver and small intestine rapidly begin to involute and in severe cases may lose as much as two thirds of their total protein. The severe involution, along with hypoalbuminemia (albumin less than 1.5 g/dl), renders the gut unable to digest or absorb nutrients; these effects of protein malnutrition become apparent more rapidly in dogs and cats than in adult humans. The effects in dogs and cats resemble those in human neonates and infants. Fatty liver and muscle wasting are also common in stressed patients that are not receiving adequate protein intake.

Ultimately, the liver fails to synthesize albumin and important enzymes and purines (the building blocks of adenosine triphosphate) even when substrate is available. From the accumulated effect of the mentioned processes, the patient starves to death; this process has been called nitrogen death.

Indications and Guidelines
Patient Selection
The onset of protein–energy malnutrition and ultimate nutritional failure is insidious; the clinical signs are not as obvious as those of a fracture or hemorrhage. As a result, clinicians have often failed to recognize the need for nutritional support of seriously ill or injured patients. Even though the nutritionally depleted state develops slowly and subtly, the result of nutritional failure can be lethal or irreversible. The patient gradually wastes away, metabolizing its vital organs for energy until death ensues; this process has been called autocannibalism.

Because the deaths of many undernourished patients are associated with more obvious causes, such as wound breakdown, general depression, and sepsis, the contribution of nutritional failure to a patient's death may not be recognized. *Establishing indications for nutritional support is therefore crucial.*

Just as nutritional failure is insidious

and more difficult to recognize than other disease states of critically ill patients, the effects of nutritional supportive therapy can be subtle and difficult to monitor. Nevertheless, such therapy can reverse the course of many diseases and restore the health of many patients.

Any patient in an intensive care unit is a candidate for nutritional support; most patients in intensive care units have increased metabolic stress along with decreased intake of nutrients. Even if the patient is overweight, the intensive care unit is not an appropriate setting for restriction of food intake because body fat cannot fulfill protein requirements. In addition, a patient with any of the following clinical signs is a candidate for nutritional support:

- A history of recent or prolonged weight loss of more than 10% of its body weight
- A history of poor appetite persisting longer than five days (three days for patients that may have high catabolic rates because of disease)
- Generalized loss of muscle mass (this loss may be independent of body fat loss)
- Generalized loss of body fat with loss of skin turgor
- Generalized weakness, lack of appetite, and lethargy persisting longer than five days or only two or three days in severely ill patients, particularly small dogs and cats
- Serum albumin below the laboratory's minimum low normal range (2.3 to 2.5 g/dl for the laboratory at the University of Georgia)
- Total peripheral blood lymphocyte counts of less than 800/μl when not in severe stress (e.g., because of high endogenous cortisol or catecholamine levels).

Nutritional support should be considered for all patients with any of the following conditions, which are known to cause the loss of large amounts of protein and energy:

- Massive soft tissue or skeletal injury
- Complex surgical procedures that result in severe postsurgical stress
- Resection of more than 70% of the small intestine (until adaptation occurs)
- Diarrhea caused by severe ulcerative colitis
- Intestinal malabsorption
- Severe urinary albumin loss attributable to glomerular disease (if potentially reversible)
- Peritonitis, pleuritis, or chylous effusion with veffective, progressive drainage
- Large open wounds or burns, with persistent exudative losses.

Nutritional support is required for patients with conditions associated with inadequate food intake and in which poor nutritional state is expected to last longer than five days. Such patients may have the following:

- Fractures of the mandible or maxilla
- Extensive oral or nasal surgical procedures
- Severe generalized stomatitis, glossitis, pharyngitis, or dental infections
- Such neurologic conditions as semicoma, coma, persistent seizures requiring heavy sedation, quadriplegia, and palsy of the fifth and eighth cranial nerves
- Megaesophagus or a disease state (e.g., myasthenia gravis) that is associated with megaesophagus
- Extensive gastrointestinal surgery (gastric paresis or ileus may be prolonged)
- Severe oropharyngeal or cricopharyngeal dysphagia
- Esophageal stricture or foreign body preventing adequate intake for longer than three to five days
- Esophageal surgery
- Stomach surgery (as with resection) or complicated dilation or torsion
- Anorexia from various medical causes (e.g., renal failure, hepatic failure, or pancreatitis)
- Severe or persistent vomiting or diarrhea
- Extensive diagnostic procedures or treatments (e.g., for pancreatitis) that necessitate longer than three days of food deprivation.

Determination of Nutritional Needs

The easiest way to determine the nutritional needs of a patient is to use the basal nutrient requirements for cats and dogs reported by the National Academy of Science.[4,5] The animal's body surface area, age, and activity level and the physiologic stress it is experiencing are also considered in estimating basal energy needs. Basal metabolic rate is proportional to body surface area, not body weight; however, body surface area is difficult to measure. Nevertheless, basal energy requirements can be estimated from body weight without using exponential functions. For a cat or dog weighing less than 2 kg, the basal energy requirement = 30 × body weight (kg) + 70. Dogs that weigh more than 2 kg require 60 kcal/kg/day, and cats that weigh more than 2 kg require 43 kcal/kg/day.

Once the appropriate basal nutrient requirement (which is expressed in kilocalories per kilogram of lean body weight) for a patient is calculated, the estimate is multiplied by the estimated lean body weight of the patient. This product is then multiplied by a factor that provides for the increased metabolic rate the critically ill pa-

tient may be experiencing. The basal nutrient requirements and estimated correction factors have been published in several texts and range from 1.1 for mild stress factors in adult animals to 1.75 to 2.0 or even higher (6.7 for severe stress [e.g., severe sepsis] in growing animals).[4-7]

The published correction factors used to estimate the increased energy requirements of ill or injured patients have been based on metabolic research primarily in rats, mice, and humans. Current clinical research is being done to determine the canine and feline correction factors, and results of these studies are not available. Until these data are published, however, the factors based on metabolic research on other species must be used. Such variables as weight gain or loss over time should be used to monitor and modify the nutritional support. The following correction factors for kilocalorie requirements have been derived from studies on humans: a 25% to 30% increase in energy requirements over basal nutrient requirements of elective surgery patients; a 30% to 40% increase for skeletal trauma patients; a 50% to 60% increase for trauma patients that have received corticosteroids; and an 80% to 100% increase for patients with sepsis. It is assumed that the same percentage increases are applicable to the requirements for other nutrients.

A more accurate method of predicting requirements of protein and other nutrients (based on protein needs) is to measure the actual total protein losses (nitrogen [g] × 6.25 = protein [g]). Total protein loss includes the albumin and urea nitrogen lost in urine, the protein lost through feces, and the protein lost in the blood, exudates, and transudate in drainage fluids.

Urine nitrogen and protein losses are most accurately measured by Kjeldahl's method, but they can also be measured reliably by the same methods used to measure serum total protein and blood urea nitrogen, respectively. Estimates of nonurinary losses are based on the estimated amount of fecal and fluid protein lost during 24 hours. If the fecal and fluid protein cannot be measured, the following data (from human studies) can be used: daily average insensible nitrogen loss is 5 mg/kg; daily average gastrointestinal (fecal) nitrogen loss is 12 mg/kg.

The estimates of nitrogen loss enable the technician to estimate whether the 24-hour nitrogen balance is positive or negative; the total daily nitrogen loss is subtracted from the total daily nitrogen intake, that is, nitrogen balance = (total protein intake − total protein losses) ÷ 6.25:

Example

The 24-hour protein intake of a 3-kg, growing cat with peritonitis was 200 ml of a polymeric liquid diet (Peptamen™—Baxter, Alternative Healthcare Division) containing 4 grams of protein per 100 ml. The protein has a biologic value of 75. The nitrogen intake is calculated as follows:

$$[4 \text{ (g protein/100 ml)} \times 200 \text{ ml} \times 0.75] \div 6.25 \text{ (g protein/g nitrogen)} = 0.96 \text{ g nitrogen}$$

The patient's dressings were weighed before and after use, and the peritoneal fluid was collected by open peritoneal drainage. From these measurements, it was estimated that the patient had lost 200 ml of peritoneal fluid. The protein content of a sample of peritoneal fluid was measured with a refractometer; the fluid contained 3 grams of protein per 100 ml. The patient therefore had lost approximately 6 grams of protein through peritoneal drainage. For diagnostic tests, 10 ml of blood was drawn from the patient. According to the refractometer, the blood contained 6 grams of protein per 100 ml. The patient therefore lost 0.6 grams of protein through blood samples. The total nonfecal, nonurinary loss of protein was 6.6 grams.

The following formula is used to calculate the nonfecal, nonurinary loss of nitrogen:

$$6.6 \text{ g of protein} \div 6.25 \text{ (g of protein/g of nitrogen)} = 1.06 \text{ g of nitrogen}$$

During the 24 hours, the patient produced 200 ml of urine; the urea nitrogen was 300 mg per 100 ml of pooled urine. The urinary loss of nitrogen is calculated as follows:

$$[300 \text{ mg} \div 100 \text{ ml}] \times 200 \text{ ml} \times [1 \text{ g} \div 1000 \text{ mg}] = 0.6 \text{ g}$$

The estimated nitrogen loss from insensible and fecal loss is calculated as follows:

$$17 \text{ mg/kg} \times 3 \text{ kg} \times [1 \text{ g} \div 1000 \text{ mg}] = 0.051 \text{ g}$$

The total nitrogen losses in 24 hours were therefore $1.06 \text{ g} + 0.6 \text{ g} + 0.051 \text{ g} = 1.71 \text{ g}$ of nitrogen.

The following calculation (nitrogen intake minus total nitrogen losses) yields the nitrogen balance:

$$0.96 \text{ g} - 1.71 \text{ g} = -0.75$$

The nitrogen balance is therefore negative; steps to increase the grams of protein administered enterally, parenterally, or both must be taken.

Methods of Nutritional Support

Planning a course of nutritional support involves choosing the degree of nutritional support (partial versus total nutritional support versus hyperalimentation) and the methods of delivery (enteral versus parenteral nutrition). The goal of partial support is to blunt the loss of visceral and muscle protein and help maintain immune function during periods of undernutrition lasting a few days to one week. Total nutritional support is used to maintain body weight (visceral and muscle protein) and normal metabolic functions.

Hyperalimentation, which is the administration of amounts of essential nutrients in excess of a patient's calculated requirements, is intended to reverse the effects of previous poor nutrition. Hyperalimentation is rarely used for critically ill patients because it is difficult to achieve and is associated with a higher incidence of complications. For most critically ill patients, the goal is to prevent further loss of muscle mass and further weakness, that is, to maintain a zero balance of energy and protein.

The following rule should be followed in selecting a method of delivery of nutritional support: if the gut works, use it. In other words, enteral feeding should be chosen whenever possible because it is easier, less expensive, and usually associated with fewer complications. It is also more physiologic, supplying trophic factors (e.g., glutamine) to the intestinal mucosa and direct intestinal mucosal nutrition, thus protecting its integrity. In critically ill or injured animals, a higher level of endotoxin absorption occurs via the gut mucosa if total nutritional support has been provided parenterally than if it has been provided enterally.

Several factors influence the choice of a method of nutritional support. The veterinary staff must consider how long the patient will require the support. A delivery method that uses as much of the gastrointestinal tract as is safely possible should be used. The patient's temperament and neurologic status may influence this safety; an unconscious or semiconscious patient is at risk for pulmonary aspiration if feed is deposited in the mouth, esophagus, or stomach.

The veterinary staff must evaluate the resources available to provide nutritional support to the patient. The hospital's facilities and the experience of its staff are important. The owner's financial commitment to the animal must also be considered as well as the owner's ability and willingness to provide continued nutritional support at home if necessary.

Whether the patient requires surgery is an important consideration. If the patient will be anesthetized for another procedure, the anesthesia may enable the placement of a catheter or an esophagostomy or pharyngostomy tube. The patient's overall condition and its ability to tolerate a general anesthetic must be assessed.

In addition, specific disease states that influence the animal's nutritional route and requirements (e.g., pancreatitis or diabetes mellitus) and the patient's tolerance of the type of support provided may affect the plan for nutritional support.

The simplest, most economical feeding method possible is recommended. The following list presents delivery methods in increasing order of cost and complexity:

- Chemically enhanced oral feeding
- Forced oral feeding
- Orogastric tube feeding
- Nasoesophageal, nasogastric, or nasoduodenal tube feeding (Figure 1)
- Pharyngostomy tube feeding
- Esophageal tube feeding
- Gastrostomy tube feeding (Figure 2)
- Jejunostomy tube feeding
- Gastroduodenostomy or gastrojejunostomy tube feeding
- Peripheral vein partial parenteral nutrition
- Central vein total parenteral nutrition.

Primarily because of cost, peripheral and central vein nutritional support are recommended only if the other methods are not feasible. Some products, however, are easy to use and economical and can be used to provide some intravenous intake. These products (3% FreAmine® III and ProcalAmine®—KenVet) are considered protein-sparing materials because they decrease to some extent the loss of muscle and visceral protein and thereby retard the patient's nutritional and protein depletion. The 3% FreAmine® III can also be given via a peripheral intravenous catheter with minimal risk of thrombophlebitis and infection. The crystalline amino acids inhibit bacterial growth in the product. Bacterial growth is a serious problem with dextrose solutions. I recommend that protein-sparing products be used for most patients that require maintenance fluids. Even though such products do not supply all of the required nutrients, providing some nutrients is certainly better than providing none.

The following cost estimates were based on records of the Small Animal Hospital of the University of Georgia. Feeding methods that require only special preparation or delivery of regular canned pet foods but not the insertion or care of a tube (e.g., large-bore pharyngostomy tube) cost $0.002 to $0.005 per kilocalorie. The cost of enteral feeding methods requiring liquid polymeric formulas (cost varies according to the type of feeding method and diet required) is approximately $0.003 to $0.006 per kilocalorie. Enteral feeding methods requiring liquid monomeric formulas cost $0.007 to $0.015. Total parenteral nutrition costs approximately $0.03 to $0.04 per kilocalorie. Costs associated with partial parenteral nutrition vary depending on the

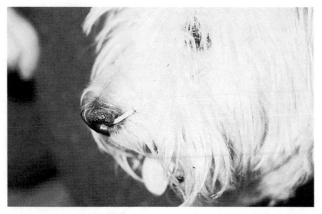

Figure 1—This 10-year-old, spayed female West Highland white terrier received nutritional support through a nasogastric tube in preparation for bowel surgery.

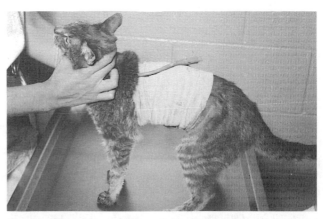

Figure 2—This one-year-old Domestic Shorthair cat required gastrostomy tube feeding for six months after ingestion of caustic toilet bowl cleaner.

amount of protein sparing that is accomplished. If only amino acids and electrolytes are provided, the cost may be only $0.01 to $0.02 per kilocalorie (e.g., 3% FreAmine® III costs approximately $8.00 and each 1-liter bottle contains 1350 kcal; the cost is therefore approximately $0.006 per kilocalorie).

The daily cost estimate for nutritional support for a 15-kg dog requiring 1000 kcal are as follows: $2 to $4 for specially prepared canned food, $7 to $15 for a liquid monomeric diet, $30 to $40 for total parenteral nutrition, and $10 to $20 for partial parenteral nutritional support (protein sparing). These costs include the cost of the materials used for administering the products but do not include the cost of placing a feeding catheter or of the required nursing care.

Other methods (e.g., partial and total nutritional support provided via intraperitoneal and intraosseous routes) are currently considered experimental. The difficulty, complication rate, and expense of these methods have not been determined.

Clinical Cases

The following two cases illustrate the use of two nutritional support methods used at the Veterinary Teaching Hospital of the College of Veterinary Medicine, University of Georgia.

Case 1

A 10-year-old, spayed female, West Highland white terrier (Figure 1) had a history of progressive weight loss and anorexia. The veterinarian suspected a colonic tumor. Nutritional support through a nasogastric tube was used for five days before surgery to improve the patient's ability to tolerate the major operation planned. After a few days of nutritional support, the dog was much more alert, appeared to feel much better, and regained much strength and energy. A clear monomeric diet, containing amino acids, essential fatty acids, and oligosaccharides, was then begun a few days before surgery to prepare the lower intestinal tract for surgery. Because the diet (Vivamex HN—Eaton Laboratories) contained no residue, the amount of fecal material decreased substantially.

Case 2

A one-year-old Domestic Shorthair cat (Figure 2) had ingested a caustic toilet bowl cleaner. A gastrostomy tube was inserted under general anesthesia at the time endoscopic examination of the esophagus was performed. Because of extensive damage to the esophageal mucosa, the gastrostomy tube was used exclusively for administration of water and food. The patient was fed a 50:50 mixture of Prescription Diet® Feline p/d® (Hill's Pet Products) and water; 1 teaspoonful (5 ml) of corn oil was added to the mixture each day. Figure 2 was taken after the cat had been fed via the gastrostomy tube for one month. The patient was maintaining its weight on four feedings per day. The owner had no problems with the gastrostomy tube or the feeding program, which was required for five additional months because of esophageal injury and scarring.

REFERENCES

1. Crowe DT: Enteral nutrition for critically ill or injured patients—Part I. *Compend Contin Educ Pract Vet* 8(9):603–612, 1986.
2. Crowe DT: Enteral nutrition for critically ill or injured patients—Part II. *Compend Contin Educ Pract Vet* 8(10):719–732, 1986.
3. Crowe DT: Enteral nutrition for critically ill or injured patients—Part III. *Compend Contin Educ Pract Vet* 8(11):826–838, 1986.
4. Raffe MR: Total parenteral nutrition, in Slatter DH (ed): *Textbook of Small Animal Surgery.* Philadelphia, WB Saunders Co, 1985, pp 225–241.
5. National Academy of Sciences: Nutritional requirements of dogs, in *Nutritional Requirements of Animals,* vol 8. Washington, DC, National Academy of Sciences, 1974.
6. Crowe DT: Understanding the nutritional needs of critically ill or injured patients. *Vet Med* 83:1224–1229, 1988.
7. Lewis LD, Morris ML Jr, Hand MS: Anorexia, inanition, critical care nutrition, in *Small Animal Clinical Nutrition.* Topeka, KS, Mark Morris Associates, 1987, chapter 5. □

Nutritional Support of Critically Ill Patients—Part II

CLINICAL NUTRITION is a regular feature of *Veterinary Technician*®. This month's feature, which is Part II of a two-part presentation, was adapted from a presentation at the International Veterinary Emergency and Critical Care Symposium in September of 1988. Part I appeared in the June 1989 issue (Vol. 10, No. 5). The author, Dennis T. Crowe, Jr., DVM, is a Diplomate of the American College of Veterinary Surgeons and is affiliated with the Department of Small Animal Medicine of the College of Veterinary Medicine, University of Georgia, Athens, Georgia.

Critically ill patients often experience increased metabolic demands concurrent with difficulty in maintaining normal intake of food. Part I discussed nutrient requirements and the indications for nutritional support. Numerous methods are used to increase the nutrient intake of critically ill patients.

Chemically Enhanced Oral Feeding

At the University of Georgia, diazepam (Valium®—Roche) and oxazepam (Serax®—Wyeth) have been used to stimulate the appetite of patients; the results of such therapy have varied. Oral or parenteral administration of benzodiazepines has been associated with stimulation of the appetite center of the central nervous system and inhibition of the satiety center by increasing the production of γ-aminobutyric acid (GABA) in the hypothalamus.

I have found that these drugs work initially, especially in cats that became anorectic as a result of polysystemic disease. After oral or intravenous administration (0.02 to 0.05 mg/kg for dogs and cats) of diazepam, many animals eat vigorously. Intravenous administration is more effective than oral administration.

The recommended oral dose of oxazepam is 0.5 to 1.5 mg/kg every 12 hours. Oxazepam is provided in 10-mg capsules; for cats, the capsule must be opened and one half to two thirds of the contents removed. Oral doses are administered 30 minutes to one hour before feeding and are not given more frequently than once every 12 hours.[a]

After initial stimulation of the appetite, benzodiazepines often leave a patient's appetite more depressed than before. The stimulatory effect on appetite also seems to decrease with subsequent doses. After several treatments, there may be no beneficial effects.

The effects of benzodiazepines on appetite varies. In some animals, no appetite stimulation is observed even after the first dose; in others, continued use has been beneficial in maintaining adequate intake.

Indication for the use of benzodiazepines for appetite stimulation should therefore be for patients with mild to moderate anorexia in which only occasional use is necessary. For example, the drugs may be used to initiate food intake or to provide supplemental nutritional intake.

Forced Oral Feeding

Forced oral feeding has been invaluable for many seriously ill or injured animals that are cooperative and strong enough to swallow food placed in the mouth. Candidates for forced oral feeding must be fully conscious and have no medical problems that preclude oral feeding. Various techniques have been useful.

A feeding syringe made by cutting off the needle end of a plastic syringe can be used to place cylindrical pieces of canned food into the back of the pharynx. As an alternative, round boluses of canned food can be placed manually in the back of the mouth, which is then held shut while swallowing is encouraged. Liquid diets can be fed with a syringe.

Such pasty materials as Nutri-Cal (EVSCO Pharmaceuticals) or peanut butter can also be used. Peanut butter contains 28% protein, and each tablespoonful [16 grams] provides 100 kcal; 16 grams of the commercial forced-feeding diet provides 75 kcal and contains 15% protein.

Orogastric Tube Feeding

Orogastric tube feeding is an excellent

---

[a]Cornelius LM: Personal communication, University of Georgia, 1988.

means of providing temporary, supplemental, enteral nutritional support. It is particularly useful for young patients and patients with oral or pharyngeal dysphagia. A 50:50 gruel of water and canned food (e.g., Prescription Diet® Feline c/d®—Hill's Pet Products) with the addition of such caloric supplements as corn oil and such protein supplements as powdered egg or milk substitutes is commonly used. If the patient refuses to tolerate the feeding tube, however, a different method of support must be chosen.

Nasoesophageal, Nasogastric, or Nasoduodenal Tube Feeding

Since the development of effective and simple techniques for placing feeding tubes through the noses of veterinary patients,[1] nasoesophageal, nasogastric, and nasoduodenal tube feeding methods have been widely used. Of these methods, nasoesophageal tube feeding is the most common.

When the esophagus is not functional (e.g., because of strictures or megaesophagus), nasogastric tube feeding is performed. If the patient is semiconscious or unconscious or aspiration is considered to be a significant risk, nasoesophageal and nasogastric tube feeding cannot be used and nasoduodenal tube feeding should be considered.

The tip of the feeding tube can be placed in the duodenum during a surgical procedure, or a weighted tube can be advanced into the duodenum with the aid of gastric peristaltic waves stimulated by the use of 0.4 mg/kg of intravenous metoclopramide hydrochloride (Reglan®—A. H. Robins). The latter method is not always successful, and the required feeding tubes (e.g., an 8-French polyurethane tube, such as Travasorb® Enteral Feeding Tube—Baxter Healthcare, Alternative Care Division) are more expensive than other nasal feeding tubes because of the mercury- or tungsten-weighted tip.

If gastric function is poor or anorexia has been long-standing, the initial feedings should be slow, continuous infusions (2 ml/kg/hr). In all cases, a complete liquid diet is necessary because the feeding tubes range in size from 5 French (Pharmaseal® Feeding Tube—American Pharmaseal) to 8 French. Commercially available polymeric diets include Criticare HN® (Mead Johnson Nutritional Division), Osmolite® HN (Ross Laboratories), Ensure® HN (Ross Laboratories), and Sustacal® (Mead Johnson Nutritional Division).

Bolus feeding (20 ml/kg) every two to four hours is usually the initial method used for nasoesophageal or nasogastric feeding. The amounts are gradually increased until the nutritional requirements can be met with feedings performed every six hours.

Large boluses cannot be fed to patients with nasoduodenal feeding tubes. For these patients, slow infusion (2 ml/kg/hr), small hourly boluses, or boluses of 2 to 4 ml/kg every two hours can be administered.

Pharyngostomy Tube Feeding

Despite occasional difficulties, pharyngostomy tube feeding is an effective means of providing enteral support to properly selected patients. The pharyngostomy tube should not pass through the pharynx cranial to the epihyoid bone (as was originally recommended) because in that location it can interfere with the function of the larynx. The tube should instead be placed as far caudally and dorsally as possible, and its placement should be performed bluntly so that the hypoglossal and glossopharyngeal nerves as well as the carotid artery and jugular vein are not damaged.[2]

If the esophagus is functional, the tip of the tube should be placed in the thoracic esophagus. Placing the tip of the tube in the stomach can predispose the patient to reflux esophagitis and gastric dilation because of the incompetence of the gastroesophageal sphincter.

With small-bore feeding tubes (i.e., 5 to 8 French), a liquid diet must be used; but a gruel of canned food can be fed through a large-bore feeding tube (i.e., 12 to 28 French). The tube should not be so large that it interferes with laryngeal function.

When the pharyngostomy tube is no longer required, the tube is simply removed and the ostomy site allowed to heal by granulation and epithelialization.

Esophagostomy Tube Feeding

I developed esophagostomy tube feeding particularly for use in cats because when pharyngostomy tubes are used, cats seem to have more complications and problems with airway interference than dogs have. Esophagostomy tube feeding has also been used for dogs as well as cats when major surgery or disease involves the pharynx or when a pharyngostomy tube might interfere with healing or compromise function.

Most of the esophagostomies I have observed were performed percutaneously with a large-bore, 10- to 14-gauge needle. A Rochester-Carmault forceps or Foerster sponge-holding forceps is inserted into the esophagus and elevated to identify the esophagus on the left side of the neck. Insertion of the needle between the parted blades of the forceps allows the surgeon to feel a definite popping sensation as the tensed mucosa of the esophagus is punctured.

A plastic polyvinylchloride (Pharmaseal® Feeding Tube [American Pharmaseal] or Pedi-Tube™ [Biosearch Medical Products]) or red rubber catheter (Sovereign Sterile, Single-Use Feeding and Urethral Catheter [Sherwood Medical]) is inserted through the needle, and the needle is then removed. Bolus or infusion feeding of liquid diets is then performed.

As with pharyngostomy tubes, when the esophagostomy tube is no longer required it is simply removed and the ostomy site allowed to heal by granulation and epithelialization.

Gastrostomy Tube Feeding

Two techniques can be used to place gastrostomy feeding tubes. A formal laparotomy can be performed in the left flank (preferably) or on the midline. After a double purse-string suture is placed in the left side of the stomach, a Foley or de Pezzer tube is placed through the left flank and into the stomach through the center of the purse-string suture. The Foley tube, if used, is expanded with sterile saline and a small amount of air.

The stomach is then fixed to the abdominal wall where the tube enters the peritoneum using a continuous suture pattern circling the gastrostomy tube. The tube is fixed to the skin and external abdominal fascia using sutures similar to those used for fixation of esophagostomy and pharyngostomy tubes. After the abdomen is closed, a dressing is used to secure the tube.

In the second method of insertion, the stomach is inflated with carbon dioxide and a Bard urologic catheter or de Pezzar tube is placed. A fiber-optic gastroscope is used to visualize the percutaneous placement of a needle inserted into the dilated stomach. A long piece of suture material inserted through the needle is grasped by the biopsy forceps of the gastroscope and pulled out of the stomach, through the esophagus, and then out the mouth.

The gastrostomy tube is carried by the suture into the esophagus and then into the stomach. The tube is then guided through the percutaneous gastrocentesis site by using an intravenous catheter and guideline technique. Once in place, the tube is pulled up snugly so that the stomach apposes the abdominal wall and the tube is fixed to the external fascia and skin as discussed.

The same diet and feeding methods used for orogastric and pharyngostomy tube feeding are used for gastrostomy tube feeding. The tube must remain in place for at least five days to allow adhesions to form between the stomach and abdominal wall.

When gastrostomy tube feeding is no longer required and at least five days have elapsed since insertion of the tube, the tube can be removed. The gastrostomy site usually heals in a few days by granulation and epithelialization. Petrolatum is used to protect the surrounding skin until the gastric drainage stops, usually within a few days.

Both techniques for placement of a gastrostomy tube require general anesthesia and carry a slight risk of peritonitis from leakage; however, both techniques have been reliable means of feeding patients for months with little aftercare. Difficulties related to tube patency are less common than occur with methods that require smaller-bore tubes. Patients have been well maintained at home and in zoos for months with gastrostomy tube feeding administered by the owner or zookeeper.

Gastroenterostomy Tube Feeding

If food cannot be deposited in the stomach because of stomach dysfunction (e.g., gastroparesis, postgastric dilation–torsion), a gastrostomy tube can be placed and used for decompression and medication and a smaller tube placed through it and led into the duodenum (or the jejunum if the function of the duodenum is impaired). The small tube is then used for feeding liquid enteral diets by drip infusion (2 ml/kg/hr) or hourly administration of small boluses.

The smaller tube is usually guided into the small intestine during abdominal surgery; but on occasion, it can be guided into the duodenum with the use of a flexible gastroscope. With this method, a separate ostomy site in the small intestine is unnecessary. If the animal vomits, however, the tube could become displaced and the tip of the feeding tube could enter the stomach. Small-bore (6- to 8-French) tubes with weighted tips are therefore preferred. After stomach function resumes, the enterostomy tube can be removed and the gastrostomy tube used for continued feeding if necessary.

Enterostomy (Duodenostomy or Jejunostomy) Tube Feeding

Enterostomy feeding has been a major factor in the recovery of many critically ill animals. Although gastroparesis is common in dogs and cats with many disease states and after general anesthesia and surgery, ileus is not. If the surgeon believes that the patient will require nutritional support after major abdominal surgery (e.g., correction of bowel obstruction), an enterostomy tube can be inserted during the procedure.

The insertion of an enterostomy feeding tube can be performed in 5 to 10 minutes, and feeding can be started as soon as recovery from anesthesia has occurred. Even though gastroparesis and mild ileus may occur after a major abdominal procedure, feeding can be accomplished through the enterostomy tube. An isotonic, iso-osmotic, monomeric enteral feeding formula (e.g., Peptamen®—Baxter Healthcare, Alternative Care Division) is preferred; but an isotonic, iso-osmotic, polymeric enteral feeding formula (e.g., Osmolite® HN—Ross Laboratories) can be used. The protein content of Peptamen® is 40 g/L, and that of Osmolite® HN is 35.1 g/L. Both products provide approximately 1 kcal/ml.

These products are best administered by gravity or pump infusion but can also be administered in hourly boluses beginning at 1 ml/kg/hr and gradually increased during 24 hours to between 2 and 3 ml/kg/hr. Some patients can eventually tolerate as much as 4 ml/kg/hr. In other patients, rates this high can result in nausea, vomiting, abdominal discomfort, and diarrhea.

Enterostomy tubes are placed as far proximally as possible in the small intestine through a purse-string suture of 4-0 monofilament nylon. Polyvinylchloride (Pharmaseal® Feeding Tube—American Pharmaseal), polyurethane (Pedi-Tube™—Biosearch Medical Products), and red rubber tubes ranging in size from 14 gauge to 6 French can be used. A needle may be needed to insert small tubes; the technique is similar to the placement of a jugular vein catheter.

The tubes must extend at least 10 to 15 cm (4 to 6 inches) in an aboral direction within the intestine. The best results are obtained if the tube can be tunneled between the subserosa and the muscularis for 2 to 3 cm before entering the lumen through the mucosa. The intestine is then sutured near the enterostomy site to the abdominal wall where the catheter exits the abdomen using continuous 4-0 monofilament material circling the ostomy site. Omentum is then wrapped around the area. Care must be taken to anchor the tube well to the material circling the ostomy site. An intravenous extension set with a stopcock is attached to the external tip of the enterostomy tube and inserted through the circumferential protective dressing at the top of the patient's back.

If intermittent hourly feedings are used, the tube should be flushed with sterile water after slow administration of the bolus. If continuous infusion is used, the catheter should also be flushed with sterile water approximately every six to eight hours. Flushing of the tube prevents occlusion, which results from buildup of coatings of the feeding formulas. Occlusion is more common when polymeric diets are used. The care of the ostomy site is the same as for other tubes (daily cleaning with 50:50 hydrogen peroxide and sterile saline and application of a triple antibiotic ointment).

When the feeding tube is no longer required, it can be removed by cutting the anchoring sutures and withdrawing the tube. The care of the ostomy site after tube removal is the same as that for other gastrostomy tubes. Healing occurs by granulation and epithelialization, and the ostomy site usually closes in a few days.

No persistent fistula has occurred in any of the approximately 50 enterostomy patients I have treated. In two of the 50 cases, the tube became dislodged and feed was deposited into the subcutaneous tissues or peritoneum. In both of these patients, the feeding tube did not extend far enough into the intestinal lumen and the tube was not anchored to external fascia. If the tube is inserted correctly and far enough (8 to 12 cm) and tube care is carefully performed, complications should be rare.

Partial Parenteral Nutritional Support

Partial parenteral nutritional support[3,4] has also been called protein-sparing nutritional support. The procedure involves administration of isotonic solutions of amino acids and electrolytes through a catheter placed in a peripheral vein.

A typical formula for partial parenteral nutrition contains the common maintenance electrolytes (potassium, chloride, sodium, calcium, and magnesium) in maintenance concentrations and approximately 30 mg/ml of crystalline essential amino acids (arginine, histidine, isoleucine, leucine, lysine, methionine, phenylalanine, threonine, tryptophan, and valine). All 10 of these amino acids are essential for dogs. Taurine, which is essential for cats, is not included. Available products were formulated for human nutrition, but manufacturers are now formulating products that more closely match canine and feline nutritional needs.

At the University of Georgia, we have used FreAmine® III 3% & Electrolytes (KenVet). This formula contains relatively high concentrations of the branched-chain amino acids valine, leucine, isoleucine, and arginine. Valine, leucine, and isoleucine can be deaminated and the carbon skeleton used as fuel by skeletal muscle as well as by the liver. This characteristic is important for patients with sepsis or hepatic disease.

Continual administration of these amino acids by partial parenteral nutrition is called protein sparing because it reduces protein catabolism. Because gluconeogenesis involving these amino acids is the preferred means of maintaining glucose levels in stressed patients, there may be less metabolic stress than occurs when hypertonic glucose solutions are used.

Products containing emulsions of soybean oil (e.g., Intralipid® 10% and 20% IV Fat Emulsion—Baxter Healthcare, Alternative Care Division) can be added to the electrolyte–amino acid products to provide energy. The breakdown of triglycerides and glycerol provides 9 kcal per gram of fatty acid. Each milliliter of a 20% fat emulsion therefore provides 0.2 grams of fat and 1.8 kcal. The major disadvantage of the fat emulsions is their cost (approximately $50.00 for 250 ml). Fat emulsions do not contribute to the osmolality of the solution.

The use of a peripheral vein for partial or total parenteral nutrition is indicated primarily for short-term support (i.e., a few days). If support will be required for longer than a few days, total parenteral nutrition should be provided through a catheter in a central vein. Long-term use of a peripheral vein for partial or total parenteral nutrition is usually associated with eventual thrombophlebitis and infection attributable to bacterial contamination. Because of these complications, catheter sites for partial parenteral nutrition are changed every 48 to 72 hours.

Regardless of whether a peripheral or central vein is used, strict aseptic technique should be followed. The sites where catheters pass through the skin should be cleaned with surgical antiseptic (I prefer chlorhexidine surgical solution) once daily, and a sterile antibacterial cream or ointment should be applied. Nonocclusive or occlusive dressing of the site is also required once daily.

Total Parenteral Nutrition

Total parenteral nutritional support is performed primarily through a jugular or external maxillary vein catheter; the tip of the catheter is placed in the cranial vena cava. Some investigators recommend the use of in-line 4- to 4.5-μm filters to decrease the chances of suppurative bacterial thrombophlebitis. In my experience, however, the most important means of prevention of thrombophlebitis are diligent aseptic care of the catheter, use of the catheter only for nutritional support, sterile mixing of the nutritional support solutions, and replacement of solutions that have been hanging for 24 hours. These measures have effectively prevented thrombophlebitis without the use of in-line filters.

The support of hospital pharmacists in the formulation and mixing of the products used for partial and total parenteral nutrition has contributed significantly to the success of these techniques at the University of Georgia. I recommend that hospital pharmacists be contacted for help whenever partial or total parenteral nutrition is required. In my experience, hospital pharmacists respond favorably to such requests. Many hospital pharmacists find

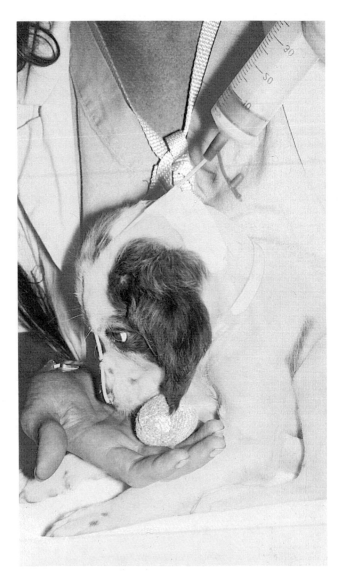

Figure 1—Two-month-old, female Brittany spaniel with a persistent right aortic arch (Case 1) being fed through a nasogastric tube on Day 5 of nutritional support. Note that the technician is distracting the patient with a toy during the feeding. The patient became more active; and therefore an Elizabethan collar was needed the next day. Surgery was performed after a week of nutritional support.

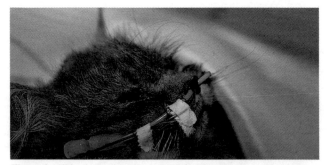

Figure 2—This three-year-old, spayed female, Domestic Shorthair cat had a chronic bowel obstruction (Case 2) and received nutritional support through a nasogastric and a nasoenterostomy tube. The 14-gauge polyethylene tube was used to administer oxygen.

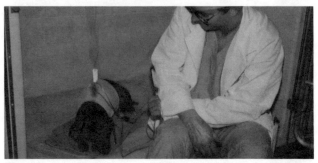

Figure 3—A middle-aged, female dachshund with septic peritonitis secondary to abscess formation in the pancreas (Case 3). A jejunostomy tube was placed during surgery. During the first 24 hours, the infusion rate was slow to avoid stimulating pancreatic secretion.

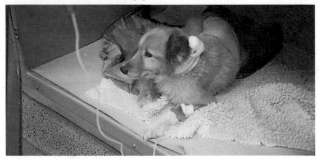

Figure 4—A 13-year-old dog recovering from surgery to remove a leiomyoma and associated fibrosis (Case 4); the lesion obstructed the common bile duct and partially obstructed the duodenum. The patient received nutritional support through a jejunostomy tube.

the provision of total parenteral nutrition to critically ill veterinary patients interesting and challenging.

At the University of Georgia, 20% Intralipid® (Baxter Healthcare, Alternative Care Division), FreAmine® III 8.5% (KenVet), 50% glucose, and a multiple vitamin infusion (Multi-Vitamin 12 Injection—Baxter Healthcare, Alternative Care Division) is used to formulate more than 90% of the infusions used for total parenteral nutrition. If total parenteral nutrition is required for longer than one week, an additional source of phosphorus and magnesium is used. With addition of the fat emulsion, the concentration of glucose in the infusion is decreased from 25% to between 15% and 17%.

When mixing the formula, it is important to add the glucose to the amino acid mixture first, then add the fat emulsion. If the fat emulsion contacts the 50% glucose solution, clumping and precipitation will occur. The phosphate-containing electrolyte salts should be added before calcium is added. Also, if the sum of the concentrations of the calcium and phosphorus salts exceeds 45 mEq/L, precipitation will result.

Total parenteral nutrition is initiated slowly. On the first day, 50% of the calculated daily energy requirement is administered (at least a 12-hour continuous administration). On the second day, 75% of the energy requirement is administered. By the third day, 100% of the calculated daily energy requirement is provided.

Blood glucose is monitored at least three times daily by refractometer or visual test strip. The turbidity of a patient's plasma (which indicates triglyceride levels) is monitored one to four times daily. The incidence of hyperglycemia and hyperosmolality is much lower if the increases are gradual and fat emulsion is used than if 100% of the energy requirement is provided on the first day and 25% glucose solutions are administered.

Clinical Cases
Case 1

A two-month-old, female, Brittany spaniel (Figure 1) underwent surgery to correct a persistent right aortic arch. Before surgery, the patient was lethargic, coughing, and exhibiting dysphagia and regurgitation. Radiographs revealed cervical and thoracic megaesophagus and pneumonia.

The patient was fed with a 6-French polyethylene (Pedi-Tube™—Biosearch Medical Products) nasogastric feeding tube for a week before surgery and for a few days after surgery. During the first two days of nutritional support, the patient was monitored for diarrhea and the size of the administered boluses was gradually increased until the patient received 40-ml boluses of Osmolite® HN (Ross Laboratories) approximately every four hours.

During the week before surgery, the patient gained strength and exhibited significant clinical improvement. The patient became more active and required an Elizabethan collar to protect the nasogastric tube.

Oral feeding was started while the nasogastric tube was still in place. The oral boluses passed into the stomach when the patient was fed in an upright position. When small boluses were fed, regurgitation did not occur.

No complications related to the nasogastric tube occurred. It was believed that the perioperative nutritional support contributed to resolution of the pneumonia and decreased the morbidity associated with the thoracic operation.

Case 2

A three-year-old, spayed female, Domestic Shorthair cat (Figure 2) had a long-term obstruction of the proximal jejunum. During the six weeks before surgery to correct the obstruction, the cat had stopped eating and had lost approximately 1.8 kg.

During surgery to correct the obstruction, an adhesion attributed to the ovariohysterectomy performed one year previously was found. The small intestine was severely distended proximal to the obstruction. The surgeon removed as much of the intestinal and stomach contents through the open proximal bowel segment as possible by a reverse milking manipulation.

While manipulating the intestine, the surgeon observed signs of hyperdynamic septic shock. The surgeon therefore decided that operative time could be saved if a nasoenterostomy tube and nasogastric tube could be placed for feeding and decompression instead of a jejunostomy and gastrostomy tube. The tip of the nasoenterostomy tube was placed in the jejunum just distal to the area of the bowel anastomosis. A 14-gauge polyethylene tube (a commercial intravenous catheter) was placed in the patient's nose to administer oxygen to treat the hyperdynamic shock.

The patient remained in the intensive care unit for several days after surgery. During the first 24 hours after surgery, 160 ml of green, foul-smelling fluid was aspirated from the nasogastric tube. As soon as the cat regained consciousness, a 5-ml/hr drip infusion of Peptamen® (Baxter Healthcare, Alternative Care Division) was begun through the nasoenterostomy tube.

The nasoenterostomy tube feeding was continued for three days. During this period, the patient's strength gradually increased. The patient was discharged from the hospital on the eighth day after surgery, at which time it was doing well.

In my experience, surgical patients that had lost more than one third of their lean body weight before surgery and did not receive nutritional support often died of such complications as sepsis, wound breakdown, or pneumonia. After this patient was treated, preoperative intravenous nutritional support for 48 to 72 hours before surgery was recommended if it is possible for all patients with chronic bowel obstructions. The immunologic functions of the reticuloendothelial system and white blood cells are significantly improved by such preoperative support in patients with significant protein–calorie malnutrition. Perhaps if this patient had received intravenous nutritional support before surgery, the septic shock observed during surgery might not have occurred.

Case 3

A middle-aged, female dachshund (Figure 3) had septic peritonitis secondary to abscess formation in the pancreas. The condition was treated aggressively; surgery was performed to remove the necrotic pancreatic tissue, abscesses, and necrotic peripancreatic tissue, which included retroperitoneal fat, omentum, and transverse fascia. A jejunostomy tube was inserted during surgery, and feeding through the tube was started after the patient regained consciousness. Intravenous administration tubing and an intravenous extension tube were used to administer the diet through the jejunostomy tube.

A monomeric elemental diet containing amino acids and monosaccharides (Vivonex® T.E.N.—Norwich Eaton Laboratories) was administered by drip infusion. To avoid stimulating pancreatic secretion, the infusion rate was 1 ml/kg/hr during the first 24 hours. During the next 24 hours, the infusion rate was gradually increased to 3 ml/kg/hr. The patient recovered.

Case 4

A 13-year-old, mixed-breed dog (Figure 4) received drip infusion (2 ml/kg/hr) of Osmolite® HN (Ross Laboratories) after surgical removal of the proximal part of the duodenum. Before surgery, the patient had icterus and was malnourished.

A possible neoplasm had obstructed the common bile duct and had partially obstructed the duodenum. The pancreas appeared to be partially atrophied but was otherwise normal. The common bile duct was reinserted into the remaining section of duodenum after resection of the tumor. The tumor was a nonmalignant mass—leimyoma and fibrosis.

The patient made a full recovery from the surgical procedure. The jejunostomy tube was removed on Day 7 after surgery, and the patient was discharged on Day 11.

I believe that nutritional support, which maintained the patient's protein and calorie intake during hospitalization, played a key role in the patient's recovery. The patient required extensive surgery and had been suffering from a negative protein-calorie balance as a result of partial obstruction of the proximal duodenum. If this patient had not received nutritional support, the risk of dihiscence of the anastomosis sites (duodenum–duodenum and common bile duct–duodenum), wound infection, sepsis, and death would have been greatly increased.

REFERENCES

1. Crowe DT, Downs MO: Pharyngostomy complications in dogs and cats and recommended technical modifications: Experimental and clinical investigations. *JAAHA* 22:493–503, 1986.
2. Crowe DT: Clinical use of an indwelling nasogastric tube for enteral nutrition and fluid therapy in the dog and cat. *JAAHA* 22:675–682, 1986.
3. Blackburn GL, et al: Protein sparing therapy during periods of starvation with sepsis or trauma. *Ann Surg* 177:588–595, 1973.
4. Blackburn GL: Parenteral nutrition, in Zaslow IM (ed): *Veterinary Trauma and Critical Care*. Philadelphia, Lea & Febiger, 1984.

Anorexia and Hospitalized Cats

The hormonal response in diseased and injured cats increases the metabolic rate, thereby causing glycogen, fat, and protein depletion to occur much more rapidly than in healthy cats.

Shirley Greene, AHT
St. Francis Veterinary Hospital
Lompoc, California

Anorexia (i.e., the lack of desire to eat) is the most common and often the first sign of illness in cats. Anorexia may result from many different medical problems. For example, facial injuries and nasal congestion can cause loss of appetite because cats depend on the sense of smell to assess palatability. Pain, stress, and fear also inhibit food intake.[1] All hospitalized cats must therefore be monitored carefully.

Cats that are not diseased, injured, growing, gestating, or lactating can survive for fairly long periods of time without eating. The hormonal response to lack of food intake in healthy cats causes the metabolic rate to slow down to (and sometimes even to fall below) basal levels. This response mechanism enables the cat to use stored body fat; body protein is thus preserved.

The hormonal response in diseased and injured cats increases the metabolic rate, thereby causing glycogen, fat, and protein depletion to occur much more rapidly than in healthy cats. In this hypermetabolic state, the cat can lose weight rapidly. With a 10% loss of body weight,

Steps in the Management of Anorectic Cats

1. The cat must be evaluated daily for weight loss. The hydration status of the animal must also be determined. Weight loss of 10% or more (that cannot be attributed to dehydration) and/or anorexia three days or more in duration are signs that nutritional support should be initiated.[2]
2. Before nutritional support is begun, fluid, acid-base, and electrolyte status should be assessed and corrected as necessary. (Potassium deficiency causes anorexia and lethargy.)[2]
3. Use the most appropriate type of support—if the gut works, use it.[2]

the cat may develop complications associated with malnutrition. A 30% to 50% loss of body weight may be fatal.[1] Major surgery, fractures, infection, and illness increase energy expenditure 25% to 75% above basal levels. Massive tissue injuries, such as those caused by burns, trauma, or sepsis, may increase energy expenditure 50% to 100% above basal levels.[2]

Sick cats lose weight differently from most species. When cats stop eating, they immediately begin to catabolize their own protein, which usually causes muscle atrophy. Sick and injured cats do not effectively use fat stores. Obese anorectic cats often remain obese in outward appearance, although they are rapidly losing weight. Such cats may feel mushy because of muscle atrophy and retention of fat stores. Loss of elasticity in the skin often results from a change in the character of the skin and subcutaneous tissue because of protein catabolism. Loss of skin elasticity in anorectic cats should not be used as a measure of dehydration. It is easy to underestimate the severity of feline weight loss based on apparent retention of fat. Hospitalized cats should be weighed daily. Because muscle weighs more than fat, marked weight loss can occur with a relatively small amount of muscle loss.[1]

Febrile cats lose weight faster than cats that are afebrile. For each one degree (Celsius) rise in temperature, metabolism is increased by 10% to 13%.[1]

Sick cats that do not eat catabolize their own stored energy and body protein, which are needed for tissue repair

and/or healing. Malnutrition exacerbates the effects of infection or other disease. A vicious cycle may ensue, as disease may convert a borderline nutritional state into a full-blown deficiency disease.

Anorexia (of even a few days in duration) associated with disease or trauma adversely affects all body systems. It thus becomes difficult for the cat to respond to treatment and be restored to health. There are few contraindications to feeding the patients (e.g., an intestinal block). Cats should not be allowed to go more than 48 hours without eating. The earlier nutritional support is started, the better the results.

METHODS OF NUTRITIONAL SUPPORT
Non–Forced-Feeding

The technician should try to stimulate the cat's interest in food. A very palatable food, such as a high-protein, high-fat canned food, should be given in small amounts. If the cat does not eat the cat food, such foods as fresh cooked chicken, canned tuna, baby food, or even smoked oysters may stimulate the cat's appetite. Warming the food enhances the aroma and palatability of many foods. If the cat's nose is clogged, cleaning the nose with nasal drops may allow the cat to smell the food, and interest in food may be stimulated.

Some cats will eat if they feel reassured. Petting and talking to the cat may make it feel more comfortable and thus encourage eating. Hand-feeding is a viable alternative.

Many cats that do not eat in the hospital will eat in the home environment; treating the cat as an outpatient should therefore be considered. If this is not feasible, having the owner come to the hospital to feed the cat often is successful.

Forced Hand-Feeding

If the cat cannot be enticed to eat, the next step is to try force-feeding. One method uses a 5-milliliter syringe. The end of the syringe is cut off, and the edges are smoothed. The open end of the syringe is pushed into a can of preferably high-calorie food. The core of food is then slowly injected into the mouth of the cat. Placing the food in the pharyngeal area stimulates the swallowing reflex.[2] Two points must be kept in mind with force-feeding.

- Most cats resent being restrained, and the stress involved may be more harmful than beneficial to critical cats.
- Cats that are extremely ill and debilitated may have an impaired gag reflex. If given too rapidly, the food may

pass into the trachea and lungs, which can result in severe aspiration pneumonia.

Another method of force-feeding is to use a high-calorie food supplement paste. The paste is placed on the nose of the cat, and many cats lick the paste off the nose. The paste also can be smeared on the roof of the mouth.

Force-feeding is most beneficial for cats that have not been anorectic for more than a few days and that are not extremely ill. Force-feeding seems to be more successful if done by the owners.

Tube-Feeding

In a severely ill and debilitated cat, tube-feeding is faster, easier, and (in most cases) less stressful than force-feeding. There are several different routes by which a cat can be tube-fed. The diet to be intubated can be used for all routes, with the exception of the jejunostomy tube. Following is a discussion on the different methods of tube-feeding, the diets, and the factors that determine how much to feed.

METHODS OF TUBE-FEEDING
Orogastric Feeding

Orogastric feeding is done with a soft rubber tube. A size 8 to 10 French urinary catheter works well. The tube should be premeasured and marked. For gastric placement, the tube is marked at the ninth intercostal space.[2] The cat should be held gently with minimal restraint. The mouth of the cat should be opened just wide enough for the tube to be passed.[1] Intubating some cats necessitates use of a mouth speculum, which should only be large enough for the tube to pass through it. The tube should be advanced slowly to avoid damaging pharyngeal and esophageal mucosa.[1] The technician must be sure that the cat has swallowed the tube and that it is not in the trachea. After the cat swallows the tube, it is advanced to the premeasured mark. Before the cat is fed, five milliliters of sterile water or saline should be instilled so the technician can be certain that the trachea has not been intubated.

Nasogastric Intubation

Most cats tolerate a nasal tube quite well, and it can usually be inserted with minimal restraint. A nasogastric tube can be sutured in place for several weeks, and the cat can eat and drink with the tube in place. Polyvinyl tubes are well suited for nasogastric feeding; however, such tubes should not be left in place for more than two weeks because they will harden in the stomach.[2]

Inserting a nasogastric tube is easy. The appropriate tube size is selected (3 to 8 French are the sizes used for cats, with 5 French being the most commonly used size). The tube is marked at the level of the ninth intercostal space for gastric placement or the seventh intercostal space for esophageal placement. Several drops of a topical anesthetic (0.5% proparacaine hydrochloride) are dropped into one nostril. The head of the cat should be kept elevated for two to three minutes. Before the tube is passed, the head of the cat should be allowed to return to a normal angle because tracheal intubation is much less likely if the head is in a normal position. The tube should be lubricated and then passed caudally through the ventral meatus and nasopharynx into the esophagus.[2] The tube is advanced to the marked point. After the tube is in position, placement should be confirmed by injecting 6 to 12 milliliters of sterile water or saline.[3] The cat will cough if the tube is in the lungs or trachea. If the technician is still uncertain of the position of the tube after instillation of liquid, a radiograph can confirm placement. The radiograph also assures the desired depth of placement of the tube. Another method to check placement is to attach a syringe to the tube and aspirate. If it is in the trachea, the tube will be difficult to aspirate; if it is in the esophagus, the plunger will pull out easily.[4] As soon as the tube is in place, it can be sutured to the skin using 3-0 nonabsorbable suture. Tape butterflies should be used to stabilize the tube; the butterflies should begin as close to the nostrils as possible. To avoid irritating the cat, the tube should not touch the whiskers.

Esophagostomy Tube

The esophagostomy tube is well tolerated by cats, and cats usually do not need an Elizabethan collar once the tube is in place. The major disadvantage of esophagostomy tubes is that the cat must be anesthetized for placement. The tube is placed in the esophagus through a stab incision in the cranial esophagus.[5] The tube is then manipulated so that the distal end of the tube is in the distal end of the esophagus. The tube is sutured in place and taped around the neck of the cat.[5] The end of the tube should be plugged with an intravenous catheter cap. Cats are able to eat easily with the tube in place.

Gastrostomy Tube

Gastrostomy tube placement has been made easier and

Blenderized Diet for Tube-Feeding[2]

1/2 can high-calorie cat food
3/4 cup water

Blend for at least one minute at high speed. Strain twice through a kitchen strainer. Adding two ounces of vegetable oil per can of food to this diet has been recommended.[5]

Liquid Diet for Cats

Combine three ounces of strained meat or egg yolk baby food with three to four ounces of water. Add one teaspoon of cooking oil and one teaspoon corn syrup. Combine all ingredients and blend well.

safer with the advent of the endoscope. Most blenderized foods and/or commercially prepared liquid diets can be fed through the gastrostomy tube, thereby making it the method of choice for chronic enteral nutrition.

Jejunostomy Tube-Feeding

The jejunostomy tube is used when nutrients must be given distal to the pylorus. Jejunostomy tube-feeding may be indicated for patients with damage or blockage to any part of the gastrointestinal tract cranial to the duodenum. The tube must be placed surgically, and only isotonic feeding solutions should be used.[1]

DIETS FOR TUBE-FEEDING CATS

Liquid diets should supply all necessary nutrients and be easily digested and used by the patient. Several commercially prepared diets for cats that are easy to use and well tolerated are currently available. There also are two recipes for diets listed in the boxes. Both types of diets have been used successfully; however, if the patient is extremely debilitated, commercial diets that have been diluted more than normal cause less initial gastric distress.

Determining Amount and Frequency

To determine the caloric needs of a sick cat, an estimate of the effect of the disease process on energy expenditure must be made. Basal energy requirement (BER) is the amount of energy expended by a healthy cat lying quietly in a warm, stress-free environment. The basal energy requirement of a healthy, unstressed cat is approximately 190 Kcal/24 hours. The basal energy requirement of the average hospitalized cat is 250 to 300 Kcal/24 hr.[5] The daily energy requirement for dogs or cats weighing more than two kilo-

grams is BER (Kcal) = $30 \times$ body wt. (kg) + 70; for dogs and cats weighing less than two kilograms, the formula is BER (Kcal) = $70 \times$ body wt. (kg)$^{0.75}$:

Cage rest	=	BER $\times$ 1.25
After surgery	=	BER $\times$ 1.25
Trauma	=	BER $\times$ 1.35
Cancer	=	BER $\times$ 1.35
Sepsis	=	BER $\times$ 1.5 to 1.7
Major burns	=	BER $\times$ 1.7 to 2.0[2]

The daily energy requirement is divided by the energy density of the diet to be used (Kcal/ml); the result is the number of milliliters per day that the cat needs. Anorectic cats, however, have various degrees of gastric contraction and decreased digestive function. Therefore, it usually is not initially possible to feed the total volume needed per day. Most nutritionists recommend starting the cat on approximately one third of the volume needed per day and slowly increasing the amount for a period of three to four days until the total volume can be tolerated. If it is physically able to eat, the cat should be offered food several times a day and be encouraged to eat during this time.

Complications

Placement of the tube is the most crucial aspect of tube-feeding. Feeding the animal too quickly may cause gastrointestinal distress, but such distress can be prevented by feeding less than 20 ml/min.[1] Flushing the tube before and after feedings keeps the food flowing and prevents it from decaying in the tube. Using the correct size of tube helps prevent esophagitis and aspiration of food. If the cat vomits, feeding must be discontinued until the cause is determined.

CONCLUSION

Anorexia is very common and is associated with many different problems in cats. It is extremely important that sick cats receive proper nutrition. The technician can play a vital role in the cat's recovery and may even determine if the cat recovers at all. The technician's duties include the following: the cat should be weighed daily, hydration status must be checked, and food intake must be carefully monitored. If the veterinarian decides that nutritional support is necessary, the technician will be responsible for administering the diet, maintaining the feeding tube, monitoring the patient, and encouraging it to begin eating on its own again.

REFERENCES

1. Pedersen NC: *Feline Husbandry*. Goleta, CA, American Veterinary Publications, 1991, pp 347–354, 317–329.
2. Lewis LD, Morris ML, Hand MS: Anorexia, inanition and critical care nutrition, in *Small Animal Clinical Nutrition. Vol III*. Topeka, KS, Mark Morris Associates, 1987.
3. Messonnie S: For anorexic patients use nasogastric intubation: Easier for you, easier on the pet. *Vet Forum*: 58, 1992.
4. Ford R: Viral respiratory infections in cats, in *Twenty-Fourth Friskies Symposium on Feline Disease and Nutrition*. Oakland, CA, 1991.
5. Norsworthy GD: Providing nutritional support for anorectic cats. *Vet Med* 86(6):589–596, June 1991.

The Care and Management of Orphaned Puppies and Kittens

William J. Monson, PhD
Vice President
Research and Development
Pet-Ag, Inc.
Elgin, Illinois

Attempting to raise orphaned puppies and kittens—as anyone who has tried knows—is a demanding, time-consuming task that requires experience, strict attention to detail, and keen observation. It is a task that can culminate in total frustration or in sheer jubilation. The husbandry and nutrition of puppies orphaned earlier than four weeks of age and kittens orphaned earlier than six weeks of age require special consideration.[1] Experience has proven that if orphan-reared puppies and kittens survive to a few months of age, they can be healthy animals with normal social behavior.

A review of the available literature demonstrates the paucity of information on raising orphaned puppies and kittens. Furthermore, there is scant technological data from which specific recommendations on care and management can be derived. This article presents information obtained during years of experience with nutrition, specific husbandry problems, and other potential complications associated with raising orphans.

Definition of *Orphan*

In practical terms, an orphan is any animal that does not have access to the natural milk of the mother. With a puppy or a kitten, the death of the bitch or the queen is not a prerequisite because insufficient quantity or quality of milk in the mother can effectively deprive the neonate of colostrum or mature milk.

Surgery, such as a cesarean section, can make it impossible for a bitch or a queen to nurse a newborn litter. Diseases affecting the mammary glands (e.g., mastitis) or postparturient uterine infections (e.g., metritis) can present potential hazards to the mother or the neonate if nursing is permitted. Puppies and kittens born in this situation are justifiably managed as orphans and are therefore included in this discussion.

Environment

Specific attention to the environment in which puppies and kittens are reared is a critical factor in the overall success of hand-rearing orphans. Bitches and queens are able to provide moist heat, stimulation of eliminatory function and circulation, mothering, security, and milk. Hand-reared puppies and kittens must be kept in a clean, warm environment with circulating moist air but without drafts.

Commercial incubators are available with heating coils embedded in hard plastic; temperature controls; high sides for partitioning; and clear, vented covers. Few individuals or veterinary practices have access to this type of artificial environment, however. In lieu of such an incubator, a box divided into compartments or smaller individual boxes can be used with equal effectiveness. The floor of the box should be covered with a soft, clean cloth or newspaper.

Environmental temperature is a critical factor, particularly during the first few weeks of life, because chilling can significantly decrease the survivability of the neonate. Neonatal kittens typically require warmer ambient temperatures than do puppies; smaller animals usually require warmer temperatures than do larger animals.[1] Heat is perhaps best provided by a covered heating pad. The pad should be positioned to allow the neonate to seek a comfort zone by moving closer to or farther from the heat source.

Heat lamps, although effective, can cause burns if left unattended. Hot-water bottles eventually cool and have obvious disadvantages. Regardless of the heat source used, a thermometer must be hung from the side of the box to monitor the environmental temperature at the orphan's level. Table I provides ambient temperature guidelines from birth through the first month of life.

When a litter of puppies or kittens is orphaned, it is possible to raise the neonates individually for the first two to three weeks of life. Although this is not essential, it provides a means of monitoring stool consistency and prevents animals from sucking on the tails, ears, paws, and genitals of siblings.[1]

Neonatal puppies and kittens are susceptible to dehydration when environmental relative humidity is low. If room air is not humidity-controlled, pans of water should be placed close to the incubator boxes. A relative humidity of 50% should help to prevent dehydration.

It is essential to provide neonates with sufficient tactile stimulation to facilitate circulation and bowel movements. An adequate supply of clean replacement towels and bedding is important. Towels moistened with warm water can be used to clean the animals' mouths and anal areas. When hand-rearing several orphans simultaneously and when more than one person is providing care, it is helpful to maintain records of activity, body weights, feeding times and quantities, temperatures, and clinical notes.

Nutrition

Clearly, one of the foremost challenges of hand-rearing orphaned puppies and kittens is meeting caloric and fluid needs. This is particularly true when dealing with a litter of newborn animals that will not have the opportunity to nurse or to consume milk from the bitch or the queen.

Normal nursing animals are afforded the milk and the delivery system that are particularly suited to the metabolic and digestive needs of the species. When a milk replacement is required, it should approximate the gross composition of the milk of the bitch or the queen. A well-formulated milk replacer will support the puppy or kitten through the critical first few weeks of life until growth, digestion, and basal metabolic functions are developed to the point that solid food can be consumed. Failure to provide a well-formulated replacer significantly affects normal metabolic and immune functions, thereby compromising the ability of the neonate to develop and thrive.

Colostrum—The First Milk

The composition of colostrum milk, the first milk nursing puppies and kittens consume, differs significantly from that of milk produced later in lactation. Colostrum is rich in maternal antibody and therefore plays a critical role in protecting neonates from disease, particularly infectious disease. Many orphans have been reared without colostrum, but these animals should be considered at risk of becoming ill during the first few weeks of life.

Composition of Milk and Milk Replacers

There are differences in the composition of natural milks and species-formulated milk replacers; there also are significant differences between natural milks of various species. Table II lists the composition of milks from various species and illustrates the importance of selecting the appropriate milk replacer for an orphaned puppy or kitten. For example, the milks from cows and goats have significantly lower protein contents than the milks from bitches and queens; used alone, cow or goat milk is not a particularly suitable replacer for puppies or kittens.

Commercially prepared milk replacers are preferred for feeding orphans[2] and are available for puppies and kittens. Such milk substitutes have compositions similar to the natural mature milk of bitches and queens, although they lack antibody. Home recipes are available but can be difficult to prepare. The following recipe can be used to prepare formula for feeding puppies.[3] Mix together these ingredients: 0.8 L of cow's milk, 0.2 L of cream containing 12% fat, one egg yolk, 6 g of bone meal, 2000 IU of vitamin A, and 500 IU of vitamin D. While heating the mixture to 104° F (40° C), add 4 g of citric acid to coagulate the casein. (The author has not evaluated this formula in feeding trials.)

The high-lactose composition of cow's milk can cause significant diarrhea in orphans, particularly puppies. This complication must be avoided when hand-rearing puppies and kittens because diarrhea can rapidly result in fluid and electrolyte losses that can lead to death if not corrected.

Daily Caloric and Water Needs

The optimum caloric intake from a balanced formula of protein, fat, and lactose is 60 to 70 calories/lb of body weight per day. Intake should be less for puppies orphaned during the first week of life and for the first few feedings of puppies orphaned when older. Less information is available about the optimum caloric intake for kittens; however, the general principles useful with puppies usually apply to kittens as well.

Specific neonatal requirements for water are not well defined. Amounts range from 2 to 3 oz/lb of body weight per day.[4,5] Feeding recommendations provided with commercial milk replacers usually meet the caloric and hydration needs of neonates.

TABLE I[a]
Temperature Guidelines for Orphans

Age	Puppies	Kittens
Birth to 7 days	85° to 90° F[b]	88° to 92° F
8 to 14 days	80°	80° to 85°
15 to 28 days	80°	80°
29 to 35 days	70° to 75°	75°
36 days and thereafter	70°	70°

[a]Used with permission from Monson WJ: Orphan rearing of puppies and kittens. *Vet Clin North Am [Small Anim Pract]* 17:568, 1987.

[b]Where a range is shown, the higher temperature is preferable for animals of the younger age.

TABLE II[a]
Composition of the Milk of Various Species

Nutrient	Bitch's Milk	Esbilac® (Pet-Ag) Bitch's Milk Replacer	Queen's Milk	KMR® (Pet-Ag) Queen's Milk Replacer	Cow's Milk	Goat's Milk
Percent solids of mature milk	24	—	18.2	—	11.9	13
Percent protein-solids basis	33	33.4	40	42.2	25.6	27.4
Percent fat-solids basis	41	44.1	28	25.0	29.9	31.9
Percent lactose-solids basis	17	15.8	27	26.1	38.7	34.2
Gross kilocalories/g solids[b]	5.7	5.9	5.2	5.0	5.26	5.34
Percent calories from protein	23.2	22.5	30.8	33.9	19.5	20.5
Percent calories from fat	64.9	66.8	48.5	45.2	51.1	53.8
Percent calories from lactose	11.9	10.7	20.8	20.9	29.4	25.7

[a]Used with permission from Monson WJ: Orphan rearing of puppies and kittens. *Vet Clin North Am [Small Anim Pract]* 17:570, 1987.
[b]Gross kilocalories calculated on the basis of 4, 9, and 4 calories/g of protein, fat, and lactose, respectively.

Feeding Techniques

Delivery

The use of a small animal nursing bottle is the preferred method of delivering milk replacer to orphans[1,2] (Figure 1). A 2-oz nurser is appropriate for kittens and small puppies. The hole in the nipple should be large enough for the milk substitute to ooze out slowly and for the orphan to effectively nurse. Older and larger animals are easier to feed with a 4-oz nurser. An eyedropper or blunted syringe is effective for orphans that are too small or too weak to nurse from a bottle. Milk must not be squeezed or forced out of the bottle while the nipple is in the animal's mouth; this practice can force milk into the lungs and can result in pneumonia or death.

Tube feeding of orphans is effective and rapid, particularly when several orphans are being fed simultaneously. Improper tube placement and handling, as well as an excessively rapid delivery rate, can result in significant injury or death, however. Appropriate training and experience is recommended before attempting to tube feed orphaned puppies and kittens.

Administration

All equipment used in feeding orphans should be very clean. The formula is always warmed before feeding; giving cold formula to orphans can lower body temperatures to critical levels.

Puppies orphaned during the first week of life that weigh between 200 and 300 g can be offered approximately 10 ml (two thirds to three quarters of a tablespoon) of milk replacer at the first feeding. Kittens weighing between 90 and 140 g should receive 5 ml of milk replacer at the first feeding. Orphans receiving milk replacer from a bottle will refuse the nipple when full.

Most people experienced in feeding orphans prefer to hold the animal during bottle feeding. The orphan's head should be tilted up and outstretched slightly while the animal is held in the feeder's palm. The bottle nipple is placed in the orphan's mouth and is pulled up and away slightly; this will elevate the head and encourage vigorous sucking.

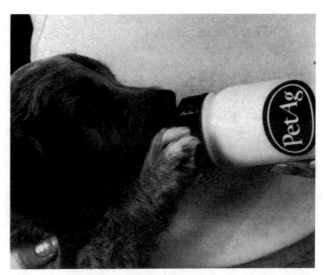

Figure 1—Milk replacer is delivered to orphaned puppies and kittens via a small animal nursing bottle.

If milk comes out of the animal's nose during nursing, the rate of feeding should be slowed. If this fails to resolve the problem, the oral cavity should be examined for evidence of cleft palate (Figure 2).

For animals orphaned during the first week of life, the actual daily intake often does not exceed 10% of the body weight for the first few days.[1] The second and third feedings should be at the same level as the first. After this, common sense and good judgment are recommended. Older and larger-breed puppies might require significantly more formula if they vigorously consume the first feeding and have a normal bowel movement. Because an orphan's digestive system must adjust to the milk replacer, it is better to underfeed than to overfeed during the first two to three days of life.

Frequency

Puppies and kittens should be fed four times daily. Ideally, feeding occurs at exact six-hour intervals; however,

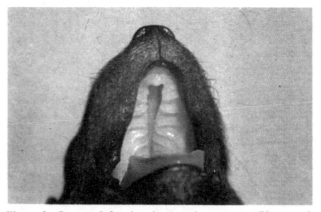

Figure 2—Severe cleft palate in a newborn puppy. (Photograph courtesy of Dr. Richard B. Ford, School of Veterinary Medicine, North Carolina State University)

the animals do well when fed at 8:00 AM, 11:30 AM, 3:30 PM, and 9:00 PM.[1] More frequent feedings of smaller volumes have been recommended, but it should be remembered that sleep is vital to neonates. Waking a neonate for feeding is stressful, undesirable, and unnecessary. Wakefulness, restlessness, and crying dictate additional feedings.

It is appropriate to increase the volume of formula offered at the rate of 1 ml (or cc) per feeding, starting 36 to 48 hours after the initial feeding. Another method used successfully involves increasing the level by 3 ml (one half to three quarters of a teaspoon) every other day. With kittens, the increase should be somewhat slower, approximately 1 ml/day or 2 ml every other day. These increases are indicated only as long as the previous feeding was voluntarily and completely consumed. If a point of refusal is reached, the feeding level should not be increased for one to two days.

Slight weight loss is fairly common during the first two to three days on milk replacer. Formula changes or significant additions should be done over a three- to four-day period by increasing the additional in increments of 25% daily.

Rate of Weight Gain

Weight gain should be monitored and recorded on a daily basis for at least the first few weeks of life. For the first five months, puppies should gain 1 to 2 g/day for each pound (0.45 kg) of anticipated adult weight. Kittens should gain 50 to 100 g/week.[2]

Introduction of Solid Food

When the eyes open and the orphan is walking, demand and tolerance for more food becomes evident. At this point, orphans can be continued on hand-feeding or provided with a self-feeding regimen. With continued hand-feeding, sufficient milk to ensure continued weight gain must be offered.

Before each feeding, the orphan should be encouraged to lap milk from a shallow bowl or saucer. The muzzle should be placed into the milk, making sure that a small amount

gets onto the tongue. Allowing the orphan to suck on a finger and then leading it to the bowl can facilitate the transition.

As soon as puppies and kittens begin lapping formula with slight or no encouragement, they can take full feedings by lapping. Puppies adjust to lapping earlier and more rapidly than kittens do. It is important to leave the bowl in the pen for no more than one hour; the bowl always should be washed with soap and water after feeding.

Solid food should be introduced as soon as lapping has been learned. Commercially prepared weaning formulas are available for kittens and puppies. A small quantity of meal-type formula is added to the milk to produce a thin gruel. This solid food in the milk enhances lapping and increases the amount of food consumed. A bowl of fresh, clean water should be provided once solid food is added.

Bottle feeding can be discontinued over a period of two to three days after lapping starts; the bottle is eliminated one feeding at a time. After feeding, puppies and kittens should be washed with a wet cloth and dried thoroughly. In general, puppies should make the transition to regular puppy food by 7 to 8 weeks of age; kittens should be on regular kitten food no later than 11 to 12 weeks of age.

Conclusions

Technicians with experience in hand-rearing orphaned puppies or kittens will recognize the value of the following key points in the successful care of orphans:

1. Avoid overfeeding, particularly during the first several days of life.
2. Use a milk replacer with a composition similar to natural milk.
3. Keep the environment, the bedding, and the feeding utensils clean.
4. Monitor weight and performance regularly.
5. Maintain an environment that is warm, draft free, and adequately humidified.
6. Keep the orphans clean of food and excrement.
7. Establish feeding frequency to permit the stomach to empty before refeeding.
8. Control diarrhea as soon as possible.
9. Make formula or ration changes slowly.
10. Start orphans on some solid food as soon as possible.

Adherence to these guidelines requires patience and attention to detail. The goals are the preservation of life and the establishment of a sound management and nutrition program. The results can be very rewarding.

REFERENCES

1. Monson WJ: Orphan rearing of puppies and kittens. *Vet Clin North Am [Small Anim Pract]* 17:567–576, 1987.
2. Lewis LD, Morris ML, Hand MS: Dogs—Feeding and care. *Small Animal Clinical Nutrition III.* Topeka, KS, Mark Morris Associates, 1987, pp 3-1—3-32.

3. Christiansen IJ: Parturition and newborn puppies. *Reproduction in the Dog and Cat*. London, Bailliere Tindall, 1984, pp 171–196.
4. Campbell DM: *Canine Pediatrics*. A Collection of Discussions from Veterinary Medicine on Nutrition in Young Puppies. Chicago, Veterinary Magazine Corporation, 1938.
5. Evans AT, Evans RH: Raising raccoons for release. Part III. Nutritional problems. *Vet Tech* 6(8):404–410, 1985.

UPDATE

An important consideration not specifically addressed above is hypothermia. A low body temperature significantly reduces the ability of the neonate to utilize formula, resulting in a greater propensity for gastric intestinal dysfunction. The neonate's normal body temperature is approximately 100° F; therefore before feeding it is important to ensure that the animal is warm and has a warm environment to stay in. Abandoned puppies and kittens are particular candidates for hypothermia.

Dehydration is another important consideration. Using an electrolyte solution as the first feeding for orphaned animals is a good practice. The electrolyte solution not only helps to restore lost body fluids but also has the effect of flushing the gastrointestinal tract prior to the introduction of the formulas.

Supplementing litters of puppies or kittens that are too large for the mother to feed assures that all the infants receive adequate nutrition and relieves the demand put on the mother. Frequently the one or two smaller infants can be fed as orphans and then returned to the mother so she can care for them. If she does not care for those being fed as orphans, they will require the special care described above.

The development of juvenile cataracts in some breeds of puppies orphaned at an early age has been a concern for many years. Research sponsored by Pet-Ag, Inc., at Colorado State University concluded that "The development of nutritional cataracts in puppies fed milk replacer formulas appears to be breed or growth rate related and influenced by the methionine and arginine content of the formulas."[1]

The appropriate additions have been made to Esbilac® milk replacer for puppies (Pet-Ag). KMR® milk replacer for orphaned kittens (Pet-Ag) has also been supplemented with amino acids.

REFERENCE

1. Ralston SL, Isherwood J, Chandler M, et al: Evaluation of growth rates and cataract formation in orphan puppies fed two milk replacer formulas. *Proceedings of the Second International Conference on Veterinary Perinatology in conjunction with the Summer Meeting of the Neonatal Society*, St John's College, Cambridge, England, July 13–15, 1991, p 56.

Preparing the Small-Animal Patient for Surgery

Teresa Raffel, AAS, CAT
Instructor Assistant, Veterinary Technician Program
Madison Area Technical College
Madison, WI

Proper preparation of the surgical site is a critical part of maintaining asepsis in surgery, but it is frequently neglected. Because the task of prepping the animal is often performed by animal health technicians, it is important that they have adequate knowledge of the necessary techniques. To efficiently prepare an animal for surgery, several factors need to be evaluated. In this article, these factors are discussed and guidelines for preparing the surgical site for general types of surgery are provided.

Preliminaries

Several parts of the preoperative preparation of the patient for surgery begin as soon as the animal arrives at the hospital. First, food is withheld from the animal for at least six hours prior to surgery. Water may be allowed until the time of surgery, or it may be taken away one hour prior to the operation. Second, the animal's general physical appearance is evaluated. A heavily soiled animal or one that has external parasites should be bathed. A bath not only improves the appearance of the animal but in the case of parasites it improves the general health of the patient. Also, the removal of gross material from the fur and skin aids in preventing possible contamination of the surgical wound. In addition, the animal should be exercised approximately one hour prior to surgery to provide the opportunity to urinate and/or defecate. If the animal cannot be exercised, the bladder can be emptied by using digital pressure or catheterization after the animal is anesthetized.

Area to Use for Prep

Preparation of the surgical site is done either in a special room that is separate from the surgical suite and is designated as a prep area, or it is done in the operating room. The advantages of having a separate room in which to do the prep are that it avoids cluttering the operating room with the surgical preparation materials and avoids contaminating the operating table and room with the mess produced during the prep. However, moving the animal to the operating room after the prep without recontaminating the operative field can be difficult. The main advantage of preparing the operative site in the operating room is that the animal can be positioned as desired and then prepped, thus eliminating the chance of contamination during transport.

Hair Removal

The first step in preparing the operative site is removing the hair. Although there are various ways to accomplish hair removal, the most common method is with an electric clipper. A No. 40 blade has been found to be the best size for adequate preoperative hair removal. Another effective tool is a straight-edged or disposable razor. Though not recommended for removal of large quantities of fur, a razor can be used after clipping if a closer shave is desired. A third method of hair removal is the use of a depilatory. Depilatories, however, have proved harsh to the skin of animals and are not practical for use in veterinary medicine.

The area to be clipped depends on the location of the surgical incision. A general rule is to clip an ample area, approximately 4 in. beyond the incision site in all directions. This amount is only a guide, and the clipping done in each case will depend on the surgery to be performed, the size of the animal, and the preference of the veterinarian. The art of clipping quickly and cleanly comes with practice, but keeping a few points in mind will help in becoming proficient.

Originally published in Volume 4, Number 5, September/October 1983

First, clipping against the grain of the hair gives a closer shave. Second, if the clipper is held as one would hold a pencil, with the blade flat against the skin, there is less chance of abrasion; abraded areas can harbor bacteria, which could contaminate the incision site. Abrasions can also be avoided by keeping the razor and clipper blades clean and sharp. Clipper burns are another hazard when removing hair. Animals with thin skin (e.g., white poodles) seem to be especially susceptible to clipper burns. Spraying the clipper blades with a commercial blade coolant when they become hot can alleviate burning.

The last consideration when removing hair is that the clip be cosmetic. An owner will immediately notice the amount of hair clipped but will not react as negatively if the cut is clean and neat, instead of irregular.

After the clipping is completed, the clipper blade should be cleaned with a brush and then lubricated. The hair removed from the animal must be vacuumed or otherwise disposed of carefully to avoid leaving loose hairs that can be picked up when scrubbing the animal. Vacuuming reduces the chance of introducing loose hair into the surgery room. A final step before starting the disinfecting part of the preparation is to empty the bladder of the animal if it did not urinate prior to surgery.

Materials

Agents used to prepare the surgical site are varied and numerous. The main reason for careful surgical site preparation is to render the skin as clean as possible. Skin cannot be sterilized, but reducing the number of normal flora to a relatively safe level for surgery decreases the chance for infection.

Soaps

There are some properties that soap used for the surgical scrub should have (Table I). Although it is difficult to find a soap that features all of these properties, there are a few commercial agents that meet many of the desired criteria.

Povidone-Iodine—Povidone-iodine[a] is an iodine

---

[a]Betadine®, The Purdue Frederick Co, Norwalk, CT 06856.

TABLE I

Desired Properties of Surgical Scrub Agents

1. Wide spectrum of antimicrobial activity
2. Long residual lethal effect against microorganisms
3. Ability to decrease microbial count rapidly
4. Quick application
5. Safe use without skin irritation or sensitization
6. Remain active and effective in the presence of alcohol and organic matter
7. Economical
8. Practical for veterinary use

complex combined with detergent and has a broad spectrum of antimicrobial activity including efficient activity against spores. It is also bactericidal, viricidal, and fungistatic and fungicidal. One fungus that can be effectively controlled with povidone-iodine is the ringworm fungus. Povidone-iodine is widely available and relatively inexpensive. It is, however, corrosive to metals, and skin reaction is fairly common. Its residual effect against gram-positive (e.g., *Staphylococcus aureus*) and gram-negative (e.g., *Escherichia coli*) bacteria is significantly better than that of hexachlorophene but is not as good as that of chlorhexidine.

Chlorhexidine—Chlorhexidine[b] is another type of solution occasionally used for the surgical scrub. This soap has been shown to be most active in alkaline conditions. Its action is bactericidal against gram-negative bacteria, and it has some action against gram-positive bacteria. Chlorhexidine has proved efficacious against 30 bacteria including *E. coli* and *Pseudomonas* sp. It has demonstrated viricidal and fungicidal activity against organisms that cause equine influenza, canine distemper, and feline viral rhinotracheitis. It has an efficient level of activity in the presence of organic material and has relatively low toxicity to tissues. In comparisons of residual activity of chlorhexidine with that of povidone-iodine and hexachlorophene, it was proved to be the most effective of the three.

Hexachlorophene—Hexachlorophene has some bactericidal activity against gram-positive organisms but is ineffective against gram-negative bacteria and fungi. This agent loses its efficacy when used with regular soap or when alcohol is used afterward. Hexachlorophene does achieve suppressive action against bacterial regrowth, but only after it has been used quite frequently. When compared with chlorhexidine and povidone-iodine, after a two-minute scrub, the largest amount of undesired regrowth was found in the area disinfected with hexachlorophene.

Solutions

Alcohol—Alcohol is often used in the process of preparing the surgical site. Though ethyl or isopropyl alcohol can be used, 70% ethanol is the recommended choice. The rapid evaporation property of alcohol makes it a desirable skin disinfectant. Alcohol is bactericidal against many gram-negative organisms but has no effect against bacterial spores. It is active against some fungal spores, but only after several minutes of exposure. Because of its ability to coagulate proteins, alcohol should not be used on open wounds or mucous membranes. It is among the best tolerated of the skin degerming agents available and can be used repeatedly without damage to the skin. Toxic effects occur only if alcohol is used on broken skin or if it is puddled under the animal.

Povidone-Iodine—Povidone-iodine is probably used most. Once applied, the brown film it produces should not be wiped off. The bactericidal activity of povidone-

---

[b]Nolvasan®, Fort Dodge Laboratories, Fort Dodge, IA 50501.

iodine is sustained by the release of free iodine as it dries and the color fades. The brown film is advantageous in that it indicates where the agent has been applied. There are disadvantages to using povidone-iodine. Even though it has a low level of free iodine, the solution can be corrosive to metals. Povidone-iodine shows no therapeutic benefit when used on open wounds.

Chlorhexidine—Chlorhexidine acetate (0.5%) with 5% isopropyl alcohol[c] solution is another alternative for final painting (spraying) of the surgical site. As with the chlorhexidine surgical scrub, this antiseptic solution has very effective antimicrobial residual activity. The blue color of the product aids in identifying the prepped area.

Benzalkonium Chloride—Benzalkonium chloride,[d] a cationic surface-active agent, is another type of antiseptic solution. It is nonirritating to tissue when used in an effective concentration and has relatively low systemic toxicity. There are disadvantages to using this agent. Its activity is antagonized by soap, pus, and tissue constituents. The film that forms after benzalkonium chloride is applied is varied in its bactericidal activity. The outer film is very bactericidal; however, the inner film surface has low bactericidal activity. The agent provides no action against spores and can occasionally cause allergic reactions.

Application of Solutions

When solutions are used as the final agent in preparing the surgical site, they can be applied by different methods. One technique is to spray the solution on from a spray bottle. This is the most convenient method, however it can be messy. Because of the misting action of the spray bottle, the flow is hard to control. An alternative to spraying is to apply the solution to a sterile gauze sponge first and then to use the sponge to apply the solution to the surgical site. This method is advantageous because the solution's activity level is increased when the agent is applied with friction. Also, sponging is less messy than spraying because the solution can be better controlled as it is applied. When applied with friction solutions dry faster than they do when sprayed. In most cases, the suppressive action of the agent is increased as the agent dries. It is also important to have the area dry before the draping process begins so as to avoid staining the drapes and to prevent any possibility of contamination through osmosis.

Applicators
Cotton

One material used as an applicator for preparing the surgical site is cotton, which is inexpensive and readily available. When used, it should be torn into small pieces, placed in a bowl, and moistened with water. Before using a piece of cotton to scrub an animal, any excess water should be wrung out. Dry cotton can be used to wipe dry the surgical site. There are, however, a few

disadvantages to using cotton. Its use can be costly if too much cotton is ripped into pieces and moistened ahead of time, because it cannot be reused and must be thrown away. Another problem is that cotton fibers often catch on hair stubble and remain in the prepped area; and the area can be contaminated in the course of trying to remove the fibers.

Gauze Sponges

Another type of applicator is the 4 × 4-in. gauze sponge. Sponges can be used if they are clean but nonsterile; however, it is recommended that they be sterile. Sponges and cotton are used in the same manner.

Sterile Scrub

The sterile scrub is done in the operating room after the animal has been positioned. When possible, it is preceded by two scrubs outside the operating room. The sterile scrub is the final scrub before the incision is made. Materials needed for a sterile scrub are a sterile basin containing 15 to 20 gauze sponges, sterile saline or water, sterile surgical gloves, and surgical scrub and solution (Figure 1).

The basin should be opened aseptically. Next, the stopper or cover should be removed from the sterile saline or water so that it is ready to pour. Using the open gloving technique, one of the sterile surgical gloves is aseptically put on. The advantage to having only one hand gloved is that the nonsterile hand is free to apply scrub agent to the sponge; pour the saline or water; and, in the case of orthopedics, to hold the limb so that it does not move while it is being scrubbed. Approximately 10 of the sponges are removed from the basin and placed on the sterile field where they will remain dry. The sterile saline or water is then poured into the basin, using the nonsterile hand, thus moistening the sponges that remain in the basin. With the gloved hand, a moistened sponge is picked up, and with the nonsterile hand the scrubbing agent is applied to the sponge. All rules of aseptic technique must be observed when disinfecting the area. The sponges can be held with the sterile hand

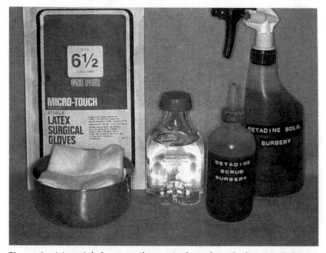

Figure 1—Materials for a sterile surgical scrub include a sterile basin containing 15 to 20 sterile gauze sponges, sterile saline or water, sterile surgical gloves, and surgical scrub and solution agents. (Courtesy of Kris Kazmierczak, RVT)

[c]Nolvaprep™, Fort Dodge Laboratories, Fort Dodge, IA
[d]Zephiran®, Winthrop Laboratories, New York, NY 10016.

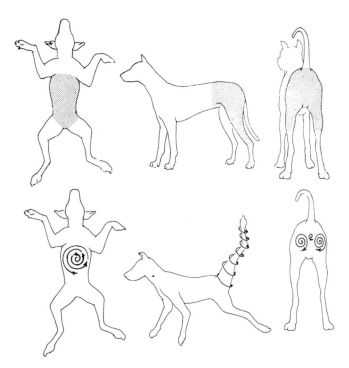

Figure 2—*Shaded areas* show section to be clipped free of hair for certain surgical procedures. *Arrows* show the direction the sponge should follow when these areas are being prepped. (From Winfield WE, Rawlings CA: *Small Animal Surgery—An Atlas of Operative Techniques.* Philadelphia, WB Saunders Co, 1979, p 17. Reprinted with permission.)

or held with sterile forceps grasped by the sterile hand.

Depending on the area of the body that requires surgery, one of three methods should be used to prep the surgical site (Figure 2). The first method, referred to as the *target pattern*, is used primarily in abdominal, thoracic, and neurologic surgeries. This scrub is begun at the proposed incision site. After concentrating on the surgical area for one minute, a circular motion in

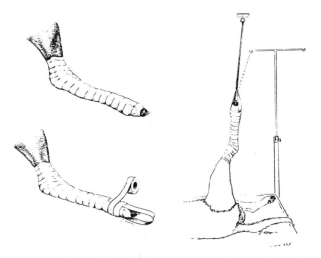

Figure 3—Proper technique for taping a limb for suspension, which is necessary prior to prepping the site for an orthopedic procedure. (From Piermattei DL, Greeley RG: *An Atlas of Surgical Approaches to the Bones of the Dog and Cat*, ed 2. Philadelphia, WB Saunders Co, 1979, p 5. Reprinted with permission.)

increasingly wider circles is started and continues until the periphery of the surgical site is reached. If the sponge becomes contaminated by hair or other gross material, it must *never* return to the already prepared incision site or surgical field. After scrubbing, the area is then wiped with a fresh moistened sponge to remove the soap. This procedure is repeated two more times; following the third scrub, alcohol may be applied. The alcohol can be left to dry, or it can be wiped dry with a fresh sterile sponge. If antiseptic solution is used, it is applied next.

A second method of prepping is used mainly for orthopedic procedures. When preparing a limb for orthopedic surgery, it is important to suspend the limb after clipping it (Figure 3). Adhesive tape or gauze should be wrapped around the area that remains unclipped. Tape is applied to the toes to form a stirrup and is secured with several more wraps of tape. The limb can be suspended from an infusion stand or from a hook in the ceiling by using a cord or adhesive tape attached to the stirrup. Once the animal is positioned and the limb is suspended, the prep can begin. Starting at the tape, but not touching it, the scrubbing is done around the leg in a circumferential pattern toward the midline. The sponge must not be contaminated by hair or other nonsterile surfaces. Once hair is reached, the sponge being used must be discarded; and if an area still needs to be prepped, another sponge is used. Usually three scrubs are done, as with the target pattern method; and an antiseptic solution is applied after the alcohol.

The third method of scrubbing is a variation of the target pattern method and is used when doing surgery in the perianal area. Scrubbing in this area is begun on one side of the anus at the center of the clipped area; the scrub is done in a target pattern. The scrubbing sponge is discarded if the anus or hair is touched. The technique is repeated on the other side of the anus. After the sides are done, the anus or most contaminated area should be scrubbed. Again, three scrubs are done, with applications of alcohol and antiseptic solution after the final scrub.

Sites of Preparation

The area to prepare for surgery will vary with the procedure being performed, the preference of the veterinarian, and the size of the animal. The following loosely structured guidelines should be varied to fit the situation at hand.

Elective Surgery

For an ovariohysterectomy, whether the patient is a cat or dog, the area to clip can be from the xiphoid process to the vulva. The clipped site should extend laterally to include the inguinal region and expose all mammary glands. Clipping this large an area allows the veterinarian to enlarge the incision if necessary. The field should be scrubbed using the target pattern.

For the castration of a dog, the clip should extend cranially to include the penis and caudally to the scrotum and inguinal region. Some veterinarians choose not to clip the scrotum because the skin is extremely sensitive and can easily be abraded. The area clipped for a castration should be scrubbed using the target pattern; the entire scrotum must be included in the scrub if it has been clipped. For feline castrations, the hair is usually plucked, not clipped, from the scrotum. Although it is important to remove as much hair as possible from the scrotum, it is not necessary to pluck beyond the scrotal area. For castration, the surgical site is not commonly disinfected in the usual manner; however, the scrotum and surrounding area may be cleansed with alcohol.

Paws of cats being declawed generally are not clipped. The feet and nails may be disinfected by the use of surgical scrub and an alcohol cleanser or by cleansing with alcohol alone.

Abdominal Preparation

For abdominal procedures, the animal is clipped cranial to the xiphoid process and caudal to the vulva if it is a female; if it is a male, it is clipped caudally to the scrotum including the hair on the penis. Laterally, the clip should extend halfway between the linea alba and the dorsal spines of the vertebrae. Male canine patients should have the prepuce flushed with a dilute disinfecting solution (1:4 povidone-iodine:tap water) prior to scrubbing the abdomen. The entire clipped area should be scrubbed using the target pattern.

Neurologic Preparation

When a dorsal approach to the cervical region is being made, the hair should be clipped cranially to the occipital protuberance and caudally to the second or third thoracic vertebra. Laterally on each side, the hair should be removed to halfway between the ventral and dorsal surfaces. If the animal is positioned on its back for a ventral approach, the area clipped should be from the mandible back to the scapulas and each side should be clipped halfway between the ventral and dorsal surfaces. In both cases the clipped area should be prepped using the target pattern. For thoracic or lumbar vertebral surgery, the area clipped should resemble a rectangle. Depending on which vertebra requires surgery, a large enough space should be clipped to allow exploration of the area. This surgical site should be prepped using the target pattern.

Thoracic Preparation

When a lateral approach is to be made, the thorax should be clipped from the spine to the ventral midline. Cranially the area clipped should extend to the neck, including the forelimb, and caudally it should extend to the diaphragm. This site should be prepped using the target pattern. If a ventral approach is to be made, the hair should be removed from the neck to the diaphragm, including the humerus of each forelimb; and it should be removed laterally on each side to halfway between the ventral and dorsal surfaces. This area should also be prepped using the target pattern.

Orthopedic Preparation

When preparing a shoulder or humerus for surgery, the hair should be clipped from the dorsal midline to the abdominal midline. The area should extend cranially to the base of the neck and caudally to approximately the sixth pair of ribs. Both sides of the limb should be clipped distally to just below the knee. For hip or femur surgery, the clipped area should extend from dorsal midline to ventral midline, as well as cranially to the last rib and caudally to the ischium. Both sides of the leg should be clipped to just below the stifle. If the elbow/knee area or below is the site for surgery, the limb should be clipped from mid-femur/humerus distally to the toes. Both sides of the leg should be clipped. Any time a limb is disinfected for an orthopedic procedure, the scrub pattern is the same. As described previously, the scrub should begin at the taped portion of the leg and continue down toward the midline.

Perianal Preparation

When clipping the perianal area for surgery, such as perineal urethrostomy or anal-sac removal, it is necessary to clip the ventral side of the tail as well as distally on each leg to the level of the stifle. Laterally each side should be clipped past the ischium. The entire area should be disinfected, as described earlier, by scrubbing each side and then scrubbing the most contaminated area last.

Open Wounds

There are a few special considerations in preparing open wounds for surgical repair. One method of protecting the wound while clipping the hair is to close the wound temporarily. This can be done with a towel clamp, Allis tissue forceps, or Michel wound clips. The biggest disadvantage to temporary wound closure is that the hair on the very edge of the wound cannot be trimmed. An alternative to temporary closure is simply to pack moist sterile sponges in the wound. After clipping an ample area (1 to 2 in.) around the wound but before removing the sponges, the edges of the wound can be trimmed using a scissors dipped in mineral oil. The oil makes the hair adhere to the scissors rather than allowing loose hair to fall into the wound. After the clipping and trimming is completed, the sponges may be removed.

For scrubbing a traumatic wound, it is especially important to consider the qualities of the available agents. Because of its ability to coagulate protein, alcohol should not be used. Although povidone-iodine is a popular choice, 2% chlorhexidine diacetate in a stable base has shown immediate and residual activity against gram-positive and gram-negative bacteria. In addition, chlorhexidine, when compared to povidone-iodine, has shown a superior residual effect as well as a higher antibacterial activity level when organic material is present. If povidone-iodine is chosen to scrub the open wound, generally only a dilute solution is used and no surgical scrub. However, if chlorhexidine is used, surgical scrub and solution can be used. After the wound has been prepared, it is advisable to wipe the wound with a sterile water-soluble lubricant jelly applied to a sterile sponge. This action helps free the wound of any remaining foreign material.

Ophthalmic Preparation

Ophthalmic surgeries are of the most delicate and fragile nature, thereby requiring special care to be taken when working with the eye. Use of a clipper to remove hair around the eye is not recommended because of the great opportunity for abrading the sensitive skin surrounding the eye. Hair removal around the eye is generally performed by trimming the hair with fine curved scissors. Applying a lubricant or mineral oil to the blades of the scissors will aid in keeping any loose hair from entering the eye. A clipper may be used to remove large quantities of hair from the ocular region such as for an enucleation. Loose hair is removed by wiping with a damp sponge, using the sticky side of adhesive tape to pick it up, or very cautiously using a vacuum. Generally, a dilute mixture (50:50) of povidone-iodine solution and sterile saline is used to cleanse the ocular region. The dilute solution can be applied to the clipped area with a cotton ball. The conjunctiva can be cleansed by applying the dilute solution to a cotton-tipped applicator and gently swabbing the area. Caution should be taken to avoid having any of the dilute mixture come in contact with the cornea. A sterile isotonic buffered irrigating solution[e] should be used to flush the eye of any debris or residual disinfecting solution. The irrigating solution can be used quite generously to ensure the removal of all unwanted material. The irrigating solution may also be applied to a cotton ball and used to remove the disinfectant from the clipped area. As with other operative sites, the clipped area and conjunctiva can be prepped and rinsed a total of three times. At the veterinarian's discretion, a final application of the 50:50 solution may be left on the clipped area.

Ear Preparation

Surgery on or near the ear requires preparation of the entire ear flap and base area surrounding the ear. All hair should be clipped from the area and must be vacuumed or wiped away. Before disinfecting the skin of the ear, the ear canal should be packed with cotton or gauze sponges to absorb any excess liquid that might flow into it. If the ear area being prepped is near the eye, a gauze sponge should be placed over the eye to protect the cornea from any scrub or solution that may splatter. Generally the area around the ear is prepped using the target pattern, and each side of the ear flap is done

separately. If the ear has been packed, the cotton or sponges should be removed after the scrub. The canal may be repacked with fresh cotton or sponges to absorb any blood that may result from surgery.

Face/Mouth Preparation

If surgery is being done on an area of the face or in the mouth, any facial hair present must be removed. Hair that is removed must be disposed of carefully. A disinfecting scrub and solution can be used on the face, but if the surgical area is near an eye, the eye should be protected with a sponge. Disinfection of the facial area should be done using the target pattern. When the mouth is the surgical site, usually a dilute solution is all that is used for disinfection. The throat can be packed with gauze sponges to absorb any excess solution or surgical blood. Before the throat is packed and the area prepped, the animal should be intubated to maintain a patent airway. Immediately after surgery the gauze sponges must be removed.

Conclusion

Animal health technicians have many choices of agents and procedures to use when preparing an operative field. The author does not recommend one product over another, rather cautions that each situation is different and therefore needs to be evaluated and approached according to individual requirements.

Acknowledgment

The author is grateful to Dr. Raymond Rudd and Dr. Daniel Richardson for their assistance.

BIBLIOGRAPHY

1. Atkinson LJ, Kohn ML: *Berry and Kohn's Introduction to Operating Room Technique*, ed 5. New York, McGraw-Hill Co, 1978, pp 222-228.
2. Blogg JR: *The Eye in Veterinary Practice—Extraocular Disease*. Philadelphia, WB Saunders Co, 1980, p 464.
3. Knecht CD, Allen AR, Williams DJ, Johnson J: *Fundamental Techniques in Veterinary Surgery*, ed 2. Philadelphia, WB Saunders Co, 1981, p 78.
4. Paul JW, Gordon MA: Efficacy of a chlorhexidine surgical scrub compared to that of hexachlorophene and povidone-iodine. *VM SAC* 5:573-579, 1978.
5. Goodman L, Gilman A (eds): *The Pharmacological Basis of Therapeutics*, ed 5. New York, Macmillan Co, 1975, p 1002.
6. Piermattei DL, Greeley RG: *An Atlas of Surgical Approaches to the Bones of the Dog and Cat*, ed 2. Philadelphia, WB Saunders Co, 1979, pp 4-6, 10.
7. Slatter DH: *Fundamentals of Veterinary Ophthalmology*. Philadelphia, WB Saunders Co, 1980, pp 171-172.
8. Swaim SF: *Surgery of Traumatized Skin—Management and Reconstruction in the Dog and Cat*. Philadelphia, WB Saunders Co, 1980, pp 125-127.
9. Tuttle JL: Pet shop sanitation. *Pet-Age* 5:6-7, 1982.
10. Winfield, WE, Rawlings CA: *Small Animal Surgery—An Atlas of Operative Techniques*. Philadelphia, WB Saunders Co, 1979, pp 14, 16-17.

[e]Dacriose, IOLAB Pharmaceuticals, Division of IOLAB Corporation, Claremont, CA.

Management of Anesthetic Emergencies and Complications

Ralph C. Harvey, DVM, MS
Diplomate, ACVA

Robert R. Paddleford, DVM
Diplomate, ACVA, ACVECC

Department of Urban Practice
College of Veterinary Medicine
University of Tennessee
Knoxville, Tennessee

Anesthesia is intended to be controlled, benign, and reversible. Anesthetic drugs produce their effects primarily by limited depression of vital processes. The inherent dangers of anesthesia as well as the debilitation resulting from the injuries

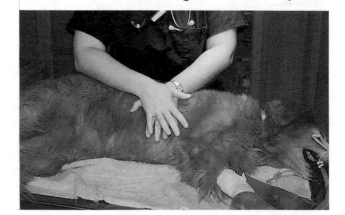

and illnesses that necessitate anesthesia and surgery predispose the patient to risks of

Originally published in Volume 12, Number 3, April 1991

serious complications and emergencies. Most anesthetic complications and emergencies are related to human error, equipment problems, ventilatory problems, or circulatory problems.

Causes of Anesthetic Problems
Human Error

Human error is ultimately responsible for most of the problems in anesthetic management. The importance of vigilance in anesthetic care cannot be overemphasized; hundreds of errors are made by *not looking* for every one error made by *not knowing*.

There is a significant degree of safety associated with familiarity. Errors are more common when the anesthetist is not familiar with the drugs or equipment being used. Miscalculation of anesthetic drug doses is a common error. The narrow therapeutic index (margin of safety between effective and toxic or lethal dose) of most anesthetic drugs makes correct dose determination or titration crucial. An absolute or relative overdose of anesthetic can cause every problem from minor excess physiologic depression to death.

An overdose of barbiturates should be managed with physiologic support of ventilation, continuous monitoring of cardiopulmonary function, and intravenous fluid therapy to speed recovery and improve cardiopulmonary function. Administration of sodium bicarbonate (0.5 to 1.0 mEq/kg) can speed recovery from pentobarbital overdose by favoring urinary elimination. The nonspecific stimulant–antagonist drug doxapram hydrochloride can be valuable in treating depression resulting from barbiturate overdose. It is administered intravenously at 0.25 to 0.5 mg/kg.

Overdoses of other anesthetics are also managed with supportive care, which is often adequate for mild to moderate overdoses. Specific antagonists are available to counteract the effects of some anesthetics. The opioid (narcotic) antagonist naloxone reverses the effects of a narcotic overdose. If the overdose is large or the narcotic lasts longer than naloxone, however, the effects of the narcotic agent may recur. Yohimbine and other specific antagonists for the tranquilizer/sedative xylazine hydrochloride are available. Yohimbine reversal of the effects of xylazine hydrochloride is particularly effective in small animals.

Nonspecific partial reversal of anesthetic depression is possible by administration of the respiratory stimulant doxapram hydrochloride. Although the net effect can be lifesaving, nonspecific reversal has been associated with residual undesirable effects (including aggression) related to

stimulation of the central nervous system. Other stimulants have been advocated to correct excessive effects of various anesthetics, but the benefits are usually limited.

Errors in administration of anesthetics also include misidentification of drugs and accidental use of the wrong medication. Anesthetics administered by an incorrect route can have serious adverse effects. Accidental extravascular injection of barbiturates can cause severe irritation and sloughing of surrounding tissue. Extravasation should be treated by infiltration with lidocaine hydrochloride and saline followed by warm compresses.

Equipment Problems

Among the most serious anesthetic complications is failure to deliver oxygen to the patient. Such failure can be caused by respiratory obstruction or misused or defective anesthetic equipment. Empty tanks or incorrectly connected gas lines and breathing circuits prevent oxygen delivery. Such problems must be recognized and corrected immediately. Empty anesthetic vaporizers or vaporizers filled with the wrong agent or overfilled are common problems. Delivery of nitrous oxide in combination with too little oxygen should be carefully avoided and is not always prevented by the fail-safe systems incorporated in modern machines.

Kinked or plugged endotracheal tubes cause respiratory obstruction. Improper cuff inflation can result in obstruction or tracheal injury or fail to prevent aspiration of vomitus. Improper placement of endotracheal tubes is common even in species that are easily intubated. Correct placement should always be verified.

Inability to fill the rebreathing bag adequately or to provide positive-pressure ventilation by squeezing the bag may indicate major leaks or disconnections. These problems can result in failure to deliver anesthetics and oxygen and substantially contribute to anesthetic gas pollution of the veterinary hospital. Stuck valves in the anesthesia machine or circuit can cause difficulty in ventilation. Inappropriate rebreathing of exhaled gases or accumulation of excessive pressure results. When patients consistently seem to be anesthetized too deeply or too lightly, the vaporizer may be out of calibration because of wear and tear or the accumulation of deposits within the vaporizer. These common problems emphasize the importance of regular inspection and maintenance of equipment.

Electrical problems in monitoring or supportive equipment may injure personnel as well as patients. Inadequately grounded or protected equipment can cause electrical burns, electrocution, or fires. Unsafe or substandard equipment should be repaired or replaced. The risk of thermal injury is so great with electric heating pads (and even with hot-water bottles) that their use for anesthetized patients is considered extremely hazardous. Circulating–warm-water blankets are a much better alternative.

Anesthetic Complications
Ventilatory Abnormalities

Hypoventilation attributable to anesthetic overdose is one of the most frequently encountered and serious complications in anesthesia. Inadequate breathing occurs with either relative or absolute overdoses of many anesthetics. Debilitated animals are more susceptible to ventilatory depression, which may occur secondary to circulatory depression and inadequate perfusion of respiratory centers, electrolyte imbalances, muscle-relaxant drugs, or thoracic injury. Support of breathing requires endotracheal intubation and positive-pressure ventilation, preferably with oxygen. The primary problem must then be identified and corrected.

Hyperventilation often results from inadequate anesthetic depth and represents an excessive response to surgical stimulation. It is important to rule out the possibility of carbon dioxide accumulation (which may result from saturated absorber granules or improper connection of the breathing circuit) as the cause of hyperventilation.

Patients that are given narcotics may pant, and effective ventilation may therefore decrease. Most often, however, panting simply represents an inconvenience to the surgeon. A less common cause of panting is hyperthermia. Erratic or jerky breathing patterns also usually indicate improper depth of anesthesia. Airway obstruction and various causes of carbon dioxide accumulation should be ruled out.

Pallor and Cyanosis

Pallor of mucous membranes is a complex sign that may be compensatory response to excessively light or deep planes of anesthesia. Reduced cardiac output attributable to anesthetic depression or increased sympathetic tone resulting from pain can cause pallor. It is important to identify the cause in order to treat the problem appropriately. Incorrect management may compound the problem and cause decompensation and immediate deterioration.

Cyanosis rarely occurs in anesthetized patients that are breathing oxygen. In order for cyanosis to develop, hemoglobin must be present in sufficient quantities and in the reduced (nonoxygenated) state. Hypoxemia that accompanies anemia therefore does not become evident through cyanosis. When cyanosis of mucous membranes or blood in the surgical field does occur, oxygen should be administered and adequate ventilation and pulse quality assured.

Circulatory Abnormalities

Bradycardia is often associated with procedures or drugs that increase the tone of the vagal parasympathetic nervous system. Difficult endotracheal intubation, deep abdominal surgical procedures, intraocular surgery, and some procedures on the neck or in the thorax can cause vagus-mediated bradycardia. Administration of atropine sulfate or glycopyrrolate effectively prevents most vagal effects. Treatment after the vagal effects become evident is often less rewarding.

Nonvagal bradycardia may result from excessive anesthetic depth or hypoxia. Bradycardia can be a serious sign of a significant anesthetic emergency. Administration of atropine sulfate and attention to possible causes are imperative.

Hypotension

Hypotension can be caused by decreased cardiac output, increased capacitance of the vasculature, or inadequate blood volume. Intraoperative fluid therapy at 10 ml/kg/hr is often adequate, but increased volumes can be necessary. Hypovolemia can be distinguished from reduced cardiac output as a cause of hypotension on the basis of patient history and clinical evaluation.

Vasodilation is a common side effect of many anesthetic drugs. The tranquilizer acepromazine maleate is hypotensive, particularly at high doses. Volatile anesthetics also cause significant vasodilation. Most anesthetics also are potent cardiac depressants, particularly at high doses. The most appropriate primary management of hypotension in an anesthetized patient is therefore to reduce the dose of anesthetic and administer fluids.

Tachycardia

Heart rates faster than 180 beats/min in dogs and 200 beats/min in cats are associated with decreased efficiency and increased cardiac work load. Tachycardia can result from fear, pain, inadequate anesthetic depth, preanesthetic excitement, or rough induction of anesthesia. Hypotension causes compensatory tachycardia. These causes of supraventricular tachycardia should be recognized and treated.

Compensatory tachycardia in response to hypovolemia and hypotension results in decreased blood flow in coronary arteries and increased myocardial work load. If other conditions contribute to hypoxia, the risk that more serious arrhythmias may develop is significant. Fluid therapy for hypovolemia, adjustment of anesthetic plane, and support measures to avoid cardiovascular deterioration are necessary.

Ventricular tachycardia is a much more serious emergency. An occasional ventricular ectopic beat is cause for concern but not necessarily indicative of patient distress. When ventricular arrhythmias become frequent or progress to ventricular tachycardia, immediate treatment is required. Ventricular arrhythmias are indicative of an irritated, hypoxic, or diseased myocardium.

Ventricular tachycardia should be treated with intravenous bolus injection of 2% lidocaine hydrochloride at a dose of 1, 2, or 3 ml in small, medium, or large dogs, respectively. This rule of thumb allows for immediate therapy without an accurate dose calculation, which could cause a life-threatening delay. Propranolol has been recommended as the drug of choice for treating ventricular arrhythmia in cats. Lidocaine hydrochloride is also effective in cats. Limitation of the total dose is more important for cats because of their smaller body size and blood volume.

Success in emergency management of ventricular arrhythmias is evaluated by continuous electrocardiographic monitoring. Bolus injections of lidocaine hydrochloride can be repeated to a total accumulated dose of about 10 mg/kg without significant risk of overdose. When two or three injections are required over a period of 15 to 23 minutes, it is necessary to convert to a continuous intravenous infusion of lidocaine hydrochloride at 30 to 80 μg/kg/min. Refractory arrhythmias may require conversion to therapy based on procainamide and/or quinidine.

Cardiopulmonary Arrest

Cardiopulmonary arrest is always an emergency. Rapid, concise, well-directed intervention is imperative to save the patient's life. It is extremely difficult for one person to provide successful cardiopulmonary resuscitation (CPR). Well-coordinated action by a team of trained personnel is necessary to provide the best chance for recovery. The entire staff of every veterinary clinic should be trained in the basic life-support techniques of veterinary cardiopulmonary resuscitation and should be ready at all times to respond to the crisis of a cardiopulmonary arrest.

It is far easier and certainly represents better patient care to prevent and avoid arrests than to treat them once they have occurred. Careful patient monitoring, particularly during anesthesia, surgery, and postoperative recovery, is crucial in avoiding cardiopulmonary arrest. Although it may not always be possible to predict the likelihood of arrest, animals showing signs of respiratory depression or hemodynamic instability should receive special attention. Other groups of patients that should be considered to be at increased risk are the very young or very old, those debilitated by disease or injury, and those with conditions or histories that might predispose them to cardiopulmonary instability.

A thorough preanesthetic evaluation not only assists in identifying high-risk patients but also helps to identify the means for avoiding potential problems. Special patient management may be indicated to correct electrolyte imbalances, hypovolemia, anemia, or other physiologic problems. Preanesthetic and presurgical preparation of high-risk patients may require a delay of varying duration to ensure that the animal is a suitable candidate to endure the inevitable stress. In emergency and life-threatening situations, however, such delays are not always possible. Clinical judgment of the veterinarian, based on all available information, determines the best course of action.

All general anesthetic agents cause some degree of cardiopulmonary depression. Their use should always be tempered with a proper respect for their ability to end life. Many safe anesthetic techniques, however, can be adapted to the special needs of high-risk patients.

Regardless of the anesthetic technique, all patients should have adequate spontaneous breathing or be provided with some type of ventilatory support. All patients should have adequate circulating blood volume. Patients with congestive heart failure require conservative fluid management, but those in hypovolemic shock require generous fluid administration. Proper attention to breathing and fluids are most valuable in avoiding cardiopulmonary arrests. These two factors, along with the possibility of absolute or relative anesthetic overdose, should receive immediate attention when any patient shows signs of cardiopulmonary deterioration.

Most cardiopulmonary arrests are unanticipated. Either they occur without the mentioned warning signs, or the signs are unrecognized until an emergency exists. It is imperative to recognize an arrest promptly and begin resuscitation. The following are the signs of cardiac arrest:

- No auscultatable heartbeat
- No palpable arterial pulse
- Gray or cyanotic discoloration of mucous membranes
- Dilated pupils
- No ventilatory attempts (except for agonal gasps)
- Unconsciousness.

Other signs of arrest may occur, and some of the listed signs may be absent or obscured in certain circumstances.

Little time exists between the arrest and the time at which definitive support and resuscitation must begin. If treatment is not initiated immediately, irreversible and often fatal changes occur within three to four minutes. The first step indicated when an arrest is suspected is to make a quick assessment of the patient's condition. If the listed signs are noted, thus verifying cardiopulmonary arrest, the next step is to call for help. This call should ideally summon all members of the team—all individuals available who can provide assistance in resuscitation.

The treatment priorities for cardiopulmonary resuscitation are known as the ABCD of cardiopulmonary resuscitation. The *A* represents the patient's airways. The oral cavity and laryngeal opening should be visually inspected to rule out obstruction by food or foreign material. The airway is then secured, if possible, by placement of an endotracheal tube. The *B* stands for breathing, which is the second priority in initiating cardiopulmonary resuscitation. Artificial ventilation is most satisfactorily provided by an anesthetic breathing circuit that delivers oxygen rather than room air. As an alternative, a self-refilling or ambulatory-type resuscitation bag may be used. Mouth-to-endotracheal tube or even mouth-to-muzzle technique may be effective (although certainly much less efficient).

The *C* represents circulation, which is provided by cardiac massage. Chest compressions are usually provided with the animal in lateral recumbency, usually with one of the resuscitator's hands on either side of the patient's thorax. Hand positions for effective cardiac massage vary with the size and conformation of the patient; but correct position is crucial to provide effective circulation and avoid irreparable damage to the liver, lungs, and other vital organs. The compressions should be quick yet slightly sustained and at a rapid rate of 90 to 120/min. Effective cardiac massage must be monitored throughout the resuscitation effort by palpation of peripheral pulse. A palpable pulse must be detected, usually over the femoral or lingual artery. If a pulse is not detected, changes in the compressive technique must be made quickly to provide a pulse.

Although internal cardiac massage is necessary in many cases to generate an effective pulse, a simple change in hand placement based mainly on size of the animal allows optimum external massage in a variety of veterinary patients. For example, one hand may encircle the sternum and provide massage by opposing force of thumb and fingers for cats and very small dogs whereas large dogs usually require both hands over the heart on one side of the thorax. Other technical modifications that might improve resuscitation include changes in patient position, abdominal binding, and simultaneous ventilation and cardiac compression. Although such adjustments may be necessary for effective resuscitation, they may entail greater risk of damage to vital organs and should be reserved for selected cases in which the standard approach is ineffective.

The *D* stands for drug therapy, which is the fourth priority in cardiopulmonary resuscitation. Rapid fluid administration is crucial in most cases. Cats generally should receive 20 ml/kg of a balanced electrolyte solution and dogs 40 ml/kg by rapid intravenous administration through a large-bore catheter. Although inadequate circulating volume is the most frequent cause of unsuccessful resuscitation, excessive fluid load and resultant pulmonary edema may be the second most common cause of failure. Therefore, once the recommended fluid load has been given the need for further fluid therapy must be carefully considered.

Cases of cardiac arrest are classified into one of three types by electrocardiographic evaluation: ventricular or complete asystole, ventricular fibrillation, or electromechanical dissociation. In addition to continued cardiopulmonary resuscitation, definitive treatment of the specific type of arrest is initiated immediately.

For patients with asystole, epinephrine injected at doses of up to 1, 2, or 3 ml of a 1:1000 concentration is recommended. Emergency drugs should be injected intravenously and circulated by cardiac massage. A jugular vein catheter is the best route for injection of resuscitative drugs. Selected drugs may be injected into the marrow cavity of long bones (intraosseous injection), sprayed into the trachea, or injected into the base of the tongue. Intracardiac injections are to be avoided when possible.

For patients with fibrillation, electric defibrillation with a direct-current defibrillator is recommended. Power settings are based on patient size and response to previous attempts. In the absence of an electric defibrillator, other therapies (including precordial chest thump or various drug combinations) have been successful. In some situations, cats and dogs can achieve spontaneous defibrillation.

Therapy for electromechanical dissociation is particularly unrewarding. This condition is indicative of deteriorating hypoxic myocardium. The prognosis is grave.

There are many areas of controversy in cardiopulmonary resuscitation. New research and continued clinical experience has led to changes in recommendations. Examples include the higher rates of cardiac compression and greatly limited indications for administration of calcium and bicarbonate during resuscitation. Further studies will provide additional understanding and thereby improve the chances for success in cardiopulmonary resuscitation. Ultimate success requires continued intensive care for at least 24 to 48 hours. Resuscitated animals are commonly unstable, and repeated arrests frequently occur.

Delayed Recovery

Delayed recovery from anesthesia is managed by recognizing possible causes and ruling out differentials. A systematic approach to potential causes provides for balanced care with correction of often multiple factors, including such factors as hypothermia, inadequate fluid support, reduced metabolism or clearance of drugs, and debilitation associated with the stress of anesthesia and surgical trauma. Deterioration resulting from a hypoxic episode must be considered.

Hypothermia

Hypothermia is among the most common of anesthetic complications. Body heat is lost with preparation of the surgical site, contact with such cool surfaces as surgical tables, breathing of dry anesthetic gases, and evaporation from the airways and the surgical field. Moderate hypothermia is a frequent problem even when attention is paid

to each of these factors. Body temperatures down to approximately 33 °C (92 °F) increase oxygen and energy requirements during recovery, but most patients can tolerate this level of hypothermia. More extreme hypothermia causes delayed recovery and reduces tissue perfusion.

Other Complications

Many other complications and emergencies can occur during or be associated with anesthesia. These include anaphylactoid reactions; hyperthermia; biochemical imbalances; and many surgical complications, such as hemorrhage and pneumothorax. Avoidance of complications and effective management of emergencies require continued vigilance and immediate appropriate actions.

■

BIBLIOGRAPHY

Eiker SW: Complications in anesthesia. *Semin Vet Med Surg* 1:204–214, 1986.

Harvey RC: Anesthetic emergencies, in Weide KD, Thomsen GM, Krout DK (eds): *Proceedings: 18th Seminar for Veterinary Technicians.* Las Vegas, NV, Western Veterinary Conference, 1989, pp 282–287.

Haskins SC: Principles of operating room emergencies, in Slatter DH (ed): *Textbook of Small Animal Surgery.* Philadelphia, WB Saunders Co, 1985, pp 389–412.

Trim CM: Anesthetic emergencies and complications, in Paddleford RR (ed): *Manual of Small Animal Anesthesia.* New York, Churchill Livingstone, 1988, pp 147–198.

Aseptic Technique

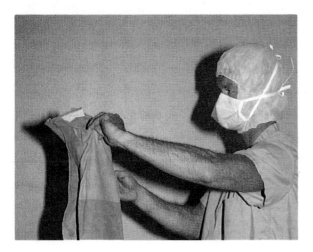

K. G. Kagan, VMD
Diplomate, ACVS
Veterinary Medicine & Surgical Specialty Practice
Charlotte, North Carolina

A critical component of surgery is the appropriate preparation of both the patient and surgeon. The principles of surgical preparation as well as general guidelines of conduct for aseptic technique are described in this article. The veterinary technician can play a key role in all preparatory aspects of surgery and surgical assistance.

PREPARATION OF THE PATIENT

Preparation of local skin for the incision is the first step in surgery. The skin is clipped or shaved over an area about two to five inches around the anticipated incision. If the operation is not a standard elective procedure, a more extensive area is prepared, which allows for a longer incision if this becomes necessary.

After clipping or shaving, the skin is prepared with an antibacterial scrub to reduce the surface bacterial levels. Care should be taken not to injure the skin when clipping or scrubbing. Scrubbing is repeated at least three times. Ideally, three preliminary scrubs should be done in the preparatory room and three final scrubs on the operation room table after

Originally published in Volume 13, Number 3, April 1992

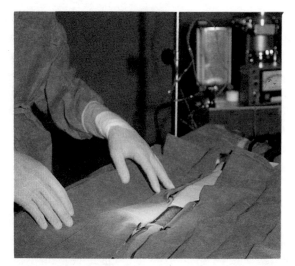

Figure 1—Incision isolated with four towels secured to the skin with towel clamps in the corners of the rectangular opening. An effective barrier between the incision site and the surrounding unprepared areas is provided.

the patient is positioned. Scrubs are performed beginning at the incision site and moving outward. A sponge or lather should never be carried from the edge of the prepared area to the center. After the scrub is completed, the skin may be coated with an antiseptic solution that is allowed to dry.

To eliminate the remaining area of the patient's body as a source of contamination, the incision site should be isolated with sterile towels. Usually, four towels are used. Each towel is folded back one-quarter and the folded edges of the four towels are placed in a rectangular fashion around the incision site. If a towel is misplaced slightly, it can be moved away from the incision but never toward the incision. If a towel is placed too far from the incision site, another towel should be placed over it rather than moving or removing the first towel. Towels are held to the skin with clamps at the corners of the rectangle (Figure 1). If a clamp is positioned improperly, it should not be removed. Another clamp should be used to hold the towel and the first clamp should be left in place.

After the towels are in place, a drape is placed over the incision site, towels, animal, and table. The drape covers all nonsterile surfaces and provides a sterile field for the surgeon (Figure 2). A fenestration in the drape is made directly over the area of the incision.

After the incision is made, the surgeon can attach a set of towels directly to the skin edges. This so-called toweling in creates the most effective barrier possible between the incision and the surrounding skin surface. Another technique for achieving a barrier is to use a self-adhering plastic film to cover the skin before the incision is made.

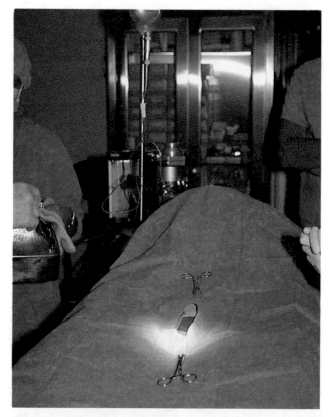

Figure 2—A sterile environment around the incision site is created by a drape that covers the patient and operating table and overlaps the instrument stand.

PREPARATION OF THE SURGEON

To control contamination, the surgeon must be almost totally covered in such a way that barriers are formed to contain contaminants and debris. Also, a sterile covering for the areas of the body that come in contact with the surgical field must be created.

Apparel

Scrub suits come in various designs. The purpose of the scrub suit is to have a clean garment that is worn only in the vicinity of the operating room. Wearing a scrub suit through daily routines before going into the operating room defeats its purpose. If a two-piece scrub suit is worn, the top should be tucked into the trousers to prevent a loose-fitting suit from touching (and thereby contaminating) the arms while scrubbing and gowning.

Ideally, street shoes should not be worn into the surgical area. Only clean shoes should be worn in surgery; a second pair of shoes should be used for daily activities in the hospital or clinic. If street shoes are used, however, shoe covers can be used to control contamination.

Surgical caps should cover all hair. Several styles are available.

Various types of hoods are available to accommodate

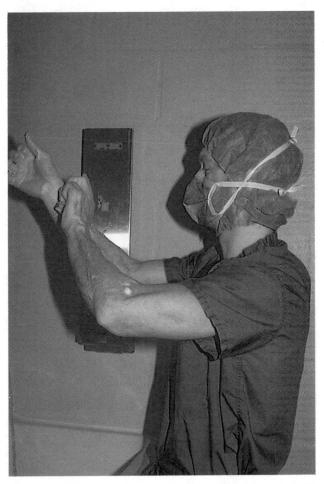

Figure 3—While scrubbing, the hands should always be held above the elbows to prevent water from carrying contaminants onto the hands and forearms.

long hair styles and beards. If a hood does not have an elastic band or tie to hold it close to the neck, the hood should be tucked in the neck of the scrub top.

Masks are worn to filter air expired from the mouth and nose. To be effective, the mask must fit snugly and the elastic bands and both sets of ties must be fastened. The upper and lower ties should not be crisscrossed because this creates a fold in the mask, which allows air to escape unfiltered from the sides of the mask. As a mask becomes saturated with moisture from the breath, effectiveness is diminished. Therefore, masks should be changed between procedures and even during long procedures. After the mask is used, it is contaminated with bacteria and should be discarded (only the ties should be handled during removal). Masks should not be allowed to dangle around the surgeon's neck by two ties.

Scrubbing

After the surgeon has put on the scrub suit, cap, mask, and if necessary hood, the scrubbing procedure of the hands and arms is begun. The purpose of the surgical scrub is to remove dirt and sebum, transient bacterial flora, and a portion of the resident flora from the hands and arms. Although the effectiveness of the traditional scrub is under question, for the foreseeable future, the current procedure will remain standard practice. Regeneration of skin bacteria begins immediately after the skin is scrubbed and disinfected. Regrowth is approximately 25% complete in 24 hours, 73% complete in three days, and 100% complete in one week.

Before starting to scrub, the cap and/or hood and mask must be in place and jewelry must be removed. Nails and cuticles should be short. If gross soil is present, it must be removed with an appropriate tool. Once the scrub is started, the hands and arms should not touch any unsterile object. If this happens, the scrub must be repeated. When arms are wet, hands are always held higher than the elbows so that water drips from the elbows and not from the hands (Figure 3).

Two types of scrubs, timed and anatomic, are available. A timed scrub is performed for 5 to 10 minutes. Hands and arms are wet and lathered to the elbow or slightly higher for about one minute and then rinsed. Soap is then applied to the hands and, using a sterile brush, the scrub begins. Fingers, hands, and arms are treated as having four sides in addition to fingertips. Each surface is scrubbed with a back and forth or circular motion, as is appropriate, for 5 to 10 minutes. At the midpoint of the scrub, the skin is rinsed and the scrub is repeated.

When an anatomic scrub is performed, the scrub proceeds from the fingertips to the elbows in an orderly progression. The fingertips, nails, and cuticles are scrubbed with at least 20 strokes. Other surfaces are scrubbed at least 10 times. The skin is then rinsed and the scrub can be repeated.

Drying

After scrubbing and rinsing, hands and arms should be dried with a sterile towel. To pick up the towel, one must bend the knees to lower the body rather than reaching down with the hand (Figure 4). Reaching down allows water from the vicinity of the elbow, an area that is contaminated, to run down to the hand. The hands and arms should be held extended, away from the body, so that the towel and arms do not come in contact with the scrub suit. To dry the arms, the towel is folded several times so that contaminated water of the proximal forearm and elbow is covered by the additional layers of towel folds. If the towel is not folded and only a single thickness is used, the towel becomes saturated and then contaminates the hands as the

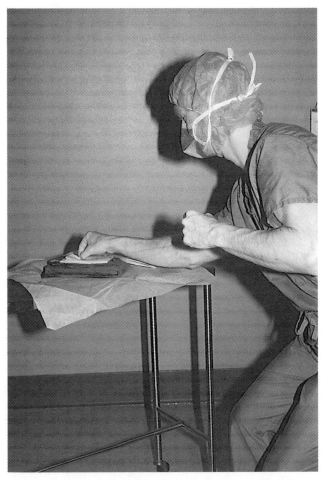

Figure 4—To pick up a sterile towel, the knees are bent to lower the body; this technique keeps the hands above the elbows and thereby avoids the possibility of water dripping from the elbow (an area that is contaminated) onto the hand.

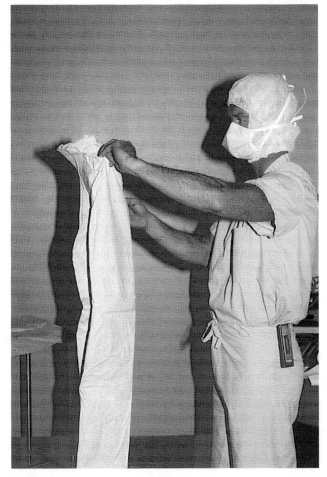

Figure 5—After the gown is picked up, the surgeon should step back away from the table before allowing the gown to unfold by gravity.

drying off procedure continues.

After the hands are dried, the surgeon may elect to take additional antiseptic steps, such as an alcohol soak or application of other antiseptics to the hands. Completion of the scrubbing and drying process is followed by the gowning process.

Gowning

Gowns provide the surgeon with a sterile surface. Most gowns are considered sterile only in front after they have been put on. The backs of gowns are considered to be sterile only when the gown is a wraparound type with front ties that have tabs; with this type of gown, an assistant can bring the ties and back of the gown around the surgeon's back and then the surgeon can tie the gown in front. Surgical gowns are folded accordion-style so that the inside of the gown at the shoulder seams is uppermost when the gown pack is opened. The gown should be picked up by the shoulders and lifted straight up until it has been removed from the wrapper. The gown should never be pulled

over the wrapper as this might contaminate the gown. Instead, the surgeon should take the folded gown up off the wrapper, step back from the table, and then, while holding the gown by the shoulder seams, allow the gown to unfold by gravity (Figure 5).

The sleeve openings should be located and the arms should be slid into the sleeves. By holding the arms extended up and out to the side, the gown can be controlled while continuing to slide the arms into the sleeves as far as but not through the cuffs. An assistant can then fasten the ties in the back of the gown and loosely fasten the neck ties.

Techniques of Gloving

Gloving can be performed by either a closed or open technique. Either technique can be done using one or two pairs of gloves. When two pairs of gloves are used, the second pair is usually a half size larger than the first. The second pair provides added protection against contamination. Also, double gloving provides protection from punctures that may occur in orthopedic procedures when working with fracture fragments and sharp edges.

It should be noted that all surgical gloves have a film of cornstarch powder added during the last steps of manufacture. The powder facilitates sliding gloves onto the hands and fingers. Before starting surgery, the surgeon and assistants should remove this film of cornstarch powder with moistened sponges. Starch granules in a wound have caused inflammation and foreign body reactions.

If performed properly, closed gloving easily provides and maintains sterility of the outside of the gloves. The procedure for closed gloving is as follows:

1. Insert the hands into the sleeves of the gown as far as but not through the cuffs. No part of the hands should be exposed.
2. With the glove fingers toward the elbow, place the palm side of the left glove on the palm side of the left gown cuff.
3. Through the gown cuff, use the left fingers and thumb to grasp the edge of the left glove cuff near the left glove thumb.
4. Through the right gown cuff, use the right hand to grasp the glove cuff 180 degrees from the glove thumb and pull it over the end of the left cuff. (At this point, the left glove cuff should cover the left gown cuff and the glove fingers will be pointing in the same direction as the surgeon's fingers.)
5. Through the gown, grasp the left gown sleeve with the opposite hand and pull it proximally. As the left hand slides through the gown cuff, the fingers are manipulated so that they slide into the glove fingers.
6. Repeat the described procedure with the right glove.

The second method of gloving, open gloving, has a disadvantage in that it is difficult to avoid contamination of the cuff when rolling the cuff over the back of the hand. It is not always possible, however, to use the closed method of gloving. For example, open gloving would be used if no assistant were present and a damaged glove needed to be changed during surgery. Moisture from perspiration would permeate the gown cuff, thereby contaminating gloves that were put on by the closed technique. Thus, it is essential that one is able to glove by the open method. The procedure for open gloving is as follows:

1. With the left hand, grasp the right glove by the folded cuff and remove it from the pack without touching the outside of the glove. Slide the right hand into the glove and leave the cuff folded down.

2. Pick up the left glove by sliding the gloved fingers of the right hand under the folded glove cuff. Avoid touching the inside of the left glove with the right (gloved) hand.
3. Slide the left hand into the glove and carefully pull the cuff over the gown cuff.
4. With the left hand, finish putting on the right glove by inserting the gloved fingers of the left hand under the right glove cuff and turning the cuff of the glove of the gown cuff.
5. Adjust the gloves so that they fit properly on the fingers and hands.

With the help of an assistant, a glove can be changed during surgery using the following closed gloving procedure:

1. The assistant takes the sterile glove from the circulating technician and opens it. The assistant holds the glove open by placing his or her fingertips under the folded cuff edge (at two points approximately 120 degrees apart) with the palm of the glove toward the surgeon.
2. The surgeon places his or her gloved fingers under the cuff at a third point, triangulating the opening into the glove.
3. The surgeon and assistant pull the glove open and over the other hand of the surgeon and the hand is pushed into the glove.
4. The surgeon and assistant maintain tension on the glove cuff until the glove cuff is up onto the sleeve of the surgeon's gown, at which time they let go.

After the gloves have been put on, an assistant adjusts the fit of the gown from the inside at the back, and the outside back tie is fastened. If an assistant ties the outside back tie, the back of the gown is not considered sterile.

GENERAL GUIDELINES FOR ASEPTIC TECHNIQUE

The limits of the sterile surgical field are:

• The top of the instrument table
• The top of the drape
• The front of the surgical gown from the tabletop to the shoulders
• The gloves and sleeves of the surgical gown (remember that the backs of most surgical gowns are considered unsterile).

Guidelines for Aseptic Technique

1. All articles are either sterile or unsterile. If there is any doubt, the article is considered unsterile.
2. Only the outside of wrappers should be touched when opening packs or instruments. Sterile packs should be opened facing away from the body.
3. Sterile articles should be handled only by sterile gloves or a sterile instrument.
4. After a sterile article is removed from a pack, it should never be returned to the sterile table or tray if contaminated.
5. Any time a linen becomes moist, it should no longer be considered a sterile barrier. (Bowls of saline should be kept in remote locations or on metal trays.)
6. Gloves punctured during the surgical procedure must be changed. An assistant who is not scrubbed pulls the glove off by grasping the gown cuff (through the glove) and pulling the glove over the hand. Then, if the gown cuff is dry, a closed gloving technique can be used. When two people are scrubbed, the replacement glove can be put on (and sterility maintained) using another of the closed gloving techniques.
7. If transfer forceps are used, they should be lifted straight out of the container so the tips do not touch either side of the container. The tips of the forceps should always point down when they are used.
8. Sterile articles being removed from a pack should be lifted up and out—they should never be pulled over the edge of the container barrier.
9. Before solutions (e.g., saline) are poured into a sterile container, a small amount of the solution should be poured into a waste container. The outside of the solution container should never touch the sterile container. Solutions should not be poured from such a height that they splash.
10. Members of the surgical team should avoid turning their backs toward sterile surfaces unless gowns wrap all the way around the back. Changing positions at the table should be done in a back-to-back manner.
11. Sterile instruments that fall below waist level or below the top of the surgery table are considered unsterile and should not be returned to the sterile tray.
12. Because the front of the gown between the shoulders and the waist is the only area of the gown that is considered sterile, hands and arms should not go above or below this area.
13. Excessive movement should be avoided during the surgical procedure.
14. Conversation should be kept to a minimum during the surgical procedure. It has been shown that bacterial contamination in the operating room increases when there is more conversation.
15. Gowned and gloved members of the surgical team not actively participating in the procedure should have hands clasped together at the level of the midchest or placed on the surgical table. If practical, the latter is preferred.

BIBLIOGRAPHY

Gayle D, et al: Re-evaluation of scrub technique for preoperative disinfection of the surgeon's hands. *Ann Surg* 155:107-118, 1962.

Kundsin RB, Walter CW: The surgical scrub—practical considerations. *Arch Surg* 107:75-77, 1973.

Leonard EP: *Fundamentals of Small Animal Surgery*. Philadelphia, WB Saunders Co, 1986, pp 89-138.

Moylan JA, Kennedy BV: The importance of gown and drape barriers in the prevention of wound infection. *Surg Gynecol Obstet* 151:465-470, 1980.

Nealon TF: *Fundamental Skills in Surgery*. Philadelphia, WB Saunders Co, 1962, pp 24-33.

Preoperative and Postoperative Care of the Orthopedic Patient

Christine Royce-Bretz, RVT
Department of Small Animal Clinics
School of Veterinary Medicine
Purdue University
West Lafayette, Indiana

Small animal fracture patients compose a large percentage of the patients in veterinary hospitals and often require long-term hospitalization and physical therapy. Veterinary technicians can significantly reduce the frequency of preoperative and postoperative complications through awareness of some basic but necessary precautions.

Initial Emergency Treatment

The majority of orthopedic injuries result from trauma. Statistics indicate that 75% to 80% of fractures result from accidents caused by cars or other motorized vehicles.[1] Care of the traumatized patient should begin at the scene of the accident[2] where the animal must be maintained until professional help is available. The initial communication between client and hospital is usually by telephone.

During this first contact, the veterinary technician should explain common first aid techniques to the client because careful handling of the animal may prevent additional trauma. Such basic techniques include using pressure bandages to stop bleeding and using rolled magazines, wood splints, and tape to immobilize a limb fracture. These simple measures, if handled properly by the client, may dramatically reduce the potential complications associated with fractured limbs. The technician should advise clients to use a belt or rope, if available, to muzzle an injured dog. Muzzling can prevent injury whenever clients must perform procedures that are uncomfortable for a pet that has been hurt and may try to bite. Clients should be cautioned that even an ordinarily docile pet may snap when in pain. The clients should then be instructed to drive carefully to the veterinary hospital to obtain professional care.

The Examination

After the patient is presented at the veterinary clinic, a thorough evaluation must be performed. This includes a complete physical examination of all body systems. Penetrating wounds of the thorax or abdomen and diaphragmatic hernias are life-threatening soft tissue conditions frequently seen in trauma patients. Orthopedic problems are rarely life threatening, however, and technicians should know what priority to give an injury. The animal's condition must be stable before radiography is attempted.

When the patient has been carefully evaluated, initial care of the wound can begin. First, the affected area is clipped and cleansed to remove gross contamination. A sterile dressing is applied to stop further contamination. Prevention of sepsis should be a constant consideration. Only sterile materials are used for wound cleansing. Use of a povidone iodine (Betadine®—Purdue Frederick) or chlorhexidine gluconate (Hibiclens®—Stuart Pharmaceuticals) scrub decreases contamination. Detergents and commercial soaps are cytotoxic and should be avoided. Sterile isotonic solution (i.e., Ringer's or normal saline) should be used to lavage the wound. Tap water is not recommended. Even though it is relatively clean, tap water is hypertonic and causes cells to dehydrate, producing interstitial edema.

Fracture Management

A fracture is defined as the destruction of the continuity of a bone. For descriptive purposes, fractures may be classified in two major groups: closed and open.[3]

A *closed fracture* is one in which there is no communication between the broken ends of the bone and the external environment. The most important goal in the management of a closed fracture is preventing an open fracture and minimizing additional soft tissue damage. The Robert Jones bandage is recommended for stabilization of fractures below the stifle and elbow and helps to prevent limb edema. Above the stifle and elbow, the Robert Jones bandage is contraindicated for fractures because the weight of the bandage may cause angular displacement of the fracture.[2] Surgical treatment of the fracture is a decision made when the patient is stable.

Infection is always possible in *open fractures* because the bone is exposed to environmental contamination. Degree of bacterial contamination has been shown to be the single most important factor in determining if a wound will become infected.[2] Contamination is not the same as infection. A contaminated wound is soiled with microorganisms. Infection is the invasion of the body by pathogenic microorganisms and the reaction of tissues to their presence. Infection begins when the host can no longer fight off the increasing numbers of organisms. Infection rates of open fractures have been reported to range from 3% to 25%.[4]

Culture and sensitivity tests (if available) are warranted in wounds that appear to have the potential for infection. A recent human study has shown that if a wound becomes infected, initial cultures are positive for the organism causing the infection in 70% of the cases.[4]

If culture and sensitivity tests cannot be performed, broad-spectrum, bactericidal antibiotics should be given. When culture and sensitivity results are known, a narrow-spectrum, bactericidal antibiotic would be indicated to minimize the emergence of resistant organisms.

Preoperative Considerations

The biggest challenge facing the veterinary technician who is handling orthopedic patients is the prevention of surgical contamination. Primary sources of such contamination are the patient, the environment, the surgical materials, and the operating room personnel.[2] Achieving asepsis in the veterinary surgery area is impossible; however, reduction of contaminants is possible and is a necessity. Surgery requires a thorough knowledge of and a strict adherence to aseptic techniques.

All materials and equipment used in an orthopedic procedure must be sterilized. The operating room should be kept spotlessly clean. Dust-collecting surfaces in the surgery room should be wiped with an alcohol-moistened cloth the morning of the scheduled surgery, with the technician paying close attention to lights and equipment that will be directly over the incision site. A heated water pad covered by a towel should be placed on the surgery table just before the procedure is begun, to prevent patient hypothermia. Although proper air ventilation is necessary in the operating room, excessive air circulation (i.e, open windows, circulating fans) is a hazard and should be minimized. Clinic personnel should avoid unnecessary traffic in the surgery area, and adherence to the general rules of surgery-room cleanliness cannot be overemphasized.

The Patient

Food should be withheld from the patient for at least 12 hours before surgery. A bath is recommended the day before surgery, especially for heavily soiled animals. Bathing of animals with fractures is not always feasible, however. It is more convenient for everyone involved if the patient is allowed to void before anesthesia. The majority of orthopedic patients should have an indwelling cephalic catheter to permit administration of preoperative and intraoperative drugs and intraoperative and postoperative fluids. Some orthopedic patients need to be catheterized before surgery to permit measurement of urine output if the veterinarian decides urine monitoring is necessary.

Renal function should be evaluated before anesthesia. Some animals survive the trauma of surgery yet emerge from the anesthetic only to become uremic and depressed because of renal failure. When a lack of intraoperative fluids is combined with poor renal function and hypotension during surgery, the end result is renal shutdown. The earlier that renal shutdown is treated, the better the patient's prognosis.

Anesthesia

Many orthopedic procedures require surgical manipulation, therefore general anesthesia is required. Orthopedic surgery usually means prolonged anesthesia time, so presurgical evaluation of the patient must be thorough and complete.

The patient should be weighed and the temperature, pulse, and respiratory rate recorded. Laboratory analyses (e.g., complete blood count, blood urea nitrogen) are often requested by the surgeon to determine the health status of the patient before anesthesia. Drugs to be used for induction and their dosages also need to be determined before anesthesia.

Preanesthetic medication, such as atropine sulfate, can be administered before induction. Following normal anesthetic induction with thiopental sodium, the animal is intubated and maintained on a gas anesthetic, such as methoxyflurane, halothane, or isoflurane. An esophageal stethoscope can be placed to monitor heart rate and respiratory rate. To prevent corneal drying, a bland ophthalmic ointment should be applied to the eyes following induction.

Patient Preparation

All surgical preparation of the patient should be done outside the surgery suite so that only clean materials and individuals, including the surgeon, enter the operating room. Bandages should be removed after the animal has been anesthetized. This prevents wound complications during anesthetic induction, especially if the animal experiences an excitement phase during the induction procedure. If the bandage is removed before anesthesia, even minimal movement by the animal could turn a closed fracture into an open one.

After induction, a wide area should be clipped with a no. 40 clipper blade to ensure an adequate surgical field. Shaving the area is not recommended. Clipped hair is then vacuumed. Often, the affected leg must be suspended by a stirrup. This is done by placing a strip of adhesive tape along the longitudinal axis of the lateral and medial side of the limb (Figure 1). The exposed ends of the longitudinal strips are joined together to make a stirrup from which to hang the leg. The adhesive tape is then wrapped around the lower part of the leg so that the foot is completely covered (Figure 2). Any unclipped hair near the hock and foot should be covered by the tape. Adhesive tape is preferred over gauze for suspending the leg, not only because adhesive tape is stronger and easier to work with but also because gauze tends to shed fibers onto the surgical field. Not every orthopedic surgical procedure requires suspension of the leg; positioning is done according to the surgeon's choice.

The surgical site and surrounding area are cleansed with a surgical scrubbing agent using a pattern that starts at the incision site and proceeds outward (Figure 3) . This type of scrub should be repeated at least three times. Next, the animal is taken into the surgery room and positioned with the leg still hung (if it was originally suspended); the leg is then prepped again. The second prep serves as a precaution and is an attempt to reduce significantly the number of

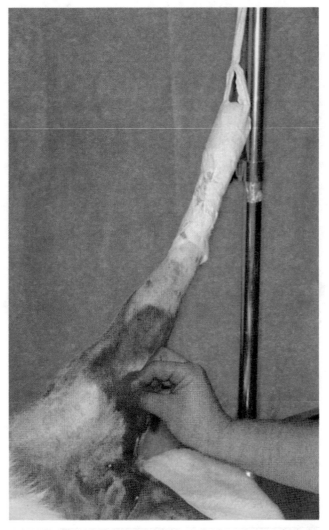

Figure 3—The surgical scrub begins at the intended surgical site and moves progressively outward.

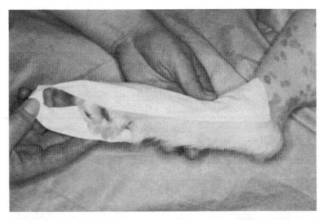

Figure 1—Adhesive tape strips applied to the medial and lateral aspects of the affected leg are joined to make a support stirrup.

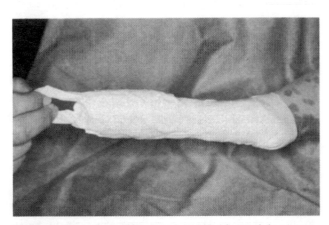

Figure 2—The stirrup (Figure 1) is secured by applying a wrap around the lower part of the leg.

organisms present at the incision site. The operative site is now ready for draping.

The drape is the principal safeguard against contamination. Drapes should be of adequate size (41 × 57 inches) to cover the entire patient and the table. The drapes should also extend from the table onto the Mayo instrument stand. Chances of contamination by moisture can be decreased by the use of water repellent drapes. Initially, the surgeon places four sterile drapes around the base of the suspended leg (Figure 4). By wrapping a sterile towel or cloth around the unsterile adhesive tape, the surgeon is free to manipulate the leg, thus decreasing the chances of contamination while applying the stockinette. The circulating nurse then grasps the tape-covered part of the foot and cuts the tape that has been suspending the leg (Figure 5). While cutting the tape, the assistant must be careful not to let any part of his or her body touch the sterile drapes or sterile personnel. The surgeon then grasps the leg through the sterile stockinette and rolls the stockinette up the leg (Figure 6).

Although the leg has been prepared in a sterile manner, the surgeon should not touch the exposed skin until the

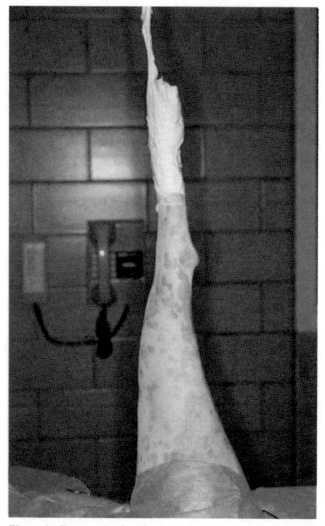

Figure 4—Drapes are placed around the base of the affected leg after initial preparation.

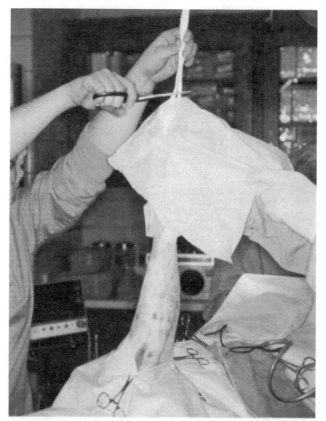

Figure 5—The limb is released from the support stirrup following the final surgical scrub but before placement of the final drapes.

stockinette has been rolled up the leg to meet the four drapes. After the stockinette is in place, the surgeon is free to grasp the limb along its entire length without fear of contact with unprepped areas. The stockinette is cut along the incision site, and the skin incision is made. A popular technique is to suture the stockinette to the subcutaneous tissue so that deeper dissection is possible with minimal risk of contamination. Some surgeons feel, however, that because stockinette is not waterproof, strikethrough will still occur if it becomes wet with blood or saline.

Instrumentation

Orthopedic instruments and appliances are among the most specialized and expensive of all surgical instruments.[5] These instruments are designed to perform a variety of different functions to bone including cutting (Figure 7A), shaping (Figure 7B), smoothing (Figure 7C), drilling (Figure 7D), or holding (Figure 7E).

Most surgical implants are made of stainless steel or cobalt-chromium material. These substances are not easily changed chemically after implantation and do not incite tissue inflammation.

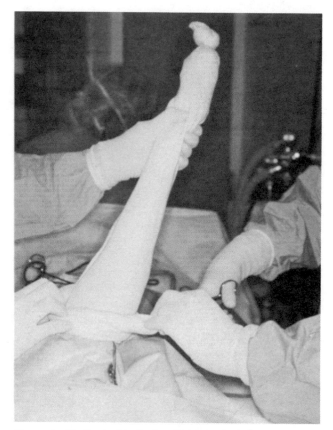

Figure 6—Sterile stockinette is rolled onto the leg.

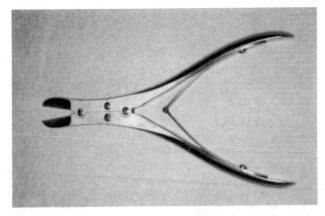

Figure 7A

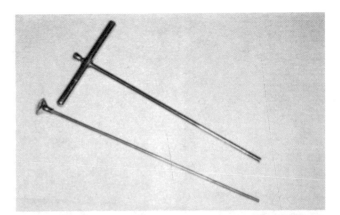

Figure 7D

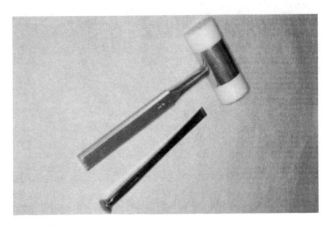

Figure 7B

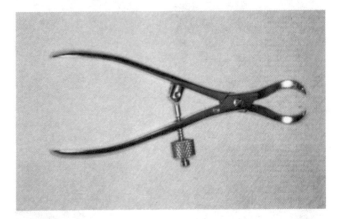

Figure 7E

Figure 7(**A** through **E**)—Selected orthopedic surgical instruments. (**A**) bone cutter, (**B**) bone chisel and hammer, (**C**) bone rasp (file), (**D**) trephine and stylet, and (**E**) bone forceps.

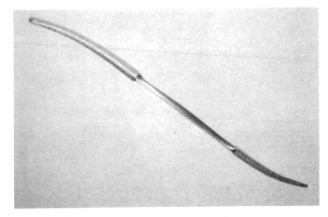

Figure 7C

Postoperative Care

Proper postoperative care cannot be overemphasized. At least every 15 minutes postoperatively, until normal parameters are reached, the patient's temperature, pulse, and respiratory rate should be recorded. Any medications administered should also be noted. The patient should not be left alone until the inhalation tube has been removed and an adequate swallow reflex has returned. Patients must be protected from self-injury when they are recovering from anesthesia.

When an external support, such as a cast, bandage, or splint, has been applied, it is imperative that it be checked frequently to ensure that circulation to the distal portion of the extremity has not been compromised.[2] The veterinary technician should look for abnormal swelling of the foot, unusual drainage or odor, and indications of excessive pain. The foot should feel warm to the touch. If the technician is responsible for the application of dressings or bandages, care must be exercised to apply even pressure over all parts of the limb being wrapped. Some postoperative swelling is to be expected, but persistent or excessive swelling may be a sign of improper bandaging. Casts and splints should not become wet; therefore, cages must be kept clean to prevent urine, feces, or saliva from soiling the external coaptation. Lack of moisture is particularly important if a plaster cast is used, because wetness causes plaster to soften and weakens its supportive action.[5] If a cast or bandage becomes wet or slips, it must be removed and a new one applied.

Physical Therapy

A veterinary technician is usually responsible for maintenance of postoperative therapy. In postoperative orthopedic care, physical therapy mainly involves controlled exercise. Exercise helps to increase circulation, improves range of motion of the limb, and improves the general "spirits" of the patient. Therapeutic exercise should also continue after hospitalization, and the technician needs to relay the instructions to owners carefully before the patient is discharged.

Conclusion

The majority of orthopedic injuries result from trauma. Proper care at the scene of the accident can decrease potential complications associated with fractures. Although fractures are rarely life threatening, certain soft tissue injuries associated with trauma are. A thorough evaluation of the patient is essential before surgery can be considered.

Infection is a constant threat in any orthopedic procedure, and much can be done to decrease chances of its development. With constant awareness of aseptic and sterile technique, postoperative complications can be kept to a minimum.

Proper postoperative care is essential. The technician must not allow the animal to injure itself, and external supports must be properly maintained. Physical therapy mainly involves controlled exercise. An exercise program, which the technician is often required to explain to the client, usually continues after hospitalization.

REFERENCES

1. Brinker WO, Piermattei DL, Flo GL: *Handbook of Small Animal Orthopedics and Fracture Treatment*. Philadelphia, WB Saunders Co, 1983, p 2.
2. Alexander JW: *Leonard's Orthopedic Surgery of the Dog and Cat*, ed 3. Philadelphia, WB Saunders Co, 1985, pp 17-25.
3. Hickman J: *Veterinary Orthopaedics*. Edinburgh, Oliver & Boyd, 1964, p 141.
4. Withrow S, Moore R: Orthopedic emergencies in small animals. *Vet Clin North Am [Small Animal Practice]* 11(1):Feb 1981.
5. Tracy DL, Warren RG: *Mosby's Fundamentals of Animal Health Technology*. St. Louis, The CV Mosby Co, 1983, pp 280-285.

Preparation of the Eye for Ophthalmic Surgery

OPHTHALMOS is a regular feature column of *Veterinary Technician*®. This month's feature was written especially for *Veterinary Technician*® readers by Cecil P. Moore, DVM, MS, Associate Professor, Department of Veterinary Medicine and Surgery, College of Veterinary Medicine, University of Missouri, Columbia, Missouri. Dr. Moore is a Diplomate of the American College of Veterinary Ophthalmologists.

The goal of surgical preparation of the eye is to eliminate microflora, including potential pathogens, from the surgical site in order to prevent postsurgical ocular infections. This column discusses surgical preparation procedures that may be used for extraocular and intraocular surgery. Before considering specific antiseptic agents and techniques pertaining to preparation of the eye, it is important to review ocular microbiology in normal and diseased states.

Ocular Microbiology

Studies of ocular microflora from normal dogs and cats indicate that aerobic bacteria are isolated from the eyes of more than 90% of dogs and approximately 40% of the eyes of cats.[1,2] This difference may reflect species variations in environment, behavior, or natural host defense mechanisms. Gram-positive bacteria predominate as the normal ocular flora of canine and feline eyes.[1-4]

In dogs, coagulase-positive *Staphylococcus* species, *Streptococcus* species, *Corynebacterium* species, and *Bacillus* species are the prevalent gram-positive isolates.[1,3,4] Of the streptococcal isolates from normal eyes, α-hemolytic streptococci are more prevalent than ß-hemolytic streptococci. The gram-negative organisms *Escherichia coli*, *Neisseria* species, and *Pseudomonas* species are less commonly isolated from normal eyes. In cats, *Staphylococcus* species are the prevalent bacterial flora of normal conjunctiva and eyelid margins.[2]

Organisms that are most common-

ly isolated from the eyes of dogs with external ocular infections are coagulase-positive *Staphylococcus* species, *Staphylococcus epidermidis*, α- and ß-hemolytic *Streptococcus* species, *Pseudomonas* species, *Proteus* species, *Escherichia coli*, *Corynebacterium* species, and *Bacillus* species.[5,6]

Similar surveys that specifically report the incidence of aerobic bacterial isolates from feline patients with external eye disease have not been published. The lack of data probably is because of the lower incidence of

bacteria in normal feline eyes and because most infectious eye diseases in cats are caused by *Chlamydia psittaci*, feline herpesvirus type 1, or *Mycoplasma* species,[7] all of which must be confirmed by special culture methods or other specialized diagnostic procedures.

Antimicrobial Agents

To reduce or eliminate surface microbes before surgery, antibiotic preparations and irrigating solutions (often with a safe and effective antiseptic

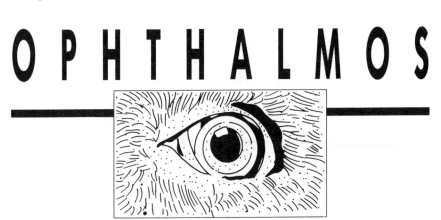

added to them) may be used on the eyelids, conjunctiva, and cornea.

Presurgical Antibiotics

Elective ophthalmic surgery should *not* be done on an infected eye. Topical and/or systemic antibiotics should therefore be given before surgery to treat ocular infections. The choice of antibiotic should be based either on culture and sensitivity results or an assessment of the organism most likely to be present (see the section on ocular microbiology).

Broad-spectrum topical antibiotics

(e.g., triple antibiotic) are routinely used one to three days before non-emergency intraocular surgery. Antibiotics that may be toxic at systemic therapeutic levels can safely be used topically. Ointments should not be used within 12 hours of intraocular surgery because vehicles and preservatives found in ophthalmic antibiotic preparations may possibly introduce irritating substances into the wound. If an ointment is inadvertently used within this period, it can probably be effectively removed before surgery by careful, repeated irrigation of the eye.

One indication for use of systemic antibiotics in patients requiring ophthalmic surgery is repair of acute trauma (e.g., laceration of the eyelids or globe) because wound contamination is assumed. Systemic antibiotics also may be used before elective intraocular surgery when the consequences of infection would seriously jeopardize the outcome of surgery.

Ocular Lavage

Gentle irrigation of the eye flushes debris and reduces conjunctival bacteria. It is important to use the appropriate amount of fluid (usually 10 to 15 ml) and to apply only low-pressure lavage to the ocular surface. Sterile physiologic saline is used most commonly as an ocular lavage; sterile distilled water is unacceptable because of its hypotonicity. Commercially prepared eye washes (Ak-rinse™—Akorn, Dacriose™—IOLAB, Eye-stream™—Alcon Laboratories), which are polyionic and buffered for ocular use, also may be used to flush the eye before surgery; such products, however, contain preservatives that may cause minor ocular irritation in some patients. These agents also should *not* be used to irrigate ruptured eyes.

Antiseptics often are added to the irrigating solution. Selection of a specific agent at an appropriate concentration is based on established safety (i.e., absence of tissue damage) and effective antimicrobial activity.

Antiseptic Solutions

Povidone-iodine solution is widely used as a cutaneous antiseptic in relatively dilute concentrations (i.e., 0.2% to 1.0%); in dilute concentrations, greater quantities of the active free iodine become available. Because the stock solution (Betadine™ Solution—Purdue Frederick) contains 10% povidone-iodine, dilutions of 1:10, 1:25, and 1:50 yield 1.0%, 0.4%, and 0.2% solutions, respectively. The advantages of povidone-iodine include a wide spectrum of activity and excellent tolerance by ocular surface tissues. Disadvantages include short residual activity and reduced efficacy in the presence of organic matter.

The effectiveness of various dilutions of povidone-iodine in eliminating resident bacterial flora in canine eyes before surgery has recently been studied.[8] Bacteria were eliminated with 1:2, 1:10, and 1:50 povidone-iodine dilutions. A 1:50 povidone-iodine solution was demonstrated to be as effective as more concentrated solutions. During surgical preparation, a 1:10 dilution may be more appropriate to cleanse the skin because of the relative abundance of organic material (i.e., keratinized epithelium and sebaceous debris) associated with cutaneous tissue. The more dilute 1:50 solution is appropriate for irrigating the ocular surface (i.e., the cornea and conjunctiva).

Chlorhexidine is an effective antiseptic solution that may be more appropriate in some situations as a cutaneous presurgical antiseptic than povidone-iodine. For example, chlorhexidine has better residual activity and is more effective in the presence of organic material[9,10]; however, because of the solution's potential for irritating the cornea and conjunctiva, it cannot be recommended for preparation for ophthalmic surgery.[11] Alcohol solutions also should *not* be used around the eyes because they may damage ocular surface tissues.

Presurgical soaps (i.e., povidone or chlorhexidine scrub soaps) should not be used around the eyes. Detergent components of these soaps may cause considerable irritation to the eye and may possibly result in chemosis, corneal erosions, or ulcers; irritation also may stimulate self-trauma. Labels of preparations simply identified as *scrub solutions* should be read carefully because these solutions may contain detergent. If there is any doubt regarding the contents of antiseptic solutions, they should *not* be used in prepping the eye for surgery.

Hair Removal

Clipping hairs from around the eye is important when preparing the surgical field. Preferred means and methods of clipping hair from the surgical field vary from surgeon to surgeon. For example, some surgeons may prefer scissors to electric clippers to remove hair. Eyelashes, tactile cilia, and longer facial hairs are most effectively removed with scissors. Some surgeons prefer to clip the hair 24 hours before surgery to minimize the inflammation of adnexal tissues that can be caused by clipping; however, if care is taken and tissues are gently handled, clipping can be done immediately after anesthetic induction and before surgery.

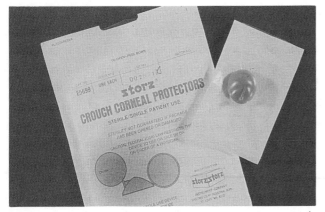

Figure 1—Crouch Corneal Protectors (Storz Instrument) are smooth, plastic shields that are individually wrapped in sterile packaging. The corneal protector is placed under the eyelids to cover and protect the surface of the eye during surgical preparation.

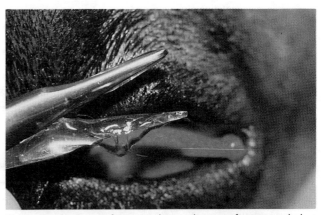

Figure 2—Placement of scissors during clipping of upper eyelashes. Sterile lubricating gel is applied to the scissor blades before the eyelashes, tactile cilia, or long facial hairs are clipped to prevent hair fragments from dropping into the eye. A corneal protector has been inserted under the eyelids before the hair is clipped.

A corneal–scleral protector (Crouch Corneal Protector—Storz Instrument) (Figure 1) can be placed under the eyelids to shield the cornea while periocular tissue is clipped and cleansed. The corneal–scleral protector is lubricated with contact lens solution to facilitate insertion, minimize frictional irritation, and keep the cornea moist. Curved scissors, lightly coated with sterile water-soluble lubricant (K-Y Jelly™—Johnson & Johnson, Surgilube™—E. Fougera & Co.) are used to clip coarse hairs that might enter the surgical field (i.e., lashes, tactile cilia, or long facial hairs). The lubricant causes cut hairs to stick to the scissor blades and thus prevents the hairs from falling into the eye (Figure 2). A clean, sharp No. 40 clipper blade (A5 Clipper™—Oster, a division of Sunbeam) is then used to shave the eyelids and periocular area.

When using clippers or scissors, rough, hasty, or careless manipulations must be avoided because abrasions, edema, or lacerations of the eyelids may result. To clip eyelid hair effectively and safely, the skin is gently stretched and the clippers are pushed slowly over the eyelid against the direction of hair growth (Figure 3). This method allows close

trimming of the hair while avoiding abrasions or other trauma that could result in postsurgical inflammation and discomfort. The area of hair to be removed varies with the specific procedure but should exceed the area that will be draped by a distance of two centimeters in all directions.

Preparation for Adnexal Surgery

Surgeons have varying preferences for the techniques and materials used for ocular surgical preparation. The following general guidelines may be followed for most ophthalmic preparation procedures. Sterile latex gloves should be worn during surgical preparation. After hair removal, the clipped area is flushed thoroughly with sterile, room temperature (or preferably warmed) saline to remove hair and debris.

Because the eyelids are very sensitive (even to minor trauma), care must be taken to avoid overzealous or rough handling during the preparation process. If eyelid tissue is not carefully handled, swelling and irritation may result; these occurrences can further complicate surgery and/or result in postsurgical self-trauma.

Periocular tissue is swabbed and

gently cleansed with a dilute (1:10) povidone-iodine solution applied to cotton or soft gauze. Starting near the eyelid margin, the periocular skin is swabbed in concentric, circular motions (Figure 4). The eyelids are swabbed three times in this manner and are flushed with sterile saline between swabbings. Absorbent towels are placed under the patient's head or a receptacle is positioned next to the head to collect the irrigation fluid.

As an alternative, baby shampoo (No More Tears™—Johnson & Johnson) may be used for cleansing the eyelids. Baby shampoo is reported to be safe and effective for cleansing the ocular adnexa. The solution is made as a 1:3 aqueous dilution.[a] Although baby shampoo should not irritate the ocular surface, contact with the cornea should be minimized and thorough rinsing of the eyelids, conjunctiva, and cornea should be done after the eyelids have been cleansed.

After the eyelid prep, the corneal–scleral protector is removed and the conjunctiva is gently irrigated with

[a]Nasisse M: Personal communication, North Carolina State University, Raleigh, North Carolina, January, 1992.

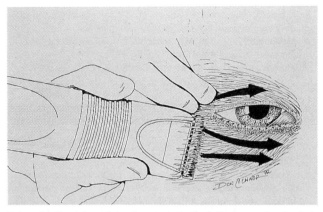

Figure 3—Illustration of the correct method of clipping periocular hair with electric clippers. Note that the skin is stretched laterally toward the base of the ear and the clippers are directed against the grain of hair growth. Placement of the corneal protector is recommended before clipping the hair (see Figure 2).

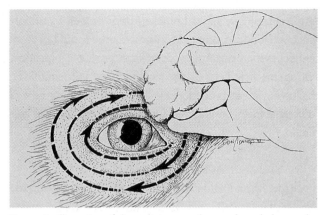

Figure 4—Illustration of the technique used to swab and cleanse the eyelids. Cotton swabs are soaked in 1:10 povidine–iodine–saline solution; and beginning near the eyelid margin, the eyelid skin is swabbed in concentric motions. As an alternate method, baby shampoo prepared as a 1:3 aqueous dilution may be used to prepare the eyelids. It is recommended that the corneal protector be left in position while the eyelids are being cleansed (see Figure 2).

1:50 povidone-iodine solution. A cotton-tipped applicator soaked in the same antiseptic solution is used to swab the conjunctival surfaces, including the recesses (fornices) under the eyelids and behind the third eyelid. Care must be taken to avoid touching or abrading the cornea. Finally, the conjunctiva and cornea are flushed with sterile saline. Sterile gauze is used to dry the skin surface before draping.

Preparation for Primary Ocular or Intraocular Surgery

For surgery that involves the surface of the eye or for intraocular procedures, a slightly different sequence is recommended than that used for adnexal surgery. After the cornea–scleral protector is inserted and the hair is removed (as previously described), the initial (first of three) eyelid scrub is done with 1:10 povidone-iodine or 1:3 baby shampoo and the corneal–scleral protector is removed.

Next, the conjunctiva is irrigated with 1:50 povidone-iodine solution and a cotton-tipped applicator soaked in the same antiseptic solution is used to swab the conjunctival

surface, with care being taken to avoid abrading the cornea. The eyelids are swabbed two additional times with 1:10 povidone-iodine or 1:3 baby shampoo, and the conjunctiva and cornea are flushed after each cleansing with the 1:50 povidone-iodine solution. Again, sterile gauze is used to dry the skin before draping.

Additional Considerations

For unilateral procedures, the eye that is not undergoing surgery (usually positioned on the side facing down) is protected by a sterile ophthalmic lubricating ointment applied in the eyelid fissure and onto the globe. The ointment, which may or may not contain antibiotics, is applied immediately after anesthetic induction.

For bilateral procedures, hair is removed from the eyelids of both eyes before the patient is positioned on the operating table. The second eye to undergo surgery is prepared and irrigated one time after the hair is clipped and immediately before the eyelid is closed (to be discussed later). Subsequent cleansing and irrigation (during the second and

third preparation) of the second eye are done immediately preceding the actual surgery.

For intraocular surgical procedures, the second eye to undergo surgery is protected by keeping the eyelids closed either with nonstick tape over the eyelids or by placing temporary tarsorrhaphy sutures in the eyelids before surgery is initiated on the first eye. This step is especially important in brachycephalic breeds in which exposure is common and may result in serious corneal ulcers. The tape or sutures should not contact the cornea. Protecting the globe in this fashion allows the cornea to remain moist without necessitating the use of ointment. The tape or suture material is removed when the patient's head is positioned for surgery on the second eye and the preparation procedure is complete. For surgical procedures involving only the eyelids or third eyelids, applying ophthalmic ointment to the other eye (instead of taping or suturing) is satisfactory.

Conclusion

Use of appropriate antibiotics and nonirritating concentrations of effective antiseptic solutions before surgery as well as adherence to standard preparation procedures should prevent unnecessary postsurgical complications (i.e., infections, iatrogenic irritation, or chemical-induced inflammation). Following these procedures will help ensure a successful outcome from ophthalmic surgery in small animal patients.

ACKNOWLEDGMENTS

The author thanks Lana L. Linton, DVM, Linda L. Collier, DVM, PhD, and Dorothy Rainwater, RVT, College of Veterinary Medicine, University of Missouri–Columbia, for their assistance in preparation of this article.

REFERENCES

1. Gerding PA, Kakoma I: Microbiology of the canine and feline eye. *Vet Clin North Am [Small Anim Pract]* 20:615-625, 1990.
2. Campbell LH, Fox JG, Snyder SP: Ocular bacteria and mycoplasma of the clinically normal cat. *Feline Pract* 3:10-12, 1973.
3. Urban M, Wyman M, Rheins M, et al: Conjunctival flora of clinically normal dogs. *JAVMA* 161:201-207, 1972.
4. McDonald PJ, Watson ADJ: Microbial flora of normal canine conjunctivae. *J Small Anim Pract* 17:809, 1976.
5. Murphy JM, Lavach JD, Severin GA: Survey of conjunctival flora in dogs with clinical signs of external ocular disease. *JAVMA* 172:66-68, 1978.
6. Gerding PA, McLaughlin SA, Troop MW: Pathogenic bacteria and fungi associated with external ocular diseases in dogs: 131 cases (1981-1986). *JAVMA* 193:242-244, 1988.
7. Martin CL: Feline ophthalmologic diseases. *Mod Vet Pract* 929-934, December, 1981.
8. Roberts SM, Severin GA, Lavach JD: Antibacterial activity of dilute povidone-iodine solutions used for ocular surface disinfection in dogs. *Am J Vet Res* 47:1207-1210, 1986.
9. Osuna DJ, DeYoung DJ, Walker RL: Comparison of three skin preparation techniques. Part 2: Clinical trial in 100 dogs. *Vet Surg* 19:20-23, 1990.
10. Phillips MF, Vasseur PB, Gregory CR: Chlorhexidine diacetate versus povidone-iodine for preoperative preparation of the skin: A prospective randomized comparison in dogs and cats. *JAAHA* 27:105-108, 1991.
11. MacRae SM, Brown B, Edelhauser HF: The corneal toxicity of presurgical skin antiseptics. *Am J Ophthalmol* 97:221-232, 1984.

Medical Nursing Care of Ophthalmic Patients

OPHTHALMOS is a regular feature of *Veterinary Technician*. The new author is Paula J. Scott Lanning, BA, RVT, Department of Small Animal Clinics, School of Veterinary Medicine, Purdue University, West Lafayette, IN 47907.

Ophthalmic patients often require special handling. Visually impaired animals must be approached slowly and spoken to gently to avoid being startled. When in an unfamiliar environment, they should be carried if possible. Blind animals should be kept on a leash when exercising, carefully led around obstacles, and continually spoken to for reassurance and localization. Visual animals often can sense that a blind animal has decreased defenses; to prevent the possibility of aggression toward the blind animal, it is best to isolate the visually impaired patient from unfamiliar animals.

Because of the nature of ophthalmic diseases, a large proportion of ophthalmic patients are very young or very old. Thus, special needs according to the age of the animal must be considered when an ophthalmic patient is hospitalized. Puppies need more frequent feedings and socialization (Figure 1). They also must be monitored more closely to prevent further trauma to the eye; they are more active than older animals, and portions of a young eye are more susceptible to damage because it is not developed completely until sixteen weeks of age. Geriatric patients can have special dietary needs, usually have to eliminate more frequently, and often have ingrained habits requiring special attention.

Restraint

Proper restraint technique is necessary to prevent damage during an ophthalmic examination or when cleaning or medicating the eye. Basic diagnostic tests can be frightening, and eye disease can be painful to the patient. The following method of restraint protects the animal and the person treating the eye.

The patient's head must be held firmly and steadily; this is accomplished best by holding the muzzle with one hand and the back of the head with the other (Figure 2).

For support, the elbow of the hand holding the muzzle should rest on the table. When restraining an animal with eye disease, it should be habitual to avoid putting pressure around the patient's neck. Increased intraocular pressure resulting from occluded jugular veins can complicate certain ophthalmic problems; for example, the increased pressure might be enough to rupture the globe of a patient with a compromised cornea.

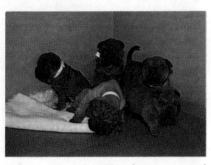

Figure 1—Shar pei puppies often are presented at a young age for entropion, or rolling in of the eyelids. The technique of lid tacking for correction of this defect is evident here.

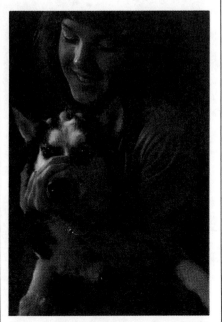

Figure 2—The proper method of restraint for ophthalmic examination.

Cleaning the Eye

Care always should be used when cleaning or medicating the eye. Commercial eyewashes are preferred over home preparations. Most companies that dispense ophthalmic medications manufacture eyewash, a solution usually containing a combination of sodium chloride, potassium chloride, boric acid, and a preservative. These are sterile, isotonic solutions made specifically for ophthalmic irrigation and are relatively inexpensive. Eyewash and other topical ophthalmic medications should not be used directly from the refrigerator because cold irritates the eye.

Cotton balls are the preferred material used to clean the eye. Because the eyelids are formed of loose connective tissue covered with thin skin, they are easily irritated by rougher materials such as gauze or paper tissues.

To clean the eyelids, moisten the cotton balls with eyewash and gently pull each lid up or down to wipe against the bony orbit. Never apply pressure directly to the globe.

To irrigate the eye, apply eyewash directly onto the globe or into the conjunctival sac. Avoid touching the tip of the bottle to the eyelids; this will contaminate the entire bottle of solution.

Medicating the Eye

There are several ways to administer drugs to the eye. The route is decided by the location at which medication is required, the frequency of medication necessary, and owner and patient compliance. Topical administration—in solution, suspension, or ointment form—is the most common route. Topical ophthalmic drugs primarily reach the eyelids, the cornea, and the conjunctiva. Some such agents will penetrate to the internal structures of the globe.

Solutions and suspensions are the easiest topical drugs to apply and have the advantage of not interfering with vision. Because the contact time is less than with ointments, drops might need to be instilled more frequently. When applying, rest the hand on the patient's head (Figure 3). This is necessary to avoid injuring the globe if the patient moves suddenly. The hand on the head should pull up the upper eyelid while the free hand pulls down the lower lid. The drop is applied from a distance to avoid contamination.

Ointments remain on the eye longer and have less loss through the nasolacrimal system. They do interfere with vision, however; and excess ointment can build up on the eyelids, causing irritation and necessitating more frequent cleaning. To apply an ophthalmic ointment, the patient's lower lid should be pulled down and a thin ribbon of ointment squeezed along the inside of the lid. Body heat and the movement of the eyelids will distribute the ointment over the eye.

Other methods of giving ophthalmic drugs (subconjunctival, retrobulbar, and intracameral injections) are beyond the scope of this article and will be discussed in future articles as they apply to specific diseases and their treatments.

Protecting the Eye

Preventing self-trauma is a vital concept in medical nursing of the ophthalmic patient. Even an animal with a painful eye might attempt to rub at it if he objects to topical medication. Another important concern is protection of the eye after ophthalmic surgery. The benefits of intraocular or eyelid surgery can be wasted if the patient is allowed to scratch or rub at sutures.

Many sources recommend taping the dewclaws as minimal protection from self-trauma. This measure alone cannot prevent an animal from rubbing its eyes on furniture or carpeting, as many are prone to do. Taping the dewclaws rarely is necessary if appropriate therapy is initiated.

Bandaging the eye offers advantages in addition to preventing self-trauma. It immobilizes the globe, helps prevent infection, and provides added warmth. The major drawback is inaccessibility of the globe to examination and medication. Because frequent evaluation and topical medication are essential in managing most eye diseases, bandaging often is not recommended.

A sturdy Elizabethan collar helps ensure that an animal will be prevented from further damaging the eye while allowing easy access to the globe. There are several brands of Elizabethan collars; most are constructed of cardboard or plastic.

The Medicollar™ (Evsco Pharmaceuticals) is made of durable cardboard lined with a thin layer of foam padding. It is lightweight and comfortable but should be used on a short-term basis only because it can be damaged by water, pet food, and toenails.

Plastic Elizabethan collars, such as the Buster™ (Jorgensen Laboratories), are the sturdiest and most practical for ophthalmic nursing care. They are offered in a variety of sizes, and each size is adjustable. Care should be taken that the collar is fitted properly; it must be large enough to prevent a hind paw from reaching the eye, but

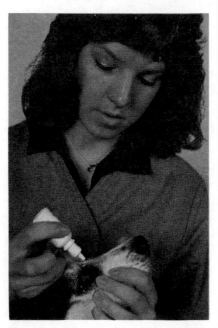

Figure 3—Application of a topical ophthalmic solution.

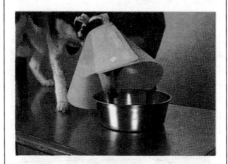

Figure 4—A well-fitted Elizabethan collar. Note that the patient has no trouble reaching its dish.

the technician must be sure that the animal is able to eat and drink while wearing the collar (Figure 4). It might be necessary to trim the outer edge if the collar is too long.

Client Education

Home nursing care of the ophthalmic patient during the course of treatment for a disease process or during the healing of a surgical case is crucial to a successful outcome. The veterinary technician often is responsible for showing the client how to clean and medicate the patient's eyes and for explaining other special instructions. Discharge instructions always should be written and given to the client as well as discussing the special care required.

Before discharging an ophthalmic patient, the technician should be certain that the owner is confident about medicating the eye. It is best to observe the owner applying topical medication before the animal is released. In addition to discussing the pet's specific problem and stressing the importance of home nursing care, the discharge instructions should describe signs that might signal a worsening ophthalmic condition (e.g., squinting, ocular discharge, and change in eye color). The owner should be made to feel welcome to call immediately if these signs are noted.

Acknowledgments

The figures appear through the courtesy of Sam Royer (Figure 1) and Mark Cap (Figures 2 through 4), Department of Medical Illustrations, School of Veterinary Medicine, Purdue University.

Coming next: The first in a series of features on medical nursing care of the glaucoma patient.

BIBLIOGRAPHY

Magrane WG: *Canine Ophthalmology.* Philadelphia, Lea & Febiger, 1965, pp 31-46.

Severin GA: *Veterinary Ophthalmology Notes,* ed 2. Fort Collins, CO, Colorado State University, 1976, pp 25-26.

Slatter DH: *Fundamentals of Veterinary Ophthalmology.* Philadelphia, WB Saunders Co, 1981, pp 45-51.

Vestre WA: *Veterinary Ophthalmology Notes.* West Lafayette, IN, Purdue University, 1984, pp 14-19.

Medical Nursing Care of Glaucoma Patients

OPHTHALMOS is a regular feature of *Veterinary Technician*. The author is Paula J. Scott Lanning, BA, RVT, Department of Small Animal Clinics, School of Veterinary Medicine, Purdue University, West Lafayette, IN 47907.

The veterinary technician can play an important role in the management of glaucoma in pets. The technician should be able to recognize clinical signs, perform basic diagnostic techniques, give treatments, and counsel clients regarding the disease process.

Glaucoma is an increase in intraocular pressure significant enough to cause damage to the eye. Glaucoma almost always causes irreversible blindness unless treated promptly and correctly.

Aqueous humor is the clear fluid that fills the anterior chamber of the eye and is responsible for maintaining the shape of the globe, nourishing its avascular structures, and eliminating metabolic wastes (Figure 1). The aqueous is secreted by the ciliary body epithelial cells; diffuses into the posterior chamber of the eye; and flows over the anterior surface of the lens, through the pupil, and into the anterior chamber. The aqueous returns to the general circulation through the trabecular meshwork of the iridocorneal, or drainage, angle—where the base of the iris and the peripheral cornea meet.

There is a delicate balance between the production of the aqueous and its outflow. If outflow is restricted, there is no feedback mechanism to decrease the production of aqueous. The intraocular pressure thus rises, and glaucoma results.

Glaucoma is classified as primary or secondary. Primary glaucoma occurs as a breed-related, often hereditary condition not associated with other ocular diseases. The restriction of aqueous outflow is caused by an inherent defect resulting in a narrow or closed drainage angle or by an interference of outflow in the trabecular meshwork or the collecting channels. Breeds with a predisposition to primary glaucoma include cocker spaniels, basset hounds, beagles, dachshunds, toy and miniature poodles, terriers, dalmatians, Siberian huskies, and Samoyeds.

Secondary glaucoma occurs as a result of any ocular condition that interferes with aqueous outflow. Ocular trauma, lens lux-ation, uveitis, and intraocular tumors are the most common precursors to secondary glaucoma seen in veterinary practice.

Diagnostic Techniques

The diagnosis of glaucoma is based on assessment of the presenting signs, history, and measurement of intraocular pressure. Gonioscopy to evaluate the drainage angle and retinal examination are performed by the veterinary ophthalmologist to establish the prognosis and to modify therapy.

Veterinary technicians should be able to recognize the clinical signs of glaucoma. Acute glaucoma causes intraocular pain that is commonly manifested as blepharospasm, elevated nictitating membrane, epiphora, photophobia, and lethargy. The conjunctival and episcleral vessels become congested. The pupil becomes dilated and unresponsive to light. The cornea appears cloudy because of the decreased function of the endothelial cells and the resultant edema of the corneal stroma (Figure 2).

Enlargement of the globe, or buphthalmos, indicates a chronic condition and an irreversible loss of vision. Even if the pressure is reduced, the eye often will remain enlarged.

The most important diagnostic test for glaucoma is measurement of intraocular pressure by tonometry. Three forms of tonometry are used in veterinary medicine.

Digital tonometry is accomplished by the examiner placing the index fingers against the patient's globes over the upper eyelids. Relative pressure is estimated by comparing the rigidity of the globes. This technique is too crude to determine pressure and therapy accurately.

Applanation tonometry measures the force necessary to flatten a constant area of the cornea by the application of a flat disk to the surface. This is the most accurate type of tonometry, but the equipment involved is expensive and usually restricted to specialty practices.

Indentation tonometry uses the Schiotz tonometer to measure the indentation of the cornea. A small, weighted plunger protrudes through a concave footplate when placed on the cornea. The plunger is attached to a rocker arm and a needle that moves across a scale. The scale reading is converted to mm Hg of pressure using a calibration table. Intraocular pressures vary slightly among breeds and individuals. The normal range for dogs and cats is 12 to 25 mm Hg. Pressures should always be taken bilaterally for comparison.

For Schiotz tonometry, the cornea is anesthetized with a topical anesthetic (proparacaine hydrochloride). The patient's head is elevated so that the instrument can be held vertically while resting on the cornea. The footplate should rest gently on the central portion of the cornea, avoiding

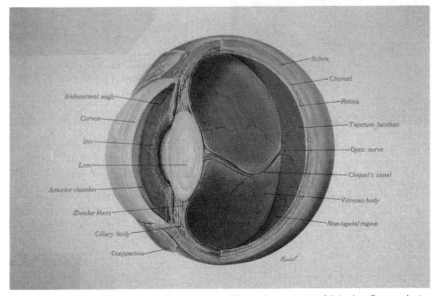

Figure 1—Anatomy of the canine ocular structures. (Illustration courtesy of Schering Corporation)

Originally published in Volume 8, Number 7, August 1987

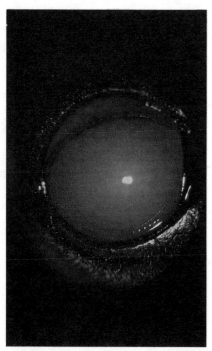

Figure 2—Acute congestive glaucoma. Note the corneal edema and the congested vessels.

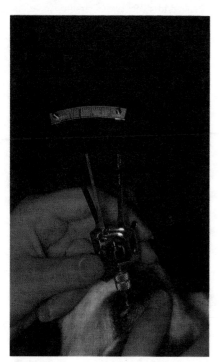

Figure 3—The Schiotz tonometer in use.

excess pressure on the globe (Figure 3). Three readings are taken and averaged. If the intraocular pressure is high, the scale reading will be less than 3 and not accu-

rate. Additional weight must be placed on the instrument, and three more readings must be taken. The Schiotz tonometer is a small, relatively inexpensive diagnostic tool that is essential to the diagnosis and management of glaucoma in a veterinary practice.

Gonioscopy is used to visualize the iridocorneal angle. A special bubble-shaped lens (the goniolens) is placed on the cornea. The curvature of the lens allows the light to bend in such a way that the angle is visible. Gonioscopy determines whether the angle is narrow or obstructed.

Ophthalmoscopy to examine the retina and the optic disk is necessary to evaluate damage resulting from the increased pressure. The extent of damage often determines whether treatment should be aimed at preserving vision or relieving pain and when surgical intervention is required.

Treatment

Initial treatment of glaucoma is often based on the stage of the disease process. The most intense medical therapy is initiated for an acute attack, when there is still a good chance of preserving vision. If treatment is not started within a few hours of onset, irreversible damage will result. Once the pressure is reduced, the cause of the glaucoma must be determined so that proper long-term medical or surgical therapy can be initiated.

Emergency therapy is necessary to open the drainage angle and to reduce aqueous production. Intravenous mannitol (1 to 3 g/kg of a 20% or 25% solution, given over 30 minutes) will decrease pressure by shrinking the vitreous, thus pulling the iris back and opening the angle. Water should be withheld from the patient during treatment. The intravenous dosage can be repeated up to four times within the first 48 hours if the patient is monitored closely for signs of dehydration.

A topical cholinergic drug, such as pilocarpine or demecarium bromide, will act to constrict the pupil. This facilitates outflow of aqueous. During an acute glaucoma attack, the drug should be given every hour until the pupil constricts, then continued at the rate of one drop every 8 to 12 hours. In cases of primary chronic glaucoma, a low dose of such a drug is prescribed indefinitely unless surgery is performed.

Carbonic anhydrase inhibitors (e.g., acetazolamide) are given orally or intravenously to decrease aqueous humor production. The prescribed dosage might require adjustment if side effects—such as panting, weakness, and vomiting—are noted.

Topical timolol maleate, a β-adrenergic

receptor blocking agent, reduces intraocular pressure by decreasing aqueous production. Pupil size is not affected, and the drug is usually well tolerated in animals. Topical steroids or oral aspirin or both also are frequently prescribed to reduce the pain and inflammation of glaucoma.

Medical therapy to control glaucoma is often unsuccessful on a long-term basis. There are several surgical alternatives available for treating the glaucomatous eye. These procedures, focusing on surgical nursing care, will be addressed in an upcoming Ophthalmos feature.

Client Education

The owners' understanding of the disease process and their willingness and ability to treat their pets are vital in the successful management of glaucoma. Veterinary technicians should explain the importance of home nursing care, how to monitor for clinical signs of an acute attack, and how to medicate properly with topical and systemic drugs.

After glaucoma is under control, medically or surgically, clients should be instructed to keep the remaining medications handy in the event of recurrence. If signs of an acute attack are noted, clients should call the clinic immediately. If clients understand dosage requirements, they should begin or increase the treatment even before the veterinarian is reached.

They also should be counseled on the importance of obtaining frequent reevaluations to check intraocular pressures.

Acknowledgments

The figures appear through the courtesy of the Department of Medical Illustrations, School of Veterinary Medicine, Purdue University, and through the courtesy of Schering Corporation (Figure 1), Dr. William A. Vestre (Figure 2), and Mark Cap (Figure 3).

Coming next: A discussion of medical nursing care of ophthalmic patients with keratoconjunctivitis sicca.

BIBLIOGRAPHY

Gelatt KN (ed): *Textbook of Veterinary Ophthalmology.* Philadelphia, Lea & Febiger, 1981, pp 390–433.

Severin GA: *Veterinary Ophthalmology Notes,* ed 2. Fort Collins, CO, Colorado State University, 1976, pp 269–276.

Vestre WA: Glaucoma in the dog and cat, in Ford RB (ed): *Schering Veterinary Clinical Classroom.* Princeton Junction, NJ, Veterinary Learning Systems Co, Inc, 1984.

Vestre WA: *Veterinary Ophthalmology Notes.* West Lafayette, IN, Purdue University, 1984, pp 115–126.

Medical Nursing Care of Patients with Keratoconjunctivitis Sicca

OPHTHALMOS is a regular feature of *Veterinary Technician*. The author is Paula J. Scott Lanning, BA, RVT, Department of Small Animal Clinics, School of Veterinary Medicine, Purdue University, West Lafayette, IN 47907.

The precorneal tear film is essential to the health of the external eye and the adnexa. The film is composed of an inner mucoid layer, a central aqueous layer, and a superficial outer oily layer. The mucoid component is produced by goblet cells in the conjunctiva. Microvilli on the corneal epithelium and the hydrophilic surface of the inner layer enhance tear adhesion to the cornea. A row of meibomian glands along the eyelid margin produces the outer oily layer. This layer acts to retard evaporation of the aqueous layer.

The majority of the tear film is aqueous in nature and is produced by the lacrimal gland, the accessory lacrimal glands, and the gland of the nictitating membrane. This serous component is responsible for the primary functions of the tear film: to lubricate the cornea and the conjunctiva and to wash away foreign matter and waste products. The precorneal tear film also supplies nutrients to the cornea and protects against bacterial infection. The latter function is possible because of the lysosomes and the leukocytes normally present in the tear film.

Keratoconjunctivitis sicca, or dry eye, is a common ophthalmic disease of dogs (cats are less commonly affected) and is the result of a decrease in the production of the aqueous portion of the tears. Acute keratoconjunctivitis sicca can be caused by inflammation of the lacrimal gland or damage to the parasympathetic innervation to the lacrimal gland. Lacrimal gland inflammation can be linked to systemic disease, for example, canine distemper virus. Damage to cranial nerve V can cause a decrease in corneal sensation, with a resultant decrease in reflex tearing.

The cause of chronic dry eye frequently is never discovered. Possible causes include congenital hypoplasia of the lacrimal gland, spontaneous or senile lacrimal gland atrophy, orbital trauma, drug toxicities, and chronic bacterial conjunctivitis. Another common precursor to keratoconjunctivitis sicca is a history of surgical removal of the gland of the nictitating membrane (the third eyelid). This outdated procedure was the common treatment for prolapse and hypertrophy of the gland ("cherry eye"). It is now known that the gland is responsible for as much as 40% of the aqueous portion of the tear film. A surgical procedure to replace and suture the gland to the periosteum of the orbital rim currently is the preferred treatment for preserving glandular function.

Regardless of the cause, the presenting signs of keratoconjunctivitis sicca are similar. Keratoconjunctivitis sicca results in the cornea and the conjunctiva being directly exposed to the environment, which leads to inflammation and possible ulceration and infection. A characteristic clinical sign is ropy mucoid discharge caused by the overproduction of the mucin layer, a compensatory response to diminished production of the aqueous layer (Figure 1).

Irritation to the patient will cause discomfort and pain leading to blepharospasm and itching or rubbing of the eye.

Depending on severity, the cornea can appear dull and lack the shine and luster of a normal cornea. The conjunctiva is reddened and swollen to varying degrees. In advanced cases, the cornea can become vascularized and eventually pigmented. At this stage, the irritation subsides and the patient no longer exhibits signs of pain because of chronic nerve degeneration.

Diagnostic Techniques

In addition to being aware of the presenting signs, the veterinary technician should perform some basic diagnostic tests. A decreased Schirmer tear test value is the most important diagnostic indication of keratoconjunctivitis sicca. The prepackaged sterile strips are 0.5 × 35 mm Whatman no. 41 filter paper (Figure 2). Before testing, excess mucous should be wiped gently from the eye with a dry cotton ball. No topical solutions are instilled so that the measurement is not artificially increased or decreased; if topical anesthetic is applied, the decrease in corneal sensation will decrease reflex tearing.

The strip should be folded at the notch at a 90° angle and inserted over the patient's lower eyelid, in contact with the globe (Figure 3). After contact for one minute, the moistened area of the strip from the notch is measured against the scale on the package. The normal measurement in dogs is 15 mm or longer. Five to 15 mm is questionable, and less than 5 mm is considered to be diagnostic for keratoconjunctivitis sicca.

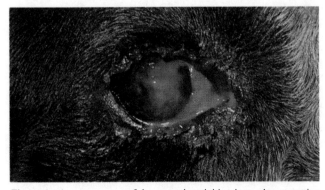

Figure 1—A severe case of keratoconjunctivitis sicca, demonstrating characteristic mucoid ocular discharge.

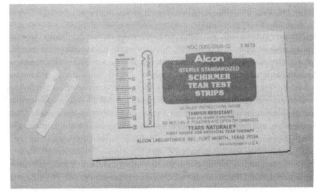

Figure 2—Prepackaged Schirmer tear test strips (Alcon Laboratories).

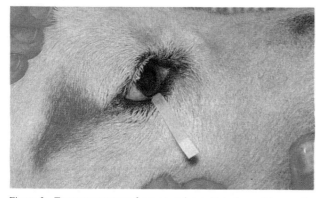

Figure 3—Tear measurement for a normal eye. Note the moisture on the strip.

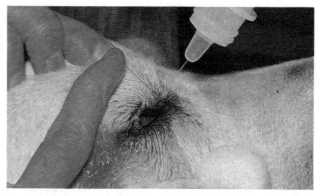

Figure 4—Staining the eye with fluorescein dye to evaluate corneal integrity.

Because of a dry eye's decreased protection, secondary corneal ulcers are common complications of keratoconjunctivitis sicca. All dry eyes should be stained with fluorescein to evaluate the integrity of the corneal epithelium. The tip of the fluorescein strip should be moistened with sterile eyewash and then placed directly on the eye. Excess stain should be flushed thoroughly using sterile eyewash (Figure 4). Several cotton balls are held under the eye to collect the excess rinse. Fluorescein stains fur, skin, and clothes a bright yellow-orange. Care also should be taken to avoid touching the tip of the bottle of eyewash directly to the eyelids after staining. A slight amount of stain will turn an entire bottle of eyewash green. A bright green stain retention on the cornea indicates an area of abrasion or ulceration. Fluorescein staining is an important procedure to perform when evaluating the keratoconjunctivitis sicca patient because the presence of corneal ulceration can change the medical therapy prescribed.

Treatment

The treatment regimen for a case of keratoconjunctivitis sicca is multifaceted and includes supplementing the tear film, stimulating lacrimation, controlling infection and inflammation, and keeping the eye and eyelids clean and comfortable.

Artificial tears can be purchased as over-the-counter products at most pharmacies. These tears contain the vehicles of topical ophthalmic drug preparations only; thus there is no chance of overdose. Solutions should be applied as frequently as possible. Lubricating ointments are used when treatment is not feasible for an extended period (three hours or more).

Broad-spectrum antibiotic ophthalmic solutions or ointments are prescribed to control or prevent bacterial infection. The frequency of use is determined by the severity of the disease or the presence of infection. Treatment generally is two to three times per day; if effectiveness is doubted, a bacterial culture and sensitivity should be performed.

Topical steroid preparations also are prescribed two to three times daily to control inflammation. If corneal ulceration is present, steroids are contraindicated because they delay healing.

Pilocarpine, used topically in the treatment of glaucoma, is a direct-acting cholinergic agent that can stimulate tear production when given orally. The drug must be mixed with food because it is bitter tasting. This is also important because undiluted pilocarpine in the canine stomach usually induces vomiting.

The oral dose of pilocarpine must be adjusted for each individual. The amount usually depends on the size of the patient. As a general guideline, one or two drops of a 1% to 2% solution once or twice daily is initiated for dogs weighing less than 15 pounds. The number of drops should be increased by one per day until early signs of overdose are noticed. Because pilocarpine is a general glandular stimulant, signs of overdose include salivation, emesis, and diarrhea. An overdose can cause tachycardia; the agent's use therefore is contraindicated in patients with concurrent heart disease.

Some function of the lacrimal glands is necessary to the success of oral pilocarpine therapy. The patient should be reevaluated a few weeks after therapy is initiated. If virtually no improvement is noticed, the pilocarpine should be discontinued. By contrast, some patients respond so well to this therapy that their conditions can be controlled with oral pilocarpine alone.

At least 30 days of intensive medical therapy is usually prescribed. In many instances, tear production will spontaneously return, allowing treatment to be reduced or discontinued. If there is no visible improvement, a surgical alternative involves the parotid salivary duct being transposed through the facial tissues and positioned in the palpebral conjunctiva. This procedure results in the eye being lubricated by saliva. If the cornea is not severely diseased, saliva is an adequate substitute for the tear film. The procedure

and the nursing care involved will be discussed in an upcoming Ophthalmos feature.

Client Education

Patients with keratoconjunctivitis sicca are rarely hospitalized. The veterinary technician's primary role in managing the condition, when diagnosed, is client education.

Proper home nursing care is essential to effective control of cases of keratoconjunctivitis sicca. Technicians should feel comfortable demonstrating to clients the proper method for medicating and cleaning the patient's eyes. The importance of frequent application of drops and ointments must be emphasized.

The effects of oral pilocarpine should be discussed, including the effects of overdose. If the client notices excessive salivation, diarrhea, or vomiting, the number of drops or the strength of solution must be reduced. By spending sufficient time discussing home nursing care, the technician can help to ensure a successful outcome of each case of keratoconjunctivitis sicca.

Acknowledgments

The figures appear through the courtesy of the Department of Medical Illustrations, School of Veterinary Medicine, Purdue University, and through the courtesy of Dr. William A. Vestre (Figure 1) and Mark Cap (Figures 2 through 4).

Coming next: A discussion of medical nursing care of ophthalmic patients with corneal ulceration.

BIBLIOGRAPHY

Buyukmihci NC: *Comparative Ophthalmology Notes.* Davis, CA, University of California, 1984, pp 89–93.

Gelatt KN (ed): *Textbook of Veterinary Ophthalmology.* Philadelphia, Lea & Febiger, 1981, pp 130–131, 317–323.

Severin GA: *Veterinary Ophthalmology Notes,* ed 2. Fort Collins, CO, Colorado State University, 1976, pp 121–123.

Vestre WA: *Veterinary Ophthalmology Notes.* West Lafayette, IN, Purdue University, 1984, pp 97–98.

Medical Nursing Care of Patients with Corneal Ulcers

OPHTHALMOS is a regular feature of *Veterinary Technician*. The author is Paula J. Scott, BA, RVT, Veterinary Ophthalmic Consulting, 8250 Bash Rd., Indianapolis, IN 46250.

The cornea is the normally transparent anterior portion of the fibrous tunic of the globe. It is composed of five distinct layers: the precorneal tear film, the epithelium, the stroma, the Descemet's membrane, and the endothelium (Figure 1). Ninety percent of the thickness of the cornea is the stroma, which is composed of collagen fibrils uniquely arranged in parallel sheets. This tissue, although hydrophilic, is normally kept dehydrated because of the pumping action of the endothelium and the epithelium. The layered arrangement, deturgescence, and lack of blood vessels and pigment all give the cornea its clarity.

A break or erosion in the superficial corneal tissue is called a corneal ulcer. The epithelial layer of the cornea is the main barrier to microorganisms; thus a corneal ulcer is highly susceptible to secondary infection. Because infection with some strains of bacteria can lead to the loss of an eye rather quickly, all corneal ulcers should be considered emergencies.

Causes

Of several possible initiating causes of corneal ulcers, the most common is trauma. Corneal scratches from cats, clippers, and plant material are common in dogs and cats. Trauma to the cornea also can result from an anatomic abnormality, such as distichiasis (an abnormal row of eyelashes), ectopic cilia, or entropion (rolling in of the eyelids). Conditions such as lagophthalmos (inability to blink effectively), prominent globes, or keratoconjunctivitis sicca can predispose an eye to corneal ulcers. Chemical insult, burns, and uncontrolled infection are other possible causes.

Diagnostic Techniques

Because the cornea is richly supplied with nerve endings, a corneal ulcer is an extremely painful condition. Patients will exhibit blepharospasm, photophobia, miosis, and epiphora in response to the insult.

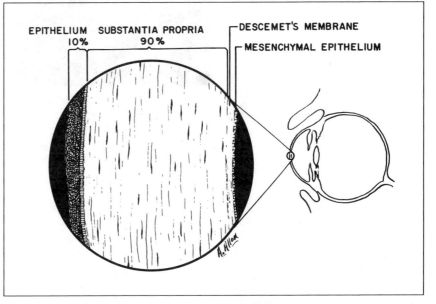

Figure 1—Schematic diagram of a cross section of the cornea.

The cornea might appear cloudy because of increased fluid uptake by the stroma (edema). Three to six days after the initial trauma, blood vessels can be visible growing into the cornea. This neovascularization is an important part of the normal healing process with deep ulcers.

Corneal ulceration is one of the most common eye diseases. Therefore, in veterinary practice, every eye causing pain should be stained with fluorescein dye. This dye is water soluble and will not penetrate intact epithelium. Where there is disruption of this layer, however, the exposed corneal stroma will stain bright green because of the solubility of the stroma (Figure 2).

The method of staining with fluorescein is relatively simple. Sterile fluorescein-impregnated strips are preferable to solutions because of the ease with which solutions can become contaminated. The strip should be moistened with sterile eyewash and then applied directly to the corneal surface. Excess stain should be flushed liberally from the eye.

This technique is used not only to detect corneal ulceration but also to outline the defect and determine its depth. If a corneal ulcer takes stain along the edges but fails to do so in the center, it is possible that the

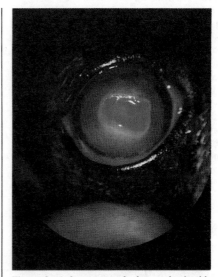

Figure 2—A large corneal ulcer stained with fluorescein dye.

ulcer has penetrated through the stroma to the Descemet's membrane. This is a very serious finding because such deep ulcers are in danger of rupture.

The diagnostics for corneal ulceration must be pursued further than merely detecting the presence of a defect in the cor-

Originally published in Volume 9, Number 3, April 1988

nea. In order to properly treat the disease, the cause must be determined. A careful history taken by the veterinary technician is an essential step in the process.

The location and character of a corneal ulcer also can help determine its cause. An ulcer on the superior third of the cornea might be caused by an aberrant eyelash or a small eyelid tumor. Ulceration under or near the nictitating membrane should alert the veterinarian to the possibility of a foreign body lodged behind the structure (Figure 3). Traumatic or infectious ulcers frequently affect the central cornea.

Treatment

In order for a corneal ulcer to heal, complicating factors must be corrected. For example, for temporary relief of distichiasis or ectopic cilia, the aberrant eyelashes should be epilated. For permanent removal, electroepilation or cryotherapy to destroy the roots is recommended. Eyelid surgery might be necessary if entropion is complicating the healing process.

Routine medical treatment of an uncomplicated corneal ulcer should begin with broad-spectrum topical antibiotics to prevent bacterial contamination. If purulent discharge is present and unresponsive to the prescribed antibiotic, a bacterial and fungal culture and sensitivity profile should be obtained. The culture should be taken at least a few hours after topical medication is applied because the preservatives in the solutions can inhibit bacterial growth. A sterile swab prepackaged with a transport medium, such as the Culturette® (Scientific Products), is ideal for this purpose (Figure 4). The cotton tip of the swab should be moistened with the transport medium just before swabbing. With the Culturette®, this involves squeezing and breaking the tip containing the material; the transport medium then moistens the swab within its sterile container. Cultures should be obtained by rolling the tip of the swab deep within the conjunctival fornix or gently across the surface of the ulcerated area. Care must be taken to avoid touching the swab to other surfaces, including the patient's outer eyelid. The swab is then returned to its plastic container and processed according to the guidelines of the individual practice. Antibiotic therapy is altered according to the results of the sensitivity profile.

To relieve the pain of a corneal ulcer, a topical cycloplegic (atropine) is applied a few times per day. This therapy controls ciliary spasms by paralyzing the ciliary muscles. To avoid alarming clients, they should be informed that the patient's pupil will remain dilated as a result of this action. Cycloplegics are contraindicated if the patient is prone to glaucoma. Topical anesthetic drops should not be prescribed for pain relief of a corneal ulcer. These agents interfere with corneal healing di-

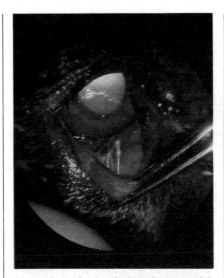

Figure 3—A foreign body (plant material) lodged behind the nictitating membrane.

rectly by delaying new epithelial growth and indirectly by removing the protective mechanisms of the eye.

During the complex healing process, rapidly multiplying corneal epithelial cells produce collagenase, an enzyme that catalyzes the destruction of collagen tissue. Corticosteroids can greatly increase the activity of collagenase, which will delay or prevent corneal healing. Topical steroids therefore should not be used as treatment for corneal ulceration. Only after the wound is completely epithelialized and stable for some time should topical steroids be prescribed, and then only if there is excessive neovascularization and possible scarring.

If edema is present in the corneal stroma, it can cause delay in the epithelium adhering to the stroma. Topical 5% sodium chloride can be added to the treatment regimen to aid in pulling fluid out of this tissue. This solution must be given at least 30 minutes apart from other topical medications because its osmotic effect will prevent corneal penetration of these drugs.

General practitioners can perform a third eyelid flap technique to protect a deep corneal ulcer. The technique involves suturing the nictitating membrane securely to the conjunctival surface of the superior eyelid so that the membrane acts as a natural bandage and supports the cornea. Although the flap should cover the cornea completely, topical therapy still will be effective.

Surgical alternatives for corneal ulcers that are in immediate danger of rupture are most successfully performed by veterinary ophthalmologists. These techniques, including the corneal graft and the conjunctival flap, will be discussed in an upcoming Ophthalmos feature.

Client Education

The technician often is responsible for

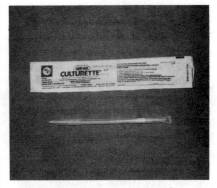

Figure 4—A sterile swab (Culturette®—Scientific Products).

demonstrating to the client the proper method of giving ophthalmic medications. The treatment regimen for corneal ulceration frequently involves alternating topical antibiotics throughout the day in addition to cycloplegics and sodium chloride solution. A sample treatment schedule worked around the client's personal schedule can be written down and explained by the technician. This simple service eliminates confusion and ensures that the patient receives the proper medication.

The technician also can prepare the client for the expected appearance of the ulcerated eye as it heals. Clients should be informed of possible complications and signs of problems. Owners of pets with severe ulcers in the process of healing are often concerned about the eye's appearance. The technician should stress the importance of neovascularization as part of the normal healing process. Although the blood vessels are unsightly and can interfere with vision, they will recede or can be removed after the cornea is healed.

Acknowledgments

The figures appear through the courtesy of Dr. William A. Vestre and the Department of Medical Illustrations, School of Veterinary Medicine, Purdue University.

Coming next: A discussion of medical nursing care of eye diseases that specifically affect cats.

BIBLIOGRAPHY

Buyukmihci NC: *Comparative Ophthalmology Notes.* Davis, CA, University of California, 1984, pp 115–152.

Gelatt KN (ed): *Textbook of Veterinary Ophthalmology.* Philadelphia, Lea & Febiger, 1981, pp 343–363.

Severin GA: *Veterinary Ophthalmology Notes,* ed 2. Fort Collins, CO, Colorado State University, 1976, pp 159–201.

Szymanski C: Diagnosis and treatment of corneal disease, in Ford RB (ed): *Schering Veterinary Clinical Classroom.* Princeton Junction, NJ, Veterinary Learning Systems Co, 1984.

Vestre WA: *Veterinary Ophthalmology Notes.* West Lafayette, IN, Purdue University, 1984, pp 90–96.

Understanding Wound Healing

Dudley E. Johnston, MVSc
Professor of Surgery
Diplomate, American College of Veterinary Surgeons
School of Veterinary Medicine
University of Pennsylvania
Philadelphia, Pennsylvania

Animal health technicians are frequently asked to assist in caring for wounds. Some of these are surgical wounds; others are accidental. They vary in shape, size, and location on the animal's body. Many questions about wounds are raised by clients in veterinary practice. The purpose of this article on the principles of wound healing is to strengthen the background knowledge of the technician for use in the areas of nursing care and client education.

The Basic Procedures in Wound Healing

Simple tissues such as fat and connective tissue regenerate completely and rapidly following injury. Skin is not a simple tissue, it is a highly complex organ containing glands, muscles, and hair follicles. In mammals, the complex organs and appendages have lost the power of regeneration, and instead damaged tissue is replaced by a fibrous scar tissue which, on the skin, is covered by regenerated and remodelled epithelium.

Injury, including every surgical procedure, is followed by *inflammation,* a vascular and cellular response capable of defending the body against foreign substances, of disposing of devitalized tissue and of initiating the repair mechanism. The changes seen after injury, and in the healing process, are the processes of inflammation. It is convenient to discuss three phases: a substrate phase, a repair phase and a maturation phase.

Phase 1: Substrate Phase

At the injured site, blood flows into the gap created by the cutting instrument, fills the space and clots, uniting the edges of the wound. At the surface, the clot dehydrates and forms the scab. A scab serves an extremely useful purpose in providing limited protection from external contamination and a surface beneath which cell migration and movement of the wound edges can occur.

Almost immediately after injury, small vessels dilate and white blood cells and other blood constituents leak into the wound. This process carries nutrients, antibodies and cells into the injured, or healing area.

Beginning about 6 hours after wounding, a natural "cleaning up" process known as *debridement* begins. The white blood cells that have migrated into the wound remove and break down cellular debris, bacteria and other foreign material.

Thus, inflammatory exudate, composed of escaping fluid from vessels, migrating white blood cells and dead tissue, accumulates in the injured area, whether or not infection is present. Surgeons want a minimal amount of this exudate, so that debridement can continue to remove all dead tissue, and proliferation can then proceed unhindered.

Phase 2: Repair Phase

Repair processes begin almost immediately after injury and proceed as fast as dead tissue, blood clots and other barriers are removed from the injured area. In uncomplicated simple wounds, debris is usually removed by the third to fifth day by which time the 3 basic healing processes, epithelial proliferation and migration, fibroblast proliferation, and capillary infiltration, can commence in the wound area.

Epithelial proliferation and *migration* are the first clear-cut signs of rebuilding. In general, the epidermal response to trauma includes mobilization of cells from the underlying dermis, migration of cells, multiplication of preexisting cells and differentiation to restore cellular function in new cells. The surface cells that have covered the incision begin to differentiate and produce keratin, leading to loosening and shedding of the scab in 5 to 6 days.

Epithelial growth and migration occurs in all wounds in the healing area, including the wounds made by insertion of sutures. If large irritating sutures are used and left in place for excessive periods, the epithelium

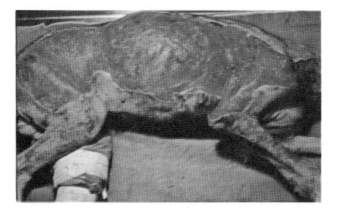

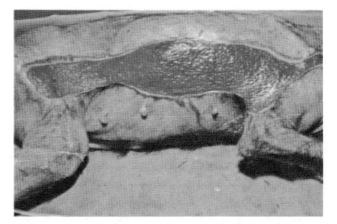

Fig 1—Healing in a open wound (*1A*). The wound bed is covered by a layer of healthy granulation tissue. Epithelialization is occurring at the edges of the wound. which is being reduced in size by contraction (*1B*).

in the suture tracts, and particularly the resulting keratin, can cause unsightly suture reactions that have been confused with abscesses caused by infection.

The second basic healing process is *fibroblast proliferation*. The fibroblast is a cell which secretes the ground substances and collagen that form scar tissue. Collagen is responsible for strength in the wound.

The third aspect of the healing process is *capillary infiltration*. New capillaries originate as bud-like structures on nearby vessels, and penetrate the wound. The new tissue formed by the fibroblasts and the bud-like capillaries constitute what is commonly referred to as granulation tissue. This network of capillaries provides large quantities of oxygen for the cells that are actively synthesizing protein in the wound.

Phase 3: Maturation Phase

The final process in wound healing is maturation of the scar. In a healing wound there is normally an overproduction of collagen fibers leading initially to a large scar. As scar formation proceeds, purposefully oriented fibers seem to become thicker and nonpurposefully oriented fibers seem to disappear.

As part of the maturation process, limited regeneration and remodelling of specialized epithelial structures of the skin, such as hair follicles and sebaceous glands, occur to some degree. The regeneration occurs after surface epithelialization is complete and is initiated by downward projections of the new epithelium into the underlying dermis. These buds mature into hair follicles and associated sebaceous glands.

Development of Strength in a Wound

In many descriptions of wound healing, the first stage is designated as a *lag phase*. It has been clearly shown that from a cellular and biochemical aspect, a lag phase does not exist; however, the term can be usefully preserved for the development of strength in a wound.

During the lag phase of 4 to 6 days, wound strength does not increase appreciably. However, even in the first 24 hours after wounding, a wound whose edges are properly brought together has some strength. This is due to the formation of a fibrin clot in the wound, and shortly afterwards, to the adhesive forces existing in the covering epithelial cells, and to some strength in the regenerating capillaries and in the newly formed ground substance.

After 4 to 6 days, strength increases significantly to reach an early maximum at 14 to 16 days. Collagen production increases rapidly beginning at day 4, with the highest rate between days 5 and 12, a lesser rate of increase between days 12 and 21, and a markedly lower rate from day 21 to day 60.

After the collagen content of a wound has stabilized, strength continues to increase, due to cross-linking and reorienting of the already formed collagen fibers. There is an almost imperceptible gain in strength for at least 2 years; however, the strength of the scar never reaches that of normal skin or fascia. The development of wound strength is an important consideration in the time of removal of sutures.

Sutures in a Wound

One of the applications of the knowledge of basic wound healing relates to the method of suturing skin wounds so that scarring is minimized. It is known that suture tracts are areas of injury and epithelium grows down these tracts to produce unsightly scars. This scarring is reduced if nonirritating fine suture material is used and the sutures are removed as early as possible. Unfortunately, if skin sutures are removed before the wound edges are stabilized by collagen, the scar tends to become widened, up to approximately the width that the skin edges were separated before the skin sutures were inserted. The suture scars and the wide skin scar are usually of minor importance in animals; however, in some reconstructive procedures they are significant.

In the usual incision in animals when good healing is desired, but moderate scarring is acceptable, the surgeon should place some absorbable subcutaneous sutures to obliterate dead space and to support the skin sutures. A nonirritating suture material such as monofilament nylon should be selected for the skin and the sutures should be removed before there is excessive growth of epithelium down the suture tracts, but after the wound has achieved a degree of tensile strength. This is usually at 8 to 10 days.

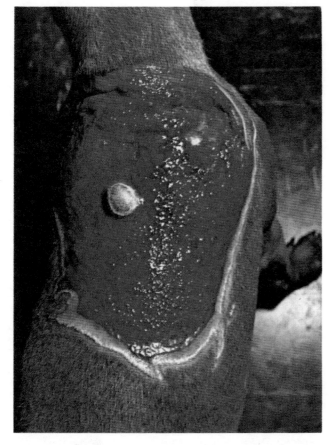 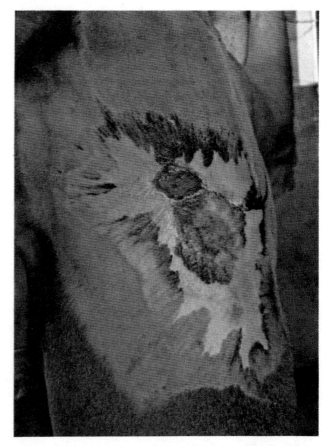

Fig 2—This open wound is allowed to close by contraction (*2A*). Closure is almost complete in 60 days (*2B*). A narrow scar of epithelium over fibrous scar tissue remains.

Healing in an Open Wound

In a full thickness skin wound in which skin edges cannot be brought together, the healing process follows the same general steps as in healing of an incised, closed wound. The same concepts apply in the development of inflammation and the subsequent phenomena. In the actual closure of the wound it is necessary to describe the regeneration of epithelium, the formation of a layer of granulation tissue in the bed of the wound, and wound contraction.

As in surgical wounds, epithelial regeneration begins by cell mobilization and migration, and by cell division at the wound edges. The wound bed is initially covered by a blood clot, later by a dried scab. The migrating epithelium moves under the clot or scab.

In large open wounds, all stages of epithelial repair are present. At the margin of the wound, thickening of the original epithelium is present. Adjacent to this and closer to the wound is the oldest part of the regenerated epithelium and several layers of cells are present. Beyond this, the advancing epithelium is eventually reduced to a single layer of flattened cells moving across the wound (Figs 1A and B). In most wounds, some degree of mutilation will be present, represented by abrasion, scratching, licking by the animal's tongue, or trauma from an ill-fitting and loose bandage. This interferes with the orderly pattern of cell migration described above.

The open wound is initially covered by a fibrin clot, then a scab following evaporation of fluid from the clot.

Following the healing pattern described previously, within 4 to 5 days after wounding, invasion of the wound bed by fibroblasts is occurring and new capillaries are being formed. This produces the typical granulating surface, which in the healthy state is flat, red and firm. New connective tissue, principally collagen, is formed in this bed.

The granulating bed is important in healing of open wounds for several reasons. The bed is extremely resistant to infection, the epithelium is able to migrate across its surface, and it is most likely that the mechanism of wound contraction is centered in the granulation tissue.

When full thickness skin is lost, there occurs a steady inward movement of the wound edges toward a central point, resulting in complete or partial obliteration of the central wound area. In wound contraction, no new skin is formed; however, the movement of the surrounding full thickness skin reduces the size of the central wound area. In many cases where the skin is loosely attached to underlying structures, as on the body of animals, the closure is virtually complete, leaving only a small scar (Figs 2A and B). In other areas, the contraction cannot reach this ideal conclusion and the scar is wider. Wound contraction is such an important aspect of the healing of open wounds that the term healing by *contraction and epithelialization* is preferred to describe this process, rather than the term *healing by granulation*.

In the incompletely contracted wound, fibrous tissue

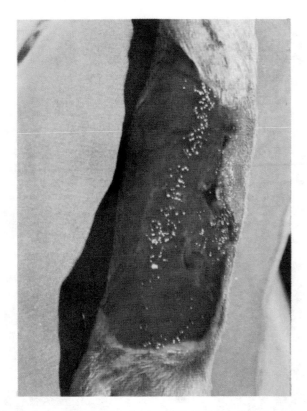
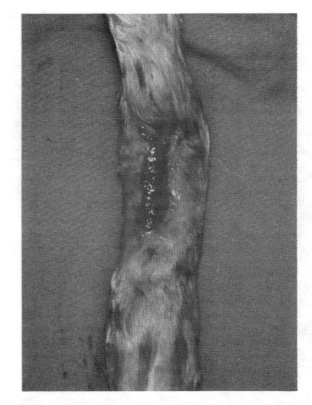

Fig 3—An open wound on the leg (*3A*) is not as likely to close completely by contraction (*3B*) as a similarly sized wound on the body. The wound is covered by epithelium which does not produce a strong surface.

formation can occur to an excessive degree. This tissue is usually poorly supplied with capillaries and presents as an unorganized mound of new tissue in the wound. This *proud flesh* can inhibit wound contraction and epithelialization, and must be controlled in order to promote wound healing.

The most likely explanation for wound contraction is that cells within the granulation tissue in the defect contract and pull the margins of the defect inward. Granulation tissue contains fibroblasts that develop characteristics typical of smooth muscle cells.

In summary, the steps in the healing of an open wound can be stated in the following way. The wound bed is quickly covered by a layer of granulation tissue over which epithelium migrates from the wound margins. While this is occurring, the granulation tissue contracts, pulling in the skin margins. The end result of wound healing by contraction and epithelialization depends to a large extent on the degree of mobility of surrounding tissue.

Once wound contraction has begun, it will continue to completion, usually in about 45 days. However, this does not always close the skin wound. On the body of an animal, closure can be almost complete and the resulting scar is minimal (Figs 2A and B). In other wounds on the body, contraction ceases before the wound is closed (Figs 1A and B). The resulting granulation tissue will cover with epithelium or it can be removed surgically and the wound closed by a reconstructive procedure (*plastic surgery*). On the limbs, contraction can sometimes satisfactorily close a wound. More commonly, there is insufficient mobility of surrounding tissue on the limbs and contraction is minimal. These wounds are left with large areas of epithelium on scar tissue (Figs 3A and B). The process of healing by epithelialization is a lengthy one and these areas are likely to be damaged by external trauma or licking.

Deformities Caused by Wound Contraction

Wound contraction is an important factor in the healing of open wounds in animals and man. It is well recognized in man, where the ill effects of wound contraction are stressed as much as, if not more than, the beneficial effects. In animals the beneficial effects predominate. However, some serious side effects have been observed in animals.

In general, two types of deformities are seen in animals associated with wound contraction. First, when a wound near the flexor aspect of a joint is allowed to heal by contraction, a web of tight skin or scar tissue can form, limiting extension of the joint. This is the so-called flexion contracture and has been seen in dogs and cats (Figs 4A and B).

The second common deformity in animals is seen at body openings, particularly the anus, so that stenosis occurs. This can follow the use of surgical excision or cryosurgery (a technique that uses very low temperatures) to treat perianal fistulae in dogs.

Systemic Factors Affecting Wound Healing

Several systemic factors have been shown to retard the healing process; however most have little clinical significance. Wound healing is delayed in animals with protein deficiency, or those that are suffering from anemia. These situations are not common clinical problems. Vitamin C deficiency can cause delayed wound healing in man. The value of supplemental

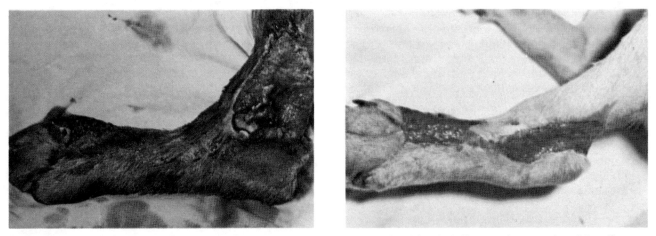

Fig 4—Wound contraction in this open wound (*4A*) has produced a severe contraction deformity (*4B*), preventing extension of the stifle.

Vitamin C in domestic animals other than the guinea pig has not been determined.

Uremia induced in the first 5 days of wound healing causes severe impairment of the healing process. After 9 days, wound healing is not affected. This can be a significant clinical problem in some animals with kidney disease.

It has been well established that, experimentally, corticosteroids delay wound healing. However, the doses are several times the usual therapeutic dose and delay in wound healing is not always seen clinically with corticosteroid therapy. The recommendation is that a wound in any animal receiving therapeutic doses of corticosteroids should be watched carefully. It is not expected that healing will be prevented. At most, a slight retardation in the rate of healing will be seen, and complete healing will eventually occur. Local application of corticosteroids can be used to prevent formation of excessive granulation tissue.

Local Factors Affecting Wound Healing

A certain amount of trauma is inevitable during surgery. Excess trauma increases the amount of debris and decreases the viability and activity of tissue. The first stages of healing are prolonged, the rate of gain of tensile strength is decreased, the possibility of infection is increased and excessive scar production can occur.

To reduce tissue trauma during surgery, incisions are made whenever possible with a scalpel. The use of scissors is reserved for dissection. Healing is delayed by prolonged pressure and tearing action of retractors, massive ligatures, and plugs of necrotic tissue from electrocoagulation.

Prolonged exposure and drying of tissue during surgery can delay healing. Also the possibility of wound infection is increased in long operative procedures.

Collections of clotted blood and serum between tissue layers interfere with wound healing. A large hematoma can exert sufficient pressure to interfere with blood supply to adjacent tissues. Free fluid in the wound encourages growth of organisms. The problem for the surgeon is that this *dead space* is deleterious

to wound healing; however, some methods to reduce dead space can be more deleterious.

Overly zealous use of buried sutures leads to foreign body reaction, strangulation of tissue, and formation of poorly draining chambers in wounds: all factors leading to increased wound infection and delay in healing. It is recommended that dead space in a wound be reduced by a combination of one or more techniques, not the use of numerous buried sutures alone. Three important techniques are the use of compression bandages after surgery (mild, comfortable pressure), drainage and the sparing use of buried sutures. Not only is the number of buried sutures kept to a minimum, but very fine material is used and the sutures are not tied so tightly that the tissues are strangulated.

If foreign material in the depths of a wound becomes infected or causes irritation, the wound rarely heals until the material is extruded or removed. This is a fascinating example of tissue intelligence designed to prevent the formation of deep and spreading infection in the body: as long as the pathway to the surface remains open, the infected foreign body does little harm. If the wound closes, a deep-seated abscess results with effects on the whole body as well as damage to adjacent structures.

A *foreign body* is described as a mass which is not normal for the tissues in which it is found. Introduced foreign bodies include the intentional types such as suture material and the metals used in bone repair, as well as the accidental type, such as grass awns.

Foreign bodies vary tremendously in their effect on tissue and wound healing. Some are virtually nonreactive and can be left in the body. Examples are stainless steel implants and lead bullets. Some organic foreign bodies such as wood, cloth and grass awns cause irritation even in the absence of infection, and must be removed.

One of the most common foreign bodies in a wound is suture material. The insertion of nonabsorbable suture material, especially braided material such as silk, into an infected wound can lead to continued infection. Absorbable suture material irritates tissue and causes exudation. Excessive exudation results when more than necessary surgical gut is used, when the suture material has a large diameter or when overly long ends are left on a suture or ligature.

Powder that is used to facilitate the donning of sterile gloves can lead to granuloma formation, and as the powder is relatively insoluble, it remains in the tissues almost indefinitely. All powders should be washed from the outside of rubber gloves before surgery.

Antiseptics and chemicals destroy bacteria but they also injure body cells. Only isotonic saline solution or preferably isotonic electrolyte solution should be applied directly to a wound. Even well-established local preparations such as 0.5% silver nitrate dressings and mafenide acetate ointment can cause epithelial regeneration to be delayed. Strong chemicals such as iodine, alcohol, phenol, etc., should not be applied directly to tissues. Antiseptics such as povidone-iodine can be used to clean an accidental wound, if diluted according to recommendations. Hydrogen peroxide is an irritant when used repeatedly in a wound.

REFERENCE

Peacock E E Jr. Van Winkle W: *Wound Repair.* 2nd ed. Philadelphia. WB Saunders Co. 1976.

UPDATE

Wound contraction is one of the significant factors in healing of open wounds in animals. Today it is agreed that the "full mechanism" is no longer a theoretical concept and that granulation tissue contains specialized cells called "myofibroblasts," which contract and pull the adjacent skin edges over the wound. Granulation tissue must be protected during wound healing.

Corticosteroids are a potent cause of delayed wound healing, and surgery may need to be delayed when large doses are used. Also chemotherapy is being used more frequently for treatment of immune disorders and cancer. In general, chemotherapeutic agents interfere with wound healing and this factor must be considered when these agents are used at the time of surgery or following it.

Additional information is available on the use of 3% hydrogen peroxide in wound care. This agent has been shown to destroy surface blood vessels in healing tissue and therefore can significantly delay healing and even cause extension of the wound if used repeatedly. In addition, it is a weak antiseptic and provides an oxygen-rich environment for only a limited time after application. In general, it has no place in wound care.

The Management of Wounds. Part I.
Practical Guidelines for Early Wound Care*

CRITICAL CARE COMPANION ANIMAL is regular feature of *Veterinary Technician®*. This month's contributing author is Steven F. Swaim, DVM, MS, Scott Ritchey Research Center, College of Veterinary Medicine, Auburn University, Auburn, Alabama.

From the beginning of time, man has instinctively poured liquids into wounds in order to kill microorganisms and enhance healing. Today, wounds are still treated with various potions and sprays as well as an array of topical medications. A basic understanding of principles of wound management significantly enhances the outcome of treatment.

Wound Lavage and How It Works

Wound lavage floats away debris and separated tissue particles; it also reduces the number of bacteria in a wound. Increasing the volume of lavage solution decreases the chance of infection. Adding antibiotics or antiseptics to the lavage is beneficial because more bacteria are exposed to the solution than are washed out. Pressurized lavage disrupts the organisms

*Adapted with permission from the proceedings of the First International Veterinary Emergency and Critical Care Symposium, San Antonio, Texas, September 1988; and the Western States Veterinary Conference, Las Vegas, Nevada, February, 1989.

present on the tissue in order for the lavage solution to wash them away.

Lavage Apparatuses

A commercial lavage apparatus consists of a lavage solution container, an intravenous administration set, a three-way stopcock, a 30-ml syringe, and an 18-gauge needle (Figure 1). By manipulating the three-way stopcock, lavage solution can easily be drawn into the syringe and delivered to the wound through the needle. Pressure of the lavage is about 7 to 8 p.s.i., which effectively lavages the wound without tissue damage.

A dental lavage apparatus (Water-Pik®—Teledyne Aquatic Corporation) has been described for wound lavage; however, its high pressure can cause tissue damage—especially in loose-skinned areas of dogs. A Water-Pik® is only indicated for lavage on badly contaminated limb wounds where the skin is more tightly attached to underlying tissue.

Plastic squeeze bottles with a fine-jet nozzle provide a good way to lavage wounds. If kept sterile, these bottles can be used several times. Plastic bottles with a trigger-type delivery mechanism have also been described for lavaging wounds. During use, the mechanism should deliver a fine stream of fluid rather than a spray.

Lavage Solutions

"...a biologically oriented surgeon would never select a solution to irrigate a wound which he would not be willing, for instance, to instill into his own conjunctival sac."[1] There are varying levels of impaired circulation associated with traumatic wounds: the most impaired circulation is near the wound surface, and less impairment occurs deeper in the tissue. Strong antiseptics for wound lavage impair the circulation even deeper within the tissue, thereby causing further tissue damage and prolonged healing time.

Povidone-iodine solution can be used for wound lavage; however, several effects are associated with its use. Because it is acidic, povidone-iodine can cause or exacerbate acidosis if used on large wounds; it may cause subclinical hypothyroidism or hyperthyroidism; it has a reduced residual activity of four to six hours because it is inactivated by exudate and blood; in vitro studies have shown that diluting povidone-iodine frees more iodine for bactericidal activity; and high concentrations of povidone-iodine may kill white blood cells and fibroblasts.

To use povidone-iodine, the wound should be cleaned thoroughly and the solution should be applied at frequent intervals during the day if it is the only topical medication being used. The povidone-iodine should be dilute

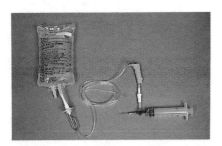

Figure 1—Wound lavage apparatus consists of a lavage solution container, an intravenous administration set, a three-way stopcock valve, a 30-ml syringe, and an 18-gauge needle. (From Swaim SF, Henderson RA: *Small Animal Wound Management*. Philadelphia, Lea & Febiger, 1990, p 15. Reprinted with permission.)

(not more than 1% solution, and an even more dilute solution may be preferable). Povidone-iodine (especially in the detergent form) can be ototoxic, so care must be taken if the solution is used to clean the ears of patients with otitis externa. A polyhydroxydine solution (Xenodine® Solution—Solvay Veterinary) may be used to treat wounds. This solution has some of the same properties as povidone-iodine.

Chlorhexidine diacetate (Nolvasan® Solution—Fort Dodge Laboratories), which has a wide bactericidal spectrum and is less affected by organic matter than povidone-iodine, is also used as a lavage solution. Chlorhexidine diacetate provides a good initial bacterial kill in addition to good residual activity; however, it forms a precipitate in saline solution. When used as a wet bandage, 0.5% solution kills bacteria but also inhibits granulation. A 0.1% solution kills less bacteria than a 0.5% solution and still inhibits granulation to some degree. At Auburn University, we use a 0.05% solution for wound lavage (1:40 dilution in water).

Hydrogen peroxide has been used to clean wounds for many years; however, it is not the best choice for wound lavage. Hydrogen peroxide has little bactericidal activity—it is more sporocidal. Hydrogen peroxide is only indicated for early lavage of dirty wounds in order to remove debris and clots.

Dakin's solution (0.5% sodium hypochlorite [Clorox®—The Clorox Company]) is once again becoming popular. The solution should be used at half strength (0.25%) or even quarter strength (0.125%). Dakin's solution reportedly reduces bacterial numbers, liquefies necrotic tissue, and stimulates granulation tissue.

Hydrophilic Compounds

Hydrophilic compounds bathe the wound from the inside out. These compounds, which act by drawing the body's own fluids up through the tissue to bathe the wound, reduce exudate viscosity in order for the exudate to be absorbed. Hydrophilic compounds should be used on smaller wounds. These compounds are contraindicated on large open wounds where the animal is already losing large quantities of fluids, electrolytes, and proteins.

One dextranomer product (Debrisan®—Johnson & Johnson Products) is composed of dextranomer beads. Fluid and debris are absorbed around the beads, and some wound products are absorbed into the beads. Debrisan® has been reported to be superior to gauze for absorption.

Copolymer flakes (Avalon® Copolymer Flakes—Summit Hill Laboratories) also absorb wound fluids. The flakes are made into a gel by adding water to the flakes. The gel is then applied to the wound. An absorbent bandage is placed over the gel to absorb the fluid that is drawn from the wound by the gel.

Systemic and Topical Antibacterials

Before manipulation of a wound and the surrounding area, a swab of the wound for bacterial culture and sensitivity should be obtained. The appropriate choice of antibiotic for a severely infected wound can more accurately be made by staining the exudate with Gram's stain to determine the predominant bacterial population of the wound. The results of culture and sensitivity tests may later alter the treatment regimen. The systemic antibiotic selected for use should be effective against the bacteria that are often present in superficial wounds, such as *Staphylococcus*, *Streptococcus*, and

Escherichia coli. Cephalosporins (e.g., cephalothin or cefazolin) can be used in early wound therapy. They should be administered as soon as possible after wound infliction, preferably during the first three hours. Antibiotic efficacy may be monitored by repeated culture and sensitivity tests. These tests may be repeated three to four days after the initial tests. If the tests yield no growth, initial therapy may be continued. A change in antibiotics should be considered when (1) culture and sensitivity test results indicate another antibiotic, (2) little change occurs in wound appearance after two to three days of initial therapy, or (3) the animal's general condition worsens and septicemia is possible.

If a wound has been thoroughly debrided and lavaged and the surgeon is confident that tissue debris or tissue of questionable viability is minimal, an antibiotic or antibacterial agent may be applied to the wound and the wound then may be bandaged. A direct smear from the wound that has been stained with Gram's stain may govern the choice of agent.

Antibiotics may be solutions, ointments, or powders. Solutions are the best form of antibiotics for wound antibiotics, and ointments are the next best form. Powders are the least desirable form of antibiotics.

A 0.1% gentamicin sulfate ointment (Garamycin®—Schering) has been proven to be effective for wound treatment. The ointment is especially effective against gram-negative bacteria.

The triple antibiotic bacitracin, polymixin, and neomycin is effective as an antibiotic ointment (Neosporin®—Burroughs Wellcome). Because these antibiotics are poorly absorbed by tissue, they should be applied early in wound management before organisms invade the tissue. These antibiotics reportedly enhance wound epithelialization.

Silver sulfadiazine (Silividone®—Marion Laboratories) is an effective topical antibacterial ointment. This ointment is effective against gram-negative and gram-positive bacteria and is especially effective against

Pseudomonas organisms. Silver sulfadiazine is used primarily for burns but can be used for other wounds. It reportedly enhances wound epithelialization.

Nitrofurazone dressing (Furacin® Soluble Dressing—Eaton Pharmaceuticals) is a common antibacterial compound that is used in veterinary surgery. Nitrofurazone dressing reportedly slows epithelialization; however, studies at Auburn University have not indicated such a finding.

Other Topical Medications

Aloe vera has become a popular topical dermatologic medication. Aloe vera contains a salicylate-type compound with antiprostaglandin effects. Prostaglandins are active in inflammation, and inflammation is a necessary stage of the wound healing process. Therefore, aloe vera should not be used on full-thickness skin wounds because it inhibits the inflammatory stage of healing and slows healing. An aloe vera preparation (Dermaide Aloe®—Dermaide Research) can be used in the early stages after a partial-thickness burn to prevent tissue ischemia by inhibiting prostaglandins and thromboxanes.

Live yeast cell derivative (LYCD) has been found to be effective in stimulating tissue oxygen consumption, epithelialization, and collagen synthesis. This over-the-counter hemorrhoid medication (Preparation H®—Whitehall Laboratories) is the commercial form of this drug. It has been used effectively at Auburn University to treat some open wounds.

An organic acid combination of malic, benzoic, and salicylic acids (Derma-Clens®—SmithKline Beecham) is commercially available for wound therapy. The acid pH of this combination reportedly enhances fluid absorption by devitalized tissue, leading to separation and subsequent removal of devitalized tissue from the wound. The low pH also discourages microbial growth.

Enzymatic debridement may be used as an adjunct to wound lavage and surgical debridement. It is indicated for wound debridement on animals that are poor anesthetic risks for surgical debridement and for debriding wounds in which surgical debridement may result in damage to healthy tissue. The enzymatic debriding agent I prefer (Granulex-V®—SmithKline Beecham) contains trypsin as the debriding agent. Part II of this two-part presentation, which will appear in an upcoming issue of *Veterinary Technician*, discusses bandaging of wounds.

BIBLIOGRAPHY

Bojrab MJ: *A Handbook of Veterinary Wound Management*. Boston, Boston Kendall Co, 1981.

Bojrab MJ: Wound management. *Mod Vet Pract* 63:867, 1982.

Lee AH, Swaim SF, McGuire JA, et al: Effects of nonadherent dressing materials on the healing of open wounds in dogs. *JAVMA* 190:416, 1987.

Lee AH, Swaim SF, McGuire JA, et al: Effects of chlorhexidine diacetate, povidone-iodine, and polyhydroxydine on wound healing. *JAAHA* 24:77, 1987.

Lee AH, Swaim SF, Yang SL, et al: The effects of petrolatum, polyethylene glycol, nitrofurasone, and hydroactive dressing on open wound healing. *JAAHA* 22:443, 1986.

Swaim SF, Henderson RA: *Small Animal Wound Management*. Philadelphia, Lea & Febiger, 1990.

Swaim SF, Lee AH: Topical wound medications: A review. *JAVMA* 190:1588, 1987.

Swaim SF: Bandages and topical agents. *Vet Clin North Am [Small Anim Pract]* 20:47, 1990.

Swaim SF: New concepts in wound management. Tijds. Voor Diergen. *J R Neth Vet Assoc* 112(suppl 1):56S–58S, 1987.

REFERENCE

1. Peacock E E Jr: *Wound Repair*, ed 3. Philadelphia, WB Saunders Co, 1984.

UPDATE

A dermal wound cleanser (Ultra-Klenz®—Allerderm, Inc.) can be sprayed on a wound to help remove debris and particulate matter. This cleanser is a mild emulsifying detergent solution that can be used on horses, dogs, and cats.

A wound treatment gel containing allantoin and acemannen (Dermal Wound Gel™—Allerderm, Inc.) can be used as a topical medication. This medication has been shown to enhance the healing of open wounds on dog paw pads, especially during the first seven days of healing.[1]

REFERENCE

1. Swaim SF, Riddell KP, McGuire JA: Effects of topical medications on the healing of open pad wounds in dogs. *JAAHA* 28:1, 1992.

The Management of Wounds. Part II.
Practical Guidelines for Wound Bandaging*

CRITICAL CARE COMPANION ANIMAL is a regular feature of *Veterinary Technician®*. This month's contributing author is Steven F. Swaim, DVM, MS, Scott Ritchey Research Center, College of Veterinary Medicine, Auburn University, Auburn, Alabama.

The basic principles of wound management were discussed in Part I of this two-part presentation. These principles include wound lavage, the apparatus and solutions necessary for lavage, and the use of systemic and topical antibacterials. Part II focuses on the techniques and materials necessary for bandaging wounds.

Bandaging Open Wounds

Some wounds should be allowed to heal as open wounds. Usually, these are large wounds, wounds that have extensive tissue damage, and/or wounds that are infected. Bandages

*Adapted with permission from the proceedings of the First International Veterinary Emergency and Critical Care Symposium, San Antonio, Texas, September 1988; and the Western States Veterinary Conference, Las Vegas, Nevada, February 1989.

play a role in the therapy of open wounds because bandages can provide a good wound-healing environment. Some naturally occurring bandages are scabs, eschars, and blisters.

In human surgery, most of the bandaging of open wounds entails bandaging split-thickness skin graft donor sites in an effort to enhance epithelialization of the wound. In veterinary surgery, the wounds usually are full-thickness, and contraction and epithelialization are necessary for adequate healing. Bandages can provide the proper environment for successful management of such wounds.

Bandages are composed of three layers: the contact (primary) layer, the intermediate (secondary) layer, and the outer (tertiary) layer. Each layer has a specific function and specific properties.

Contact Bandage Layer

When a wound has traumatized and contaminated or infected tissue, the contact layer should adhere to the tissues. The wound should be surgically debrided and flushed with copious antibacterial lavage solution. Debride-

ment is completed with an adherent contact layer bandage. The contact layer should be a wide, open-mesh gauze sponge that has no cotton filler.

Dry-to-dry bandages should be applied to wounds that have loose necrotic tissue, foreign material, and a copious low-viscosity exudate that does not aggregate. Although these bandages become wet as wound fluid is absorbed, they should be dry when first applied. As fluid evaporates from the bandage, the bandage returns to a dry state. Dry-to-dry bandages remove fluid and debris and provide a dry environment, which retards bacterial growth. The primary disadvantage is the pain induced at the time of bandage removal. Moistening the contact layer with lidocaine just before removal may reduce the pain.

Wet-to-dry bandages are another type of adherent bandage. Adherent contact layer bandages are indicated for wounds with loose necrotic tissue, foreign material, and a viscous exudate (coagulum). These bandages are applied wet to reduce the viscosity of exudate so that it can be absorbed. After the absorbed fluid has evaporated

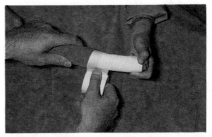

Figure 1—Taping a tightly rolled hand towel. (From Swaim SF, Henderson RA: *Small Animal Wound Management*. Philadelphia, Lea & Febiger, 1990, p 78. Reprinted with permission.)

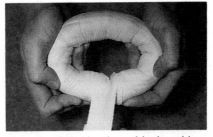

Figure 2—Taped hand towel is shaped into the form of a doughnut. (From Swaim SF, Henderson RA: *Small Animal Wound Management*. Philadelphia, Lea & Febiger, 1990, p 78. Reprinted with permission.)

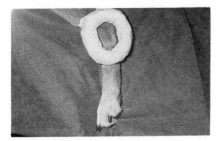

Figure 3—Doughnut-shaped bandage is taped in place with the hole over an area that is susceptible to the formation of decubital ulcers. (From Swaim SF, Henderson RA: *Small Animal Wound Management*. Philadelphia, Lea & Febiger, 1990, p 78. Reprinted with permission.)

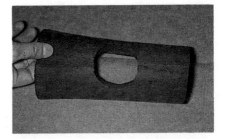

Figure 4—A piece of foam rubber pipe insulation that is split lengthwise. Note the hole, which will accommodate the olecranon area. (From Swaim SF, Henderson RA: *Small Animal Wound Management*. Philadelphia, Lea & Febiger, 1990, p 78. Modified with permission.)

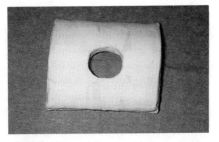

Figure 5—Two pieces of pipe insulation taped together.

Figure 6—Thick cast padding placed over the flexion surface of the radiohumeral joint.

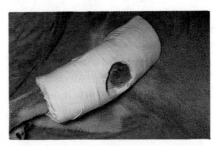

Figure 7—Cast padding and foam rubber pads taped in place, with the hole in the pads over the olecranon area. (From Swaim SF, Henderson RA: *Small Animal Wound Management*. Philadelphia, Lea & Febiger, 1990, p 78. Reprinted with permission.)

and the bandage is dry, it is removed. The advantages of wet bandages are that (1) water-soluble antibacterial compounds can be incorporated into the bandage; (2) the viscosity of exudate is reduced, which improves absorption; (3) eschars are softened; (4) necrotic tissue and debris are removed; and (5) an environment that is conducive to wound healing (i.e., a moist environment) is provided. The disadvantages of wet bandages are that (1) the moist environment is also conducive to bacterial growth; (2) the possibility of tissue maceration exists if the bandage is too wet; (3) if cold fluids are used to wet the bandage, discomfort may result; (4) bacteria can be carried inward toward the wound if the bandage is too wet; and (5) the animal will experience some discomfort if the bandage is removed after it has dried.

Nonadherent contact layer bandages should be used when wounds are in the repair stage of healing. These bandages allow absorption of excess fluid and retention of some fluid to enhance wound healing. Nonadherent bandages are available commercially. They can also be prepared by autoclaving gauze sponges with petrolatum, but this method results in inconsistent coating of the sponges with petrolatum. In addition, petrolatum has been demonstrated to slow wound epithelialization.

Polyethylene glycol–soaked sponges can be used as nonadherent bandages. These sponges do not interfere with epithelialization. A nonadherent bandage that has the additional benefit of being antibacterial can be made by using sponges coated with nitrofurazone ointment with a polyethylene glycol base (Furacin®—Norden Laboratories).

Intermediate Bandage Layer

The main function of the intermediate bandage layer is to absorb and store deleterious agents. The secondary bandage layer should be absorbent; be thick to provide storage of wound fluid, padding, and some immobilization; and remain in contact with the contact layer. This layer should not be applied with excessive pressure. The relative dryness provided by the secondary layer helps retard bacterial growth.

Outer Bandage Layer

The primary function of the outer bandage layer is to hold the other layers in place. Materials that can be used for this layer include nonstretch gauze, two-way stretch material, and adhesive tapes. Adhesive tapes can be porous, waterproof, or elastic. I prefer porous tape. Such tape allows evaporation of fluids from the underlying bandage layers; however, exogenous liquids (e.g., urine) may also be carried inward through the bandage. Waterproof tape keeps exogenous fluid out of a bandage but also may retain fluid within the bandage, which causes tissue maceration. Elastic tapes are used for pressure bandages.

Pressure Bandages

Pressure bandages should be used to control minor hemorrhage (24 to 48 hours), passive edema, excess granulation tissue, and movement. Cotton, gauze, and tape do not make good pressure bandages. Elastic bandages apply dynamic pressure but should be used with caution. Excessive pressure can impinge on nerves and impair circulation, resulting in slough. Signs of impending problems associated with the use of pressure bandages include swelling and/or hypothermia of tissue distal to the bandage, dryness, odor, staining of the bandage over a bony prominence, and/or licking and chewing.

Pressure Relief Bandages

Doughnut-shaped bandages and pipe-insulation bandages can be used to relieve pressure over convex surfaces and to help provide a good wound-healing environment. To construct a doughnut-shaped bandage, a hand towel should be rolled tightly and tape wrapped around the roll (Figure 1). The rolled towel is then formed in the shape of an appropriately sized doughnut to fit around the wound. After cutting the towel to the proper length, the ends are taped together to form the bandage (Figure 2). The bandage is centered over the wound and taped to the surrounding skin (Figure 3).

Pipe-insulation bandages can be used over the olecranon to prevent pressure on this area. Two or three pieces of foam rubber pipe-insulation of an appropriate diameter and length are split lengthwise, and a hole is cut in the center of each piece (Figure 4). The pieces are stacked together and taped (Figure 5). Cast padding is used to pad the cranial surface of the radiohumeral joint (Figure 6). This area is padded well, and a piece of metal splint material can be placed over the padding to help prevent flexion of the joint. The foam rubber pad is placed with the hole over the olecranon. The cast padding, splint, and foam rubber padding are taped in place (Figure 7). The bulky padding and splint on the flexion surface of the radiohumeral joint preclude joint flexion and prevent the patient from lying in sternal recumbency. This, in combination with the foam rubber padding around the olecranon, prevents the patient from placing pressure on the olecranon area. Because these bandages tend to slip distally, particularly in obese dogs, a spica-type bandage around the thorax and fixation of the pipe-insulation bandage to the spica-type bandage may be necessary.

Occlusive Bandages

Occlusive bandages maintain a moist environment, which improves epithelialization. The drawback, however, is that the moisture and heat that are retained promote bacterial growth. An occlusive bandage material that is available for veterinary use is Dermaheal® (Solvay Animal Health). It should be used on wounds that have a good granulation tissue bed and minimal fluid production. Another occlusive bandage is BioDres® (Dermatologics for Veterinary Medicine).

BIBLIOGRAPHY

Bojrab MJ: *A Handbook of Veterinary Wound Management.* Boston, Boston Kendall Co, 1981.

Bojrab MJ: Wound management. *Mod Vet Pract* 63:867, 1982.

Lee AH, Swaim SF, McGuire JA, et al: Effects of nonadherent dressing materials on the healing of open wounds in dogs. *JAVMA* 190:416, 1987.

Lee AH, Swaim SF, Yang SL, et al: The effects of petrolatum, polyethylene glycol, nitrofurazone and hydroactive dressing on open wound healing. *JAAHA* 22:443, 1986.

Swaim SF: Bandages and topical agents. *Vet Clin North Am [Small Anim Pract]* 20:47, 1990.

Swaim SF: New concepts in wound management. *Tijdschr Voor Diergeneeskd* 112(Suppl 1):56S–58S, 1987.

Swaim SF: The effects of dressings and bandages on wound healing. *Semin Vet Med Surg (Small Anim)* 4:274, 1989.

Swaim SF, Henderson RA: *Small Animal Wound Management.* Philadelphia, Lea & Febiger, 1990.

Swaim SF, Wilhalf D: The physics, physiology and chemistry of bandaging open wounds. *Compend Contin Educ Pract Vet* 7(2):146, 1985.

UPDATE

Calcium alginate wound dressing (C-Stat®—KenVet) can be used as the contact bandage layer. The portion of this felt-like dressing that is over a wound interacts with the wound fluid, forming a sodium alginate gel over the wound. This gelling process wicks fluid into the overlying dressings while maintaining a moist environment that enhances wound healing. The gel is washed away with saline when the bandage is changed and a new dressing is applied. The gel has no antibacterial properties as such, but it is possible that bacteria become entrapped in the gel and are washed away when the bandage is changed.

A foam sponge bandage (Hydrasorb® Foam Sponge—KenVet) is available for veterinary use. It absorbs excess wound fluid while maintaining a moist wound environment without a gel forming over the wound. The dressing is nonadherent.

When applying a wrap-around pressure bandage, it should be remembered that the amount of pressure within the bandage is dependent on four factors: (1) the tension applied to the dressing at the time of the application, (2) the number of layers applied, (3) the degree of overlap between successive layers, and (4) the curvature of the bandaged area. The smaller the diameter, the greater the resultant pressure is likely to be. When bandaging a limb, care should be used when moving from an area of larger diameter to one of smaller diameter.

BIBLIOGRAPHY

1. Swaim SF: Bandaging open wounds: What is new? *Proceedings of the Third International Veterinary Emergency and Critical Care Symposium,* 1992, pp.443–447.

Bandage Management in Small Animals

Kristine Kazmierczak, RVT
Instructor, Anesthesia
Veterinary Technology Program
Purdue University
West Lafayette, Indiana

In veterinary medicine, wound protection and support are two principal reasons for using bandages. Properly applied and managed, a bandage can reduce healing time, prevent secondary wound infections, and provide comfort and relief to the patient. On the other hand, a bandage that has been improperly applied or is incorrectly maintained may actually be detrimental to the patient's well-being. This article describes the basic principles of bandage management in small animals, techniques for identifying and preventing potential problems, and methods of home care for bandages.

Indications

Although all situations vary, there are specific indications for the use of bandages in small animal patients (Table I). A bandage can be used to maintain the proper environment for wound healing by keeping the wound clean and free of contaminants. If the animal is confined to a cage, the bandage can prevent contamination from urine, feces, or water. A bandage can also be used to prevent the patient from chewing and licking the affected area. As a protective covering, bandages can prevent secondary infections that would delay healing. Support can be provided to injured tissues, or edema associated with fractures or blunt-trauma injuries can be controlled by a bandage. On occasion, it is necessary to provide temporary support to a severely injured or fractured extremity while the patient's immediate treatment needs are attended to. Properly applied and maintained, limb bandages can provide substantial relief from pain, control edema, and prevent self-induced wound trauma. In other instances, such as following surgical repair of a fractured leg, a bandage may be applied to limit limb use during the first postoperative hours. Additionally, a bandage can be applied to secure a catheter for administration of fluids. This is most commonly seen with neck bandages to secure jugular vein catheters and limb bandages for cephalic vein catheters during intravenous therapy.

When large areas of skin have been undermined or large areas of tissue have been removed resulting in the formation of tissue dead spaces, a bandage can be strategically applied to prevent the development of seromas. Drains placed into major body cavities can also be secured to the patient with a bandage.

Bandage Materials

The bandaging materials most commonly used in veterinary medicine are gauze sponges, gauze, elastic gauze, roll cotton, adhesive tape, elastic tape, roll padding, nonadhering sponges, and nonadhering elastic wrap. The trade names and manufacturers of the materials used most often are listed in Table II.

The type and purpose of a bandage will determine the combination of materials to be used. For example, to prevent development of a postoperative seroma, the bandage may consist of gauze sponges placed along the incision line for absorption, roll cotton and elastic gauze to hold them in place, followed by either elastic tape or elastic wrap for mild pressure. In the case of a granulating wound, the same bandaging materials can be used except that nonadhering gauze sponges should always be used in place of gauze sponges. Nonadhering sponges lessen the disturbance of a granulating tissue bed each time the bandage is changed.

Originally published in Volume 3, Number 6, November/December 1982

TABLE I
INDICATIONS FOR BANDAGING

1. To protect a wound from the environment
2. To prevent self-trauma
3. To provide support to tissues
4. To control edema
5. To maintain a proper environment for healing of an open unsutured wound
6. To restrict use of a limb
7. To support indwelling catheters and drains
8. To prevent seromas

General Concepts of Bandaging

Application and care of the bandage are important factors if the bandage is to achieve the desired results. When bandaging a limb, the most important rule is to apply the bandage material spirally to prevent pressure rings. A pressure ring can develop if bandaging materials have been applied in a tight, circular fashion or if a bandage has slipped from its original position. If bandaging material encircles a part of the body and causes a constriction, severe edema can occur within 24 hours.[4]

A bandage has not been applied too tightly if it is possible to slip two fingers under the edge of the bandage (Figure 1). This should always be checked. It is particularly important when bandaging the head and neck region, the thorax, the abdomen, and the limbs. This also applies when securing an intravenous catheter; if the bandage is too tight, venous circulation becomes obstructed and the fluids will not flow. When the limbs have been bandaged, the toes should be checked at least twice daily for signs of edema or coldness. If this occurs, adequate blood flow may have been interrupted by the bandage. The bandage should be removed or loosened and the patient rechecked.

There are important precautions that must be taken when using certain bandaging materials or when ban-

TABLE II
BANDAGE MATERIALS

Materials	Registered Trade Name	Manufacturer
Adhesive tape	Zonas®	Johnson & Johnson Products Inc.
	Orthaletic-Porous®	Parke-Davis
	Curity® Standard Porous	Kendall Corp.
Elastic gauze	Kling®	Johnson & Johnson Products Inc.
	Stretch Gauze	Parke-Davis
	Kerlix® Rolls	Kendall Corp.
Elastic tape	Elastikon	Johnson & Johnson Products Inc.
	Conform®	Kendall Corp.
	J-Flex	Pitman-Moore
Gauze	Absorbent Gauze Roll	Parke-Davis
	Gauze Roll	Kendall Corp.
	Nu-Gauze®	Johnson & Johnson Products Inc.
Nonadhering sponges	Release™	Johnson & Johnson Products Inc.
	Micro Pad™	3-M
	Telfa® Ouchless	Kendall Corp.
	Adaptic®	Johnson & Johnson Products Inc.
Roll cotton	Absorbent Cotton	Parke-Davis
	Red Cross Cotton	Johnson & Johnson Products Inc.
	Curity® Cotton Roll	Kendall Corp.
Roll padding	Sof-Rol®	Johnson & Johnson Products Inc.
	Specialist® Cast Padding	Johnson & Johnson Products Inc.
	New Webril® Orthopedic	Kendall Corp.
Self-adhesive elastic wrap	Vet-Wrap®	3-M Co.
	Coban®	3-M Co.
Sponges	Topper®	Johnson & Johnson Products Inc.
	Gauze Sponge	Parke-Davis
	Unisorb®	Parke-Davis
	Kerlix®	Kendall Corp.
	Sof-Wick®	Johnson & Johnson Products Inc.
Stretch bandage	Ace®	Becton Dickinson
	Dyna-Flex®	Johnson & Johnson Products Inc.
	Rediflex®	Parke-Davis
	Tensor® Elastic Bandage	Kendall Corp.

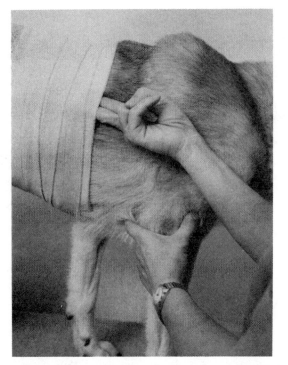

Figure 1—Two fingers slipped under the edge of the bandage ensure that it has not been applied too tightly.

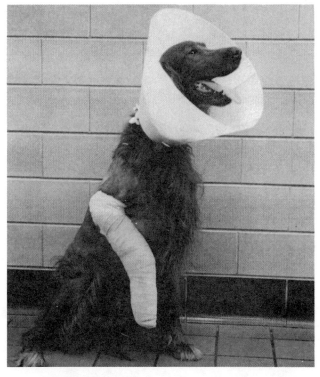

Figure 2—An Elizabethan collar can prevent the animal from chewing the bandage.

dages have been applied to certain body areas. When applying elastic tape, it should first be pulled off the roll in 6- to 12-inch increments and then applied to the underlying material. If it is applied with too much tension it can cause problems in the various body parts: peripheral limb edema may occur, dyspnea can result from a tight thoracic bandage, and difficulty swallowing or eating can stem from an improperly applied head or neck bandage.

Chafing caused by thoracic and abdominal bandages occurs most often in the axillary and groin areas. Talcum powder, medicated powder, or baking soda can be applied to relieve the irritation. Chafing may be prevented if the powder or baking soda is applied to the dry skin in the areas where the bandage is first applied.

The animal should be prevented from chewing, licking, or scratching the bandage. An Elizabethan collar (Figure 2) or side brace (Figure 3) may be necessary. Hobbles (Figure 4) can be used to prevent scratching at a thoracic, abdominal, head, or neck bandage. Persistent efforts by the patient to remove a bandage may be a signal that the bandage is causing substantial discomfort.

The reader is referred to Reference 1 for detailed instruction on the application of bandages.

Bandage Management
Limb

Indications for bandaging a limb include postoperative immobilization following fracture repair, protection

Figure 3—A side brace can prevent self-mutilation of a bandage in the pelvic or groin area.

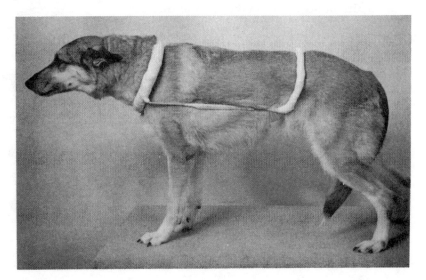

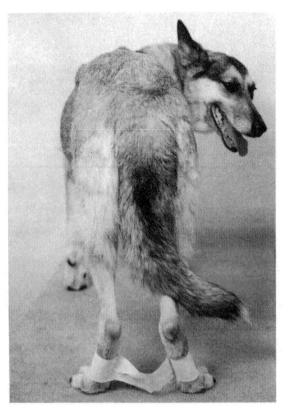

Figure 4—Hobbles can be used to prevent the animal from scratching at an abdominal, thoracic, or head and neck bandage.

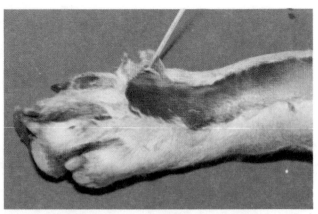

Figure 5—Gangrenous necrosis resulting from a bandage applied too tightly. Note superficial epithelial sloughing.

of a granulating wound, or stabilization of a limb during intravenous fluid therapy. A bandage commonly applied for temporary stabilization of a fracture until an animal is capable of undergoing surgery is a modified Robert Jones bandage. This bandage consists of several layers of roll cotton compressed tightly with elastic gauze and elastic tape. It should be noted that this is the only type of bandage in which elastic gauze and tape are applied tightly. The layers of cotton prevent constriction of the limb.

When bandaging the thigh, knee, upper forelimb, or elbow, the entire limb should be included. Application of the bandage should begin at the paw and continue proximally in a spiral fashion. This allows for even distribution of pressure along the limb and maintains venous return from the paw.

To ensure that the bandage has not been applied too tightly, two fingers should be slipped under the proximal end of the bandage. The toes should be checked twice a day for edema, coldness, or an offensive odor, all of which are warning signs of decreased venous return (Figure 5).

If the bandage has slipped from its original position due to the animal's movement or chewing, it may cause a pressure ring. If the bandage has slipped or the toes become edematous, remove it immediately.

Keeping a limb bandage dry and clean can be difficult when exercising a patient outside. A wet or soiled bandage is an excellent environment—warm, dark, and moist—for the growth of contaminate bacteria. Wound infection subsequent to moist dermatitis can result. Complications stemming from contaminated bandages can be avoided by taping a plastic bag around the limb while the animal is exercised outside. The protective cover can then be removed when the animal is returned inside. It is not advisable to use a rubber band to secure the bag, since it can slip and act as a pressure ring. If the bandage becomes wet, it should be removed immediately and a dry dressing should be reapplied.

Paw

The paw is normally bandaged following declawing of cats, dewclaw removal on dogs, or repair of lacerations to the toes or footpads.

To ensure that venous return from the paw is maintained, two fingers should easily slip under the proximal end of the bandage. Tape should be applied spirally to prevent pressure rings. When bandaging the paw, the accessory pad should also be included in the bandage. A small piece of cotton under the pad helps prevent irritation (Figure 6). Chafing can occur if the bandage is applied just under the accessory pad.

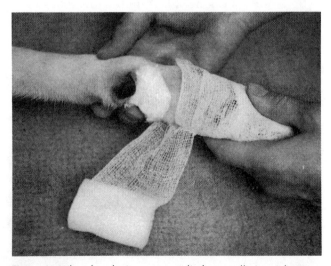

Figure 6—When bandaging a paw or limb, a small piece of cotton placed under the accessory pad can help prevent irritation due to skin-to-skin contact.

Head and Neck

The head and neck may be bandaged after ocular surgery, repair of an aural hematoma, or cervical-spinal' surgery; or to secure placement of a pharyngostomy tube or a jugular vein catheter.

Care must be taken not to restrict respiration or the ability to swallow or eat, or to impair vision (this may be unavoidable under certain circumstances). Again, to ensure that the bandage is not too tight, it should be easy to slip two fingers under each end of the bandage. If the bandage is too tight, the animal will show signs of dyspnea or difficulty swallowing, or it may scratch at the bandage. To correct this problem, the bandage can be cut to relieve the tension. Tape can then be placed over the cut bandage without any tension. This saves having to replace the entire bandage.

If the bandage loosens, it most frequently slips caudally. If this occurs, it should be removed immediately because it can restrict respiration.

Occasionally an animal will scratch at the bandage for no reason but to remove it. It may be necessary to put hobbles or an Elizabethan collar on the animal to prevent removal of the bandage.

Thorax

The thorax is most routinely bandaged when securing a chest drain, stabilizing fractured ribs, or protecting excessive wounds in this area.

The major concern when bandaging the thorax is to not impair respiratory movement. The tightness of the bandage can be checked by slipping two fingers under either end of the bandage. When applying the tape (especially elastic tape), it should be pulled off the roll and then placed onto the animal without any tension. If the animal shows signs of dyspnea, the bandage must be removed immediately. It may be too tight.

A common reason for failure of thoracic bandages is slippage of the bandage toward the abdomen. To help prevent this, the tape should be adhered to 1 to 1½ inches of hair at the cranial and caudal edges of the bandage. If the animal scratches at the bandage in an attempt to remove it, hobbles will be necessary.

Abdomen

Indications for bandaging the abdomen include radical mastectomy, surgery requiring radical dissection of the abdominal region, hernia repair, surgery that requires placement of a drain, or securing a gastrostomy tube (a tube placed into the stomach through the abdominal wall for feeding purposes).

To prevent the bandage from slipping caudally, it must be taped securely to the hair at the cranial end or even up on the chest. It should be easy to insert two fingers at either end of the bandage. If the bandage is too tight, it can impair respiration or cause discomfort.

When an animal is confined to a cage and is recumbent, a bandage can easily become contaminated with urine and feces. This can be avoided by placing the animal on a special cage rack. The rack elevates the animal 2 to 3 inches above the cage floor and allows for drainage of urine and feces (Figure 7).

In bandaging the abdomen of a male dog, the prepuce must not be included. The bandage should not interfere with the dog's ability to urinate (Figure 8).

Pelvis and Groin

A mastectomy, repair of perineal hernias, abscesses, wounds with drain placement, or pelvic surgery are a few of the situations requiring bandaging in the pelvic and groin area. This is perhaps the most difficult area to bandage.

The bandage should not be applied tightly. This is checked by slipping two fingers under the cranial edge of the bandage and where the bandage encircles the legs. Severe edema can occur in the legs, vulva, or scrotum if the bandage is too tight.

The bandage must not include the vulva, prepuce, scrotum, or anus (Figure 9). It should in no way impair the animal's ability to urinate or defecate. The bandage should be checked at least twice a day for dryness. If it becomes soiled with urine or feces, it must be changed. Placing the animal on a rack may aid in keeping the bandage dry.

To prevent the bandage from slipping caudally, apply tape to 1 to 1½ inches of hair around the cranial edge of the bandage.

Tail

Occasionally, the tail needs bandaging, such as with partial tail amputation, granulating wounds, or tumor removal. The major problem in tail bandaging is in securing the bandage. In animals with long tails, it may be necessary to apply the bandage 1 inch on either side of the lesion, or to the entire tail. In animals with docked tails, tape should be applied loosely around the tail head.

An Elizabethan collar or side brace may be necessary to prevent the animal from chewing the bandage off.

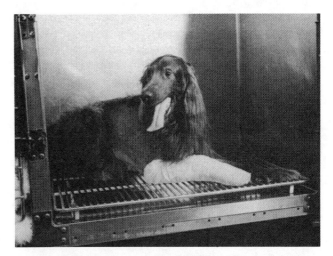

Figure 7—Elevating an animal on a rack allows for urine and feces drainage and helps keep the bandage dry.

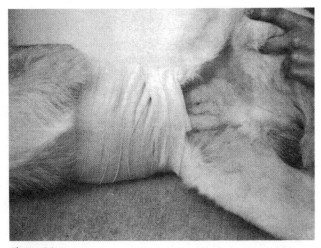

Figure 8A

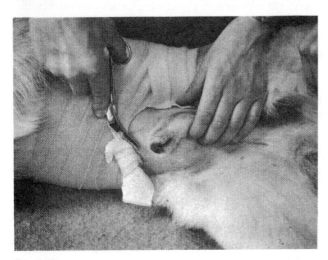

Figure 8B

Figure 8—(**A**) After the abdomen has been bandaged, (**B**) an opening should be cut in it to expose the prepuce.

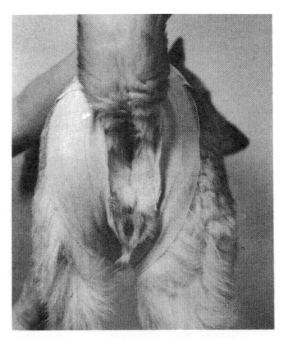

Figure 9A

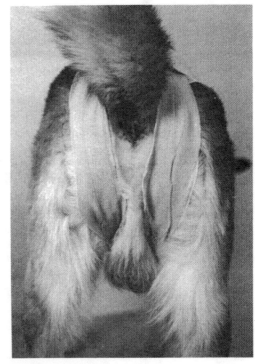

Figure 9B

Figure 9—When bandaging the pelvic and groin area, the anus should be exposed (**A**). Also, the vulva on a female (**A**) and the scrotum on a male (**B**) should be exposed.

Wound Healing

The process by which a wound can heal is divided into three general categories. First-intention healing occurs when the edges of the wound, after being brought into apposition, heal without complications and with minimal scar formation. An uncomplicated ovariohysterectomy incision is an example of first-intention healing. Bandaging may or may not be necessary; however, if a bandage is used, it should be changed every four to five days up to the tenth postoperative day.

A wound that heals by second-intention heals by wound contraction and epithelialization. Road abrasions, burns (chemical or thermal), and subcutaneous injections of certain drugs (e.g., barbiturates) are examples. As the wound heals, granulation tissue develops between the wound edges. Since these wounds require more time to heal than wounds that heal by first intention, bandages are often used to prevent contamination. Bandages should be changed every two to three days.

Third-intention healing is a two-step process. The wound is allowed to partially heal. It is then debrided, and the skin edges are surgically apposed. The new wound then heals by first-intention. These wounds are usually contaminated and require daily cleansing and protection. The bandage covering this type of wound should be changed at least daily for the first five to seven days to observe its progress. As healing progresses, the the bandage may be changed every two to three days until the time of surgery.

Although some wounds will heal without the aid of a bandage, other wounds, depending on location and severity, require a bandage. A bandage may be needed to prevent self-mutilation, prevent seroma formation, collect exudate from a draining wound, or protect an open, unsutured wound from contamination. The frequency with which the bandage is changed depends on the type of wound and the veterinarian's assessment of its progress.

Client Education

When an animal is discharged, the owner must be informed of how to properly care for the bandage and how to recognize complications. The client should be instructed to do the following:

1. Keep the bandage clean and dry. A plastic bag can be taped over the bandage when the animal is outside and removed when indoors so that the bandage can *breathe*.
2. Keep the animal relatively confined, and exercise it only on a leash.
3. Prevent mutilation.
4. Observe for edema, coldness of the toes, or an offensive odor from the bandage twice a day.
5. Notify the veterinarian immediately if any problems are observed.

Home-care instructions can be printed with the name of the clinic, the veterinarian, and the phone number and given to the client upon discharge of the patient. The veterinary technician can review this information with the client at the time that the animal is discharged.

Acknowledgment

The author is indebted to Dr. Richard B. Ford, School of Veterinary Medicine, North Carolina State University, for his editorial assistance; to Dr. Daniel C. Richardson, School of Veterinary Medicine, Purdue University, for the use of his photograph in Figure 5; and to Richard Kinsell, pharmacist, Purdue University, for his help with Table II.

REFERENCE

1. Knecht CD, Allen AR, Williams DM, Johnson JH: *Fundamental Techniques in Veterinary Surgery*, ed 3. Philadelphia, WB Saunders Co., 1987.

Physical Therapy in Small Animal Medicine Part I

Marsha Moore, RVT
Southway Animal Hospital
Marion, Indiana

Jan Rasmussen, RVT
Instructor, Clinical Veterinary Technology
Department of Small Animal Clinics
Purdue University
West Lafayette, Indiana

The veterinary technician assumes numerous roles within a small animal practice. Responsibilities include performing laboratory tests, assisting in surgery, educating clients, taking radiographs, and, one of the most important responsibilities, providing nursing care to small animal patients. The physical and mental well-being of the patient is dependent on the quality of care it receives, whether its condition is caused by trauma, disease, or surgery. High-quality nursing care is essential whether specific rehabilitation is needed or not.

Physical therapy is an excellent form of treatment which can expedite the rehabilitation process. Although physical therapy is used extensively in human medicine, it is underutilized in veterinary medicine. This article will acquaint the veterinary technician with the basic modes and uses of physical therapy, emphasizing management of the recumbent patient.

Physical therapy is the treatment of disease by physical agents such as light, heat, cold, water, electricity, massage, and mechanical agents.[1] When physical therapy is properly administered, it can expedite healing of injured tissue, prevent disability, and help restore normal function. Physical therapy can be utilized for the rehabilitation of animals with diseases of bones, muscles, joints, nerves, and skin, and dislocations, fractures, arthritis, paresis, paralysis, infections, and decubital ulcers. Physical therapy increases physical strength, improves mental status, and decreases hospitalization time, which reduces the cost to the animal's owner.[2-4]

Many modes of physical therapy are easy to perform and inexpensive. Others are complicated and require expensive equipment. No matter how simple or extensive the therapy is, the most important factor determining its quality is the person administering it. A good therapist must have a great deal of patience and an optimistic attitude. He or she must have a genuine interest in each animal and its welfare. In order for the therapy to be of optimum value, the technician must be able to make careful observations which will aid in assessing the progress of the patient.

Massage

The simplest form of physical therapy is massage; it requires no equipment and is easy to do. In massage, the hands and fingers are used to manipulate the soft tissues of the body.

The primary objective of massage is to increase blood flow through the massaged tissues. Massage also enhances the flow of lymph from tissue spaces, providing quicker elimination of wastes and more nutrients to the site. Massage can decrease the likelihood of *fibrosis,* which is an abnormal formation of adhesions between connective tissue layers;[5] the friction and pressure produced cause a mechanical stretching and dissipation of the fibers under the skin. Massage can loosen and stretch contracted tendons. It also has a beneficial effect on the nervous system and the peripheral nerves[2] because it is relaxing.

A massage medium may be used to facilitate the therapy. Lubricants are used to soften skin or scar tissue and to reduce friction. Some commonly used media are mineral oil, cold cream, olive oil, and petroleum jelly. Powders such as talc or baby powder are used more frequently than lubricants in veterinary medicine because they provide the same effect and are easier to remove. It is important to place the medium on the hands and then massage it into the animal's skin rather than applying it directly to the skin. The media should not be applied to open wounds. At the conclusion of the massage session, the lubricant can be removed with isopropyl alcohol.

There are five factors that the therapist must consider when administering massage.[2] These are

1. Direction of the stroke
2. Pressure of the stroke
3. Duration of the massage
4. Rate and rhythm of the stroke
5. Frequency of massage

The factors will vary depending on the size of the animal and the area treated, the condition of the animal, and the animal's response to and progress with the treatment.

Specific conditions that massage can benefit are

- Tight and contracted tendons, ligaments, and muscles
- Subacute and chronic traumatic and inflammatory conditions
- Peripheral nerve injuries
- Scar tissue
- Subacute and chronic edema

Specific conditions for which massage is contraindicated are

- Acute or inflammatory processes of soft tissues, bones, and joints
- Fractures
- Sprains
- Foreign bodies under the skin
- Hemorrhage or lymphangitis
- Advanced skin diseases

There are three basic types of massage techniques: effleurage, pétrissage, and friction.[2] Whichever method is used, the animal's tolerance level for pain must not be exceeded.

Effleurage, or stroking, is a gentle massage which precedes either pétrissage or friction massage. Effleurage accustoms the animal to the touch of the therapist, allowing it to relax before a deeper form of massage is applied. The patient is massaged from the periphery of the limb or affected area to the center. Effleurage can be done with a light or heavy stroke, but uniform pressure is required. A light stroke at a rate of 15 strokes per minute should be applied for a sedative effect. A heavy stroke at 5 strokes per minute should be applied to enhance draining of veins and lymph channels. The length of time that effleurage should be administered depends on the animal's condition and size. In general, a 10-minute session should prepare the animal for more extensive massage therapy.

Pétrissage, a second type of massage, is also called *kneading* or *compression*. Pétrissage is used primarily on muscle groups, individual muscles, or a part of a muscle to enhance circulation and stretch muscles, tendons, adhesions, and contractures.[2] The muscle is compressed from side to side as the hands move up it, always in the direction of venous return (toward the heart). The procedure should be gentle and never forceful enough to cause protective contraction of the leg.

The third type of massage is *friction*. It is used to aid absorption of local effusions and loosen superficial scar tissue and adhesions. In friction massage, the skin is moved over underlying tissue in small, circular, rhythmic motions while pressure is applied across the tendon or adhesion to encourage collagen to be laid down in the proper direction. The frequency and duration of friction massage varies with the animal's condition and size.

Exercise

Another simple and relatively inexpensive form of physical therapy is exercise. Therapeutic exercise is used to strengthen, improve, or maintain the function of the musculoskeletal system. Exercise can aid in improving the debilitated animal's balance, stability, coordination, and cardiovascular and respiratory function. Two important effects of exercise are increased endurance and increased range of motion of the limbs.[6]

There are two types of exercise used in physical therapy of small animals—passive and active.

Passive Exercise

Passive exercise can be employed for the benefit of the patient that is paralyzed or very weak or that has fractures. Passive exercise is accomplished by a therapist with no activity on the part of the patient. Each affected joint is put through its normal range of motion 5 to 10 times per treatment without any muscle contraction by the animal. This type of exercise helps prevent joint freezing and disuse atrophy. Passive exercise can also be used on postoperative patients, an example being a patient with intervertebral disk disease.[6] Intervertebral

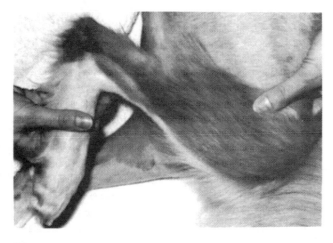

Figure 1A

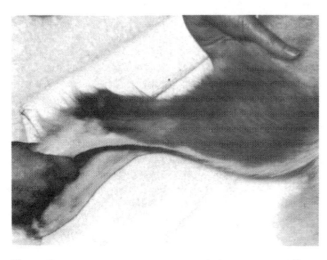

Figure 1B

Figure 1—(**A** and **B**) The technique used to support the rear leg during passive exercise therapy is illustrated.

disk disease patients should have the hindlimbs flexed and extended for 10-minute sessions several times daily (Figure 1A and B). There should never be any forced motion out of the animal's normal range of motion when using passive exercise.

Active Exercise

The most beneficial form of exercise is active exercise. Active exercise entails voluntary muscle contraction by the patient and includes many types of exercise from walking to swimming. Some patients may be willing to exercise on their own, but the reluctant patient may require some stimulation and support.

Many devices are available that provide the added support and assistance the nonambulatory animal needs. One such device is an exercise cart. This type of cart is available commercially (Figure 2) or it can be constructed from inexpensive aluminum rods and lawn mower wheels (Figure 3).[6] The cart supports the animal's torso, thereby allowing limb movement and exercise for patients that are unable to support their own

weight. Carts are especially useful in rehabilitation of patients with temporary posterior paralysis.

If an exercise cart is not available or is not well tolerated by the patient, a sling can be made with bath towels (Figure 4). The towels should not be allowed to pull against the top of the thigh because this will impede leg motion. Tailing exercise (Figure 5) can also be used intermittently with the exercise cart to prevent dependency of the animal on the cart. Care must be taken to grasp the tail at the base to prevent injury with this method.

Underwater Exercise

Another method of providing support for an animal with motion difficulties is with underwater exercise. This is indicated for the patient that has difficulty standing and balancing. The physical properties of water buoyancy and hydrostatic pressure provide the animal with support. Water movement or turbulence can be added to create a massage effect.

Buoyancy provides a lifting effect. The animal's body, when immersed in water, weighs less than it does out of water. Thus, voluntary exercise becomes possible for an animal that would otherwise be unable to stand. The animal may be able to stand and walk sooner than it would if underwater therapy were not done.

Hydrostatic pressure is the force felt on the body when immersed in water. Molecules of water *push* on the part of the animal's body that is immersed. The hydrostatic pressure increases with the depth of the water. Because of this pressure, thoracic expansion may be compromised; therefore, underwater exercise must be used with caution in patients with respiratory or cardiac insufficiencies.

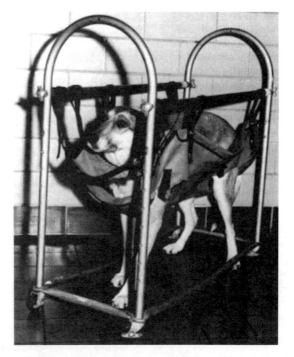

Figure 2—A dog with posterior paresis is supported in an exercise cart.

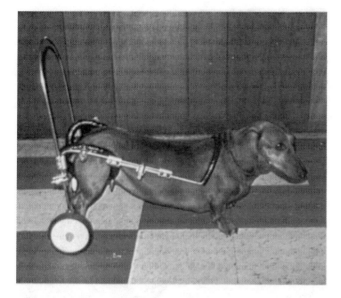

Figure 3—A custom-made cart is used to exercise a dachshund with intervertebral disk disease.

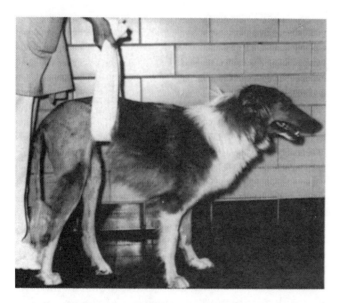

Figure 4—A collie with a pelvic injury is exercised using a bath towel as a sling.

The temperature of the water should be 102° to 105°F.[7] With warm-water therapy the animal gains as well as produces heat during the exercise period. These two combined factors cause an increase in peripheral blood supply due to dilatation of the superficial blood vessels. This, in turn, causes increased heart and metabolic rates.

Animals undergoing underwater therapy must never be left unattended—the possibility of drowning should always be kept in mind. If the patient has a neck or extremity weakness, a sling arrangement should be used for support.

Another patient safety consideration is fear. If the patient is afraid of water, the first few therapy sessions should concentrate on acclimating it to the water.

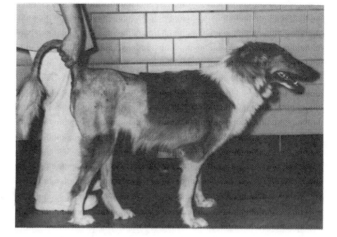

Figure 5—Animals with neurological deficits in the rear legs can be exercised by *tailing*.

A patient with an elevated temperature should not be treated with warm-water therapy until its temperature has been normal for at least 72 hours.

A povidone-iodine concentrate can be added to the water to decrease the possibility of transmitting infections from one animal to another.[8] The concentrate can also help prevent urine scald, infection of decubital ulcers, and superficial pyodermas.

Whirlpools—The *whirlpool* is an important mode of underwater exercise that is created by turbulence or movement of water. This can be accomplished with an electric turbine ejector and aerator (Figure 6), which circulates an air and water mixture. Portable agitators are available and are adaptable for use in almost any tank, bathtub, or pool. Stainless steel tanks are made commercially and are practical for veterinary hospitals because they are easily cleaned and disinfected; however, a bathtub can work just as effectively.

A nonskid surface should be placed on the bottom of the tub for the weight-bearing patient. The water temperature should be from 102° to 105°F. The turbine

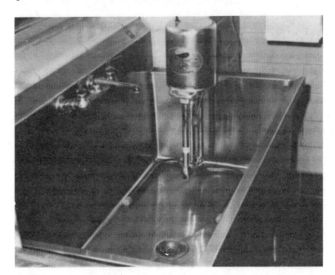

Figure 6—An electric turbine ejector in a bathtub can be used to provide whirlpool therapy.

must be grounded and left off until the water is in the tank and the patient is safely positioned in the tub. The air and water control valves can be adjusted to the desired pressure, direction, and height of water. Contrary to popular belief, the turbine should be directed so that the water is emitted in a direction *away* from the affected area of the patient's body. After each therapy session the water should be drained and the tub disinfected.

The whirlpool treatments should be scheduled after the animal has eliminated feces and urine to avoid contaminating the whirlpool bath. In general, the length of the treatment should be about 20 minutes; it should not exceed 30 minutes.[8]

The effects of whirlpool baths are the same as those of underwater exercise. In addition, whirlpools combine the effects of gentle massage and superficial heat. The swirling action of the water helps to clean and debride damaged tissues, thereby combating infections. Dirt, pus, and necrotic tissue are removed. Scar tissue is softened. Metabolism, respiration, and the mobility of extremities are increased.

Whirlpools are indicated for patients with the following conditions:

- Fractures in the late stages of healing
- Arthritis
- Stiff joints
- Adhesions
- Dislocations
- Muscle spasms
- Amputations
- Subcute and chronic inflammatory disease
- Diseases associated with decubitus
- Dermatological disorders[9]

In treating animals with dermatological disorders, the water aids healing of affected skin by removing exudates, crusts, scales, bacteria, and debris by cleansing wounds and fistulas. The whirlpool therapy also allays pain and pruritus associated with skin disorders. The water softens the keratin of the skin and promotes epithelialization.

Whirlpool therapy is contraindicated for animals affected with any of the following conditions:

- Peripheral vascular disease
- Acute injuries
- Acute inflammation
- Recent surgery
- Acute edema
- Fever
- Marked circulatory disturbances
- Cardiac or respiratory disorders

Patients with circulatory disorders may have decreased ability to dissipate heat. The technician must be extremely careful with these patients to avoid overheating.

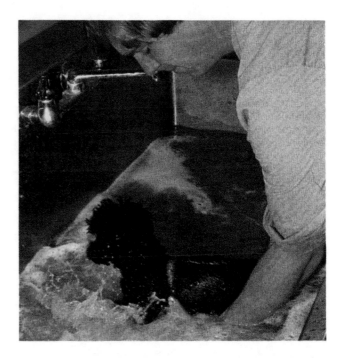

Figure 7—Swimming is an excellent form of physical therapy that can be administered in the hospital or at home.

Swimming—Swimming is good exercise for those animals that require more extensive exercise for rehabilitation or that are in the end phase of the rehabilitation period. With swimming, the animal is forced to move continuously and the decreased gravity pull allows the animal to increase its range of motion.

Small patients can swim in a bathtub in the veterinary hospital and continue the therapy at home under owner supervision (Figure 7). Children's wading pools offer an inexpensive alternative for larger patients. For bigger pets, a larger pool is necessary.

This article is the first in a two-part series on the use of physical therapy in small animal medicine and the role of the veterinary technician in physical therapy. Part II of this article will describe additional methods of physical therapy and management of the recumbent animal.

REFERENCES

1. Wittick WG: *Canine Orthopedics.* Philadelphia, Lea & Febiger, 1974, pp 441-448.
2. Downer AH: *Physical Therapy for Animals.* Springfield, IL, Charles C Thomas, 1978.
3. Downer AH: Physical therapy in the management of long bone fractures in small animals. *Vet Clin North Am* 5(2): 157-164, 1975.
4. Hoerlein BF: *Canine Neurology.* Philadelphia, WB Saunders Co, 1974, p 342.
5. Gartland JJ: *Fundamentals of Orthopedics.* Philadelphia, WB Saunders Co, 1974, p. 407.
6. Trotter EJ: Canine intervertebral disk disease, in Kirk RW (ed): *Current Veterinary Therapy V.* Philadelphia, WB Saunders Co, 1974, pp 666-673.
7. Downer AH: Underwater exercise for animals. *Mod Vet Pract* 60:115-118, 1979.
8. Downer AH: Whirlpool therapy for animals. *Mod Vet Pract* 58:39-42, 1977.
9. Muller GH, Kirk RW: *Small Animal Dermatology.* Philadelphia, WB Saunders Co, 1976, pp 182-185.

Physical Therapy in Small Animal Medicine Part II

Marsha Moore, RVT
Southway Animal Hospital
Marion, Indiana

Jan Rasmussen, RVT
Instructor, Clinical Veterinary Technology
Department of Small Animal Clinics
Purdue University
West Lafayette, Indiana

Part I of this two-part series on physical therapy discussed some basic modes of physical therapy. This article will describe additional physical therapy methods. Special emphasis will be placed on management of the recumbent animal.

Pretreatment Considerations

Before administering therapy to an animal, the therapist should review its history and medical status, noting any special precautions that should be taken. The therapist should discuss the prescribed treatment with the veterinarian to ensure that the proper treatment is administered. The patient's attitude should also be evaluated before treatment. The aggressive, depressed, or frightened animal requires special consideration.

The patient should be examined and any open wounds, scars, edema, or new skin formation noted. If the patient is to receive postoperative therapy, a waiting period of three to seven days may be mandatory to allow healing at the incision site; this allows a fibrin seal to cover the wound.[1]

Before initiating therapy, all the necessary equipment should be readied. Machinery should be warmed up and electrical devices properly grounded. An emergency kit should be kept close in case any complications develop.

During therapy, the technician should try to relax the patient and keep it positioned as comfortably as possible. Padding and support may be needed. Collars, splints, and bandages should be removed. The therapist should stay with the patient during the therapy. If the patient becomes restless or overheated or if any other adverse condition develops, the therapy should be discontinued immediately. When the therapy has been completed, the animal should be cleaned if necessary, dried com-

pletely, and examined for any unusual conditions that may have developed from the therapy such as edema, erythema, or pain.

The patient's progress or lack of progress should be charted after each treatment. Record keeping is important because the animal's condition and response to therapy will determine the number and length of future treatments. If improvement is not noted in three to five days after the initiation of therapy, the therapy should be modified or discontinued.[2]

Cold Therapy

Cold therapy is a method of physical therapy that can be easily used in veterinary practice. Cold can be applied by convection or, more commonly, by conduction. It is administered with cold packs, cold water, or ice. Cold therapy is indicated within the first 48 to 72 hours following an injury.

Cold temperature therapy decreases tissue temperature. It reduces pain and muscle spasms. It is also theorized that cold decreases nerve conduction and creates mild analgesia at the site of administration.[3] In addition, cold therapy causes local vasoconstriction and decreased capillary blood flow, thereby decreasing the amount of edema.

There should be only enough blood in the traumatized area to allow clotting, hold tissues together, fill in the dead space, and eventually act as a framework for healing.[1] Excess blood at the site can cause pain, necrosis, and delayed healing. Excess blood must go through the process of clotting, organization, degeneration, and absorption before healing can continue. Cold therapy applied within the first 24 hours following injury can greatly reduce the hemorrhage volume into the tissue spaces. Ideally, any cold therapy should be applied in the first 48 hours following injury.

Cold Packs

Commercial cold packs are manufactured for use in human medicine but they can be adapted to animals since they come in various sizes and forms. One type of cold pack is the disposable instant pack, which is activated by squeezing the pack, which breaks an inner bag, mixing the contents and causing an immediate drop in temperature. The pack remains at a temperature of 20°F for approximately 45 minutes.

Reusable cold packs are also available. These are in a liquid form, and they do not harden even if frozen. This type of pack can be bulky and heavy, so it should not be applied to a fracture site. Both instant and reusable packs should be applied with a damp towel between the animal's skin and the cold pack. Application time is usually 5 to 20 minutes. In an acute condition, the pack should be applied on an alternating schedule as follows: on for 5 to 20 minutes, then off for 45 minutes.

The easiest and least expensive form of cold therapy is to simply apply ice to the affected site. The ice should be in a plastic, leak-proof bag wrapped in a towel. A washcloth or towel soaked in ice water can be used on injuries in areas of the body to which the ice cannot conform, e.g., joints and bony prominences.

Cold packs used by drug companies for shipping drugs and vaccines can also be used for cold therapy. These packs stay frozen longer than water does and they are reusable (Figure 1).

Cold Water Immersion

Immersion of the injured limb in cold water (60°F) is another effective means of administering cold therapy.[3] Only the affected areas should be immersed in the water. Moist cold therapy should not be applied to open

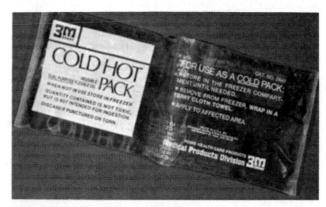

Figure 1—Commercial hot and cold packs are available. The pack shown here is a combination pack (hot and cold) for either use.

wounds unless a disinfectant is added to the water.

Cold immersion should be done for no longer than 20 minutes at a time. Large wounds should not be immersed because delayed healing may result.

Cold water immersion is used specifically for the rehabilitation of muscles, ligaments, tendons, joints, and burns and to decrease swelling and muscle spasms. It should be used for acute traumatic inflammatory conditions. Cold water immersion should be used in cases where heat has been applied with no result.

Heat Therapy

Heat is a commonly used form of physical therapy which can be applied in many forms. Three types of heat are used: radiant, conductive, and conversive. Radiant heat is applied with infrared lamps. Conductive heat is applied via hot packs and whirlpools. Conversive heat is an indirect form of heat applied in the form of microwaves and ultrasound.

The purpose of heat therapy generally is to increase tissue temperature, causing analgesia and sedation of the affected tissues. The resulting vasodilatation and increased circulation of blood to the injured site enhance the movement of phagocytes, oxygen, antibiotics, and nutrients to the area.[4] This results in increased metabolism and lymph flow. Heat relieves pain, relaxes muscle spasms, and promotes wound healing. It usually relaxes the animal, increasing its sense of well-being.

Contusions and sprains are two specific conditions that benefit from heat when it is applied 48 to 72 hours after trauma has occurred. Animals with bursitis, tendinitis, impaired circulation, or noninflammatory edema have decreased resistance to heat and should not be given heat therapy.[4]

Radiation Heat

Heat can be applied to the superficial tissues with heat radiation. Energy is transmitted to the skin and superficial tissues, which absorb the rays and convert them to heat.

Long-wave rays are emitted by all heated bodies and by items such as heating pads and hot water bottles. Long-wave rays only penetrate the tissues about 2 mm, being absorbed mostly in the upper skin layers, and they are therefore not recommended for therapy.

Short-wave rays, emitted by generators or lamps, are the most effective rays used in physical therapy. These rays are capable of penetrating the tissues up to 5 to 10 mm, influencing blood vessels, lymph flow, nerve endings, and subcutaneous tissues.

Infrared radiation is a powerful modality of radiant heat therapy. Severe burns can occur in animals receiving heat therapy from ultraviolet light (sunlamps). Infrared radiation should be used cautiously, particularly in animals with impaired circulation or over healing skin and scar tissue. It should be avoided in very old or very young patients.

Conductive Heat Therapy

Conductive heat refers to heat that is transferred from one object to another when two objects of unequal temperatures contact each other. Heat is transferred from the object with a higher temperature to the object with a lower temperature. Hot packs are the commonest method of applying conductive heat.

The principles of applying hot packs are similar to those used in applying cold packs. A protective layer of toweling should be used between any hot pack and the skin surface. The skin should be checked every few minutes. If it feels hot or appears red, an additional layer of toweling should be added. Hot packs should never be applied over new skin or scar tissue.[4]

Commercial hot packs are available. One type is a reusable pack filled with silica gel. When it is heated to 170°F, the pack retains heat for 20 to 30 minutes, which is the usual maximum application time. The pack should be covered with a towel to delay cooling. It must be kept constantly wet or it becomes unusable. Units are available for heating the water and storing the packs. The packs will last for years if used with care.

Instant, nonreusable packs are also available. These are activated by breaking an inner bag and shaking the pack to mix the contents.

Warm whirlpools at about 100°F are another form of conductive heat therapy. They provide a superficial moist heat which is more effective in relieving pain and muscle spasms than dry heat is.[2] Whirlpool therapy was discussed in Part I of this article.

Conversive Heat

Conversive heat is indirect heat energy that results from the conversion of one energy form to heat in the body tissues.[5] Ultrasound is a mode of conversive or deep-heat therapy that provides deeper heat than radiation therapy. It consists of mechanical vibrations that are identical to acoustic or sound vibrations except for their frequency and mode of emission. The frequency of ultrasound waves, which is over 20,000 cycles per second, makes them inaudible to the human ear.[6]

Ultrasound waves are transferred from the machine where they are produced to the treatment area by a hand-held transducer. When the transducer is applied to the animal's skin there are air pockets between it and the skin. Because of the reflection of the ultrasound, the waves bounce back to the transducer if the air is not removed. To eliminate a space, a *coupling medium* such as mineral oil[a] is used. For best results the animal's hair should be clipped from the area before treatment.

There are three techniques for administering ultrasound therapy. One is the contact technique; this is used on smooth, muscular surfaces with a coupling medium, which is usually a gel. The weight of the transducer or the light pressure being applied should not cause any pain.

---

[a]A commercial gel is available for use as a coupling medium.

The second way to administer ultrasound therapy is under water. This technique is used to treat very uneven surfaces, such as the olecranon or the stifle, where good transducer-body contact is impossible. Only the area of treatment need be immersed in water.

The cushion technique is the third method of ultrasound administration. This technique is used for application over bony prominences or curvatures that prevent good transducer contact yet cannot be submerged in water. For this type of administration, a plastic bag filled with tepid water is placed between the transducer and the skin, and the skin has gel on it.

Ultrasound is used for a variety of neuromuscular and musculoskeletal conditions to soften scar tissue and to reduce pain of neuromas and degenerative joint disease. It is also used to treat arthritis and bursitis.[7] The chief danger in using ultrasound is burns. The animal should never feel any pain or discomfort during the treatment. Ultrasound should not be used over the eyes, spinal cord, brain, growing bone, heart, anesthetized areas, ischemic areas, tumors, reproductive organs, acutely infected areas, or areas previously exposed to x-rays.

Care of the Recumbent Animal

The rehabilitation or recovery of a patient depends on its care. Patient care is a primary responsibility of the veterinary technician. The type of patient requiring the greatest amount of attention is the recumbent, cage-confined animal. The importance of enthusiastic nursing care and generous amounts of affection cannot be overemphasized. Many patients have special needs for rehabilitation. It is the responsibility of the veterinary technician to recognize and attend to these needs. A physical therapy program may be needed to expedite the recovery period.

It is vital that the cage-confined patient have the desire to recover. The first step in rehabilitation is to show interest in and compassion for the patient. Personal contact is very important. The technician should relate to the patient as a friend.[8] To establish this type of relationship, the technician should talk to the animal in a pleasant tone, addressing it by name.

Cleanliness is of the utmost importance. This can be a challenge with the patient that has fecal and urine incontinence. A soft, dry surface must be provided for the animal to lie on. Synthetic sheepskins (Figure 2), foam cushions, blankets, or water mattresses help prevent the formation of decubital ulcers or *pressure sores* (Figures 3 and 4). Decubital ulcers are caused by ischemic necrosis of the skin and muscles resulting from prolonged recumbency. The ulcers heal very slowly and can become severely infected. The common sites of decubital ulcer development are illustrated in Figure 5.

Although soft bedding decreases the development of decubital ulcers, a concentrated effort must be made to prevent them. Thick, tenacious ointments such as zinc oxide may be applied to protect the sites from irritation

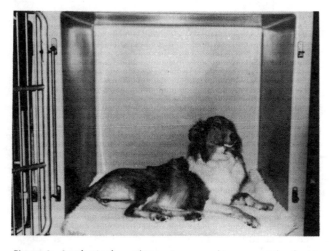

Figure 2—Synthetic sheepskin mats are used to prevent the development of decubital ulcers.

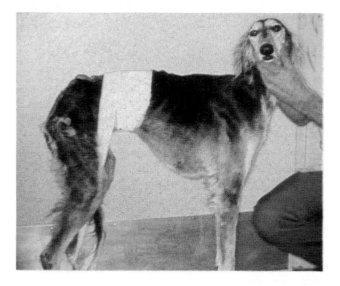

Figure 3—Decubital ulcers like this one on the hip can occur within two to three days.

from moisture, especially urine.[8] The coat must be kept clean and dry. The animal should be turned every two to three hours. Exercise carts and padded rings or doughnut bandages can be used to protect the bony areas that are most susceptible to decubital ulcer development (Figure 4).

The patient should never be left unattended in the exercise cart, especially if it is unaccustomed to it. Some patients are frightened of the cart and may struggle to escape, injuring themselves in the process. The patient is in a standing position in the exercise cart. This position improves circulation and respiration in addition to relieving pressure on the lateral bony prominences. The length and frequency of use of the exercise cart will depend on the patient's physical condition and attitude.

Whirlpool therapy seems to improve the condition of recumbent animals because it cleanses them, improves circulation, decreases decubital ulcer development, and promotes healing of those decubital ulcers that they

have. Complete drying is mandatory following bathing and whirlpool therapy.

Personally supervised exercise is an important part of patient care. If possible, the patient should be taken outdoors to defecate and urinate. The patient's urinary and bowel habits should be observed because many paralyzed animals have urine retention and require special care to prevent cystitis. The bladder should be completely emptied three to four times daily. Manual expression of the bladder is effective in most females. If the urine is concentrated, bloody, or odorous, it should be cultured for bacteria. The bladder should be flushed with sterile saline and infused with the appropriate medication via a catheter.[9]

Manual expression of the bladder is not easily accomplished in the male. The bladder should be catheterized using a small-sized catheter to reduce irritation and trauma. Urinary catheterization must be done using a sterile, well-lubricated catheter. Some veterinarians

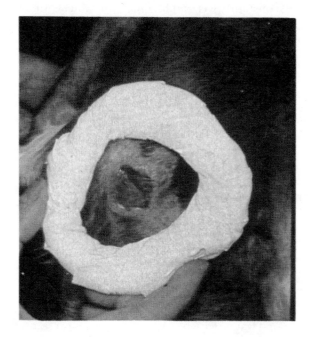

Figure 4—A metal ring wrapped with tape and cotton can be used to protect decubital ulcers and prevent them from worsening.

COMMON SITES OF DECUBITAL ULCER FORMATION

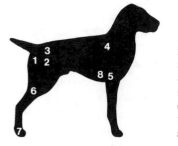

1. tuber ischii
2. major trochanter
3. tuber coxae
4. acromian of scapula (shoulder)
5. lateral epicondyle of humerus
6. lateral condyle of tibia (stifle)
7. sides of the 5th digits
8. sternum

Figure 5—The most common sites for decubital ulcer formation in recumbent dogs are shown.

prefer to use an indwelling urinary catheter if the patient is unable to urinate. The risk of catheter-induced urinary tract infection is much greater with an indwelling catheter than with repeated intermittent catheterization, though.[10]

Good nutrition is imperative for the recumbent animal. Forced feeding and watering might be necessary if the patient refuses or is unable to eat and drink.

The animal should be discharged as soon as possible, because familiar surroundings enhance recovery by improving the animal's sense of well-being and security. At home, activity and appetite should increase.

Most clients are willing to participate in the rehabilitation program at home. Therapy should be demonstrated to the client so that he or she understands how to administer it. The importance of maintaining the treatment schedule should be stressed to the client, because if the animal does not receive the required therapy, there could be a relapse in its condition. Complete, written home-care instructions concerning diet, exercise, medication, and treatment should be provided. Frequent communication with the client is necessary to monitor the animal's condition at home. Many animals will need to return to the hospital for additional checkups and treatment.

The veterinary technician can play a vital role in a physical therapy program. Besides providing high-quality nursing care, the technician can administer many modes of physical therapy and provide client education and communication.

REFERENCES

1. Swain SF: *Surgery of the Traumatized Skin: Management and Reconstruction in the Dog and Cat.* Philadelphia, WB Saunders Co, 1974, pp 70-83.
2. Downer AH: Physical therapy in the management of long bone fractures in small animals. *Vet Clin North Am* 5:157-164, 1975.
3. Downer AH: Cryotherapy for animals. *Mod Vet Pract* 159(9):659-662.
4. Downer AH: Conductive heat therapy. *Mod Vet Pract* 60(7):525-527, 1979.
5. Marone PV: Orthopaedic rehabilitation, in Gartland JJ (ed): *Fundamentals of Orthopaedics*, ed. 2. Philadelphia, WB Saunders Co, 1974, pp 407-420.
6. Downer AH: *Physical Therapy for Animals.* Springfield, IL, Charles C Thomas, 1978.
7. Downer AH: Ultrasound therapy for animals. *Mod Vet Pract* 57(7):526, 1976.
8. Hoerlin BF: *Canine Neurology.* Philadelphia, WB Saunders Co, 1974, pp 505-508.
9. Bailey CS, Holliday TA: Diseases of the spinal cord, in Ettinger SJ: *Textbook of Veterinary Internal Medicine: Diseases of the Dog and Cat.* Philadelphia, WB Saunders Co, 1975, pp 401-455.
10. Lees GE, Osborne CA: Urinary tract infections associated with the use and misuse of urinary catheters. *Vet Clin North Am* 9(4):713-727, 1979.

URINE COLLECTION IN CATS AND DOGS. PART I.

NATURAL MICTURITION,

MANUAL COMPRESSION, &

CYSTOCENTESIS

Sharon Philip, AHT

Knutsford, British Columbia

Urinalysis is a quick and easy diagnostic test that requires little equipment but provides a wealth of information about the patient. Often, the most difficult part of the procedure is specimen collection. The method of collection is equally as important as the method

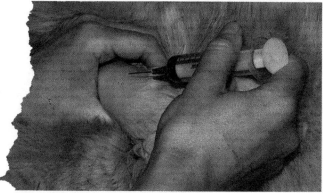

of analysis. If the collection method is inappropriate for the required test, the

Originally published in Volume 10, Number 10, November/December 1989

urinalysis results may be invalid.

There are four methods of collection: natural micturition or free flow, manual compression of the urinary bladder, urinary catheterization, and cystocentesis. Part I of this two-part presentation explains natural micturition, manual compression, and cystocentesis. Part II will detail urinary catheterization. Each method has its advantages, disadvantages, and appropriate uses for diagnostic testing or treatment. Regardless of the method chosen, particular care should be taken to prevent iatrogenic trauma or infection of the urinary tract.

If possible, the urine should be collected in the morning to obtain the most concentrated specimen of the day.[1,2] An appropriate vessel that is sterile and free of chemical contamination should be used for collection. If the client is requested to collect the sample, an appropriate container should be provided.

Urinalysis should be performed within 30 minutes of collection of the specimen.[1,2] If immediate processing is not possible, the specimen may be stored in the refrigerator in an amber bottle for as long as two hours. This storage method reduces the degradation of the urine constituents by light and chemical reactions.[1,2]

Natural Micturition

Collection of naturally voided urine is the safest and easiest method provided that the patient is cooperative. Collecting naturally voided urine from male dogs is not usually problematic. Collecting from female dogs is more difficult, however; and the method is not at all practical for collecting urine from either male or female cats. One advantage of this method is that clients can collect naturally voided urine from patients at home. Instructions and a proper container should be provided.

Natural micturition specimens may be used for routine urinalysis to screen patients for abnormalities of the urinary tract and other body systems. If a chemical strip test is all that is required, this method is satisfactory. If a microscopic examination is to be included, however, the specimen will be contaminated with cells and bacteria from the lower urinary tract, skin, and hair and may also contain such environmental contaminants as dust and pollen.[1-3]

Contamination can be reduced by obtaining a midstream specimen.[1-4] Such specimens are obtained by collecting the initial portion of the sample in a separate container or allowing it to fall to the ground. The midstream void is then collected separately. When the midstream technique is followed, the initial portion of urine can flush out some contamination; on occasion, however, the technique backfires when the patient only provides a small sample. To ensure that some specimen is collected, the two-vessel system is recommended.[1,4]

Natural micturition does not provide appropriate specimens for culture and sensitivity studies because of contamination. As mentioned, this method is usually inappropriate for collection of feline urine, but it is possible if the cat is hospitalized overnight. All bedding and paper should be removed; and a clean, dry, preferably stainless steel litter pan should be placed in the cage. An alternate method is to use shredded plastic as litter. It must be appreciated that this method is only useful as a vague screen because the urine could be hours old and contaminated with feces by morning.

Bladder Expression

In bladder expression, the bladder is located by abdominal palpation and then steady, gentle, digital pressure is applied until the animal is forced to urinate.[1,5] As with natural micturition, a midstream sample is preferred.[3] For this method to be successful, the animal must be small enough for the bladder to be compressed with one hand and the bladder must be relatively full. For these reasons, it is generally used on cats and small dogs. Although the risk of iatrogenic infection is low, iatrogenic trauma to the bladder and kidneys is a concern.[1-3]

Considerable digital pressure may be required to overcome the urethral sphincter of the normal, healthy bladder. Pressure may cause intravesicular bleeding, which is detrimental to the patient and contaminates the specimen with blood.[1-3,6]

Bladder expression is best used for incontinent patients that have full bladders and are dribbling urine. The urinary bladders of such patients should be manually compressed several times daily to prevent urine scalds.[6]

Bladder expression is contraindicated when the animal has cystitis, urethral blockage, or a history of any recent bladder trauma.[1,2,6] Not only does the resultant contamination by debris from the lower urinary tract interfere with culture and sensitivity studies, but there is the added risk of rupture of the bladder. An unhealthy bladder can be very friable; even a small amount of digital pressure may cause bladder rupture or, at the very least, backflow of contaminated urine into the renal pelvis.[1]

Cystocentesis

In cystocentesis, the bladder is located by palpation, a sterile needle is inserted into the bladder, and urine is aspirated with a syringe. Because it avoids contamination from

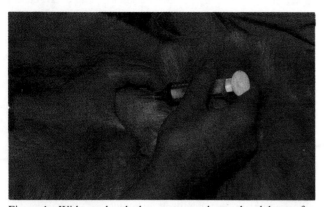

Figure 1—With one hand, the operator palpates the abdomen for the bladder and stabilizes the bladder against the ventral abdominal wall. The operator must be able to palpate the bladder when performing cystocentesis.

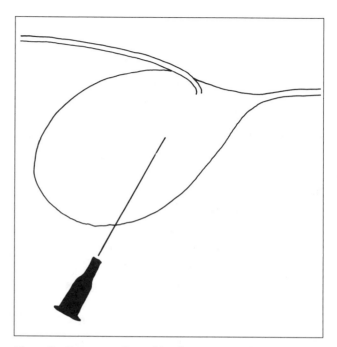

Figure 2—Correct needle position for cystocentesis. Inserting the needle in the trigone of the bladder rather than in the vertex ensures that the needle will stay in position as urine is withdrawn and the bladder collapses.

the lower urogenital tract, cystocentesis is the preferred method of urine collection when the veterinary staff is testing for urinary tract infection.[1-3,6] If done properly, the procedure is less traumatic than catheterization and rarely requires chemical restraint.

For cystocentesis to be performed, the bladder must be palpable. The usefulness of this method in large or obese patients is therefore limited. Although it is not feasible for large canine breeds, cystocentesis does work well for small dogs. The method is ideal for cats because usually their bladders are easily palpable and because (unlike catheterization) the procedure does not require sedation.

The following are potential hazards of cystocentesis:

- The bladder may tear or surrounding structures may be injured if the animal struggles.
- Urine may leak into the peritoneal cavity if the needle is withdrawn while the bladder is still fairly full or if too much pressure is applied to the bladder while the needle is in place; in either event, peritonitis may result.
- Hematuria might occur, or the needle might become contaminated if it is inserted through a loop of bowel.[3]

To perform cystocentesis properly, cats and small dogs should be restrained in lateral recumbency. Good restraint is very important. If cystocentesis is attempted on a large dog, the animal should be restrained in a standing position to facilitate palpation of the bladder.

The ventral midline of the abdomen of cats and female dogs should be clipped and scrubbed with antiseptic and rinsed well. An antiseptic solution should then be applied. For male dogs, the abdomen should be clipped lateral to the penis to avoid the superficial veins of the glans[6]; the

abdomen should be scrubbed with antiseptic and rinsed, and antiseptic should be applied.

The operator's hands should be washed thoroughly. With one hand, the operator palpates the abdomen for the bladder and stabilizes the bladder against the ventral abdominal wall (Figure 1). This is probably the most uncomfortable part of the procedure for the patient. The operator must be able to identify the bladder. If the bladder is not large enough to be located, the procedure should be postponed. Attempting the procedure when the location of the bladder is uncertain may result in contamination of the needle if it passes through a loop of bowel before reaching the bladder. Such attempts may also result in unnecessary puncturing of structures other than the bladder.[1,3]

A 22-gauge needle that is 2 to 3 cm long (approximately 1 to 1.5 inches) is inserted through the abdominal wall into the trigone of the bladder at a 45° angle (Figures 1 and 2). Inserting the needle in the trigone of the bladder rather than in the vertex ensures that the needle will stay in position as urine is withdrawn and the bladder collapses.[1,7] It is also important that the needle be at a 45° rather than 90° angle (Figure 3) so that an oblique needle track will be created.[1,3,7] An oblique track provides a better seal when the needle is withdrawn, thereby decreasing the risk of urine leakage into the peritoneal cavity. Such leakage can cause peritonitis.

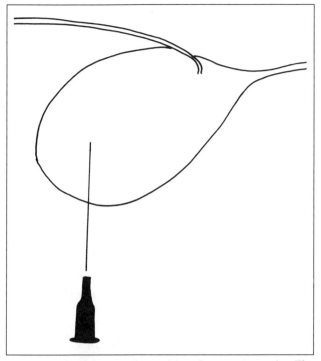

Figure 3—Incorrect needle position for cystocentesis. The oblique track created by the correct position provides a better seal when the needle is withdrawn, thereby decreasing the risk of urine leakage into the peritoneal cavity.

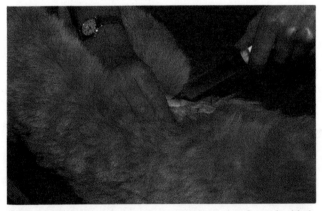

Figure 4—Correct technique for aspirating urine from the bladder. If too much pressure is applied to the bladder, urine may leak into the peritoneum. The operator should withdraw as much urine as possible but allow a small amount to remain in the bladder.

Urine is aspirated into a sterile syringe. Care is taken not to apply too much pressure to the bladder or urine may leak around the needle out of the bladder (Figure 4). The operator should withdraw as much urine as possible but allow a small amount to remain in the bladder. If the bladder is very full and only a small amount of urine is withdrawn, the puncture site is subjected to pressure and leakage may occur. Some urine, however, should be left in the bladder to prevent the sharp point of the needle from damaging the bladder mucosa. After urine is aspirated from the bladder, digital pressure on the bladder is released and the needle withdrawn.

Summary

The appropriate method of urine collection depends on the diagnostic tests to be carried out and the size and temperament of the patient. Choosing the right method ensures the validity of the diagnostic procedures as well as safety and comfort of the patient. Part II will examine the techniques for urinary catheterization in cats and dogs.

■

REFERENCES

1. Osborne CA, Stevens JB: *Handbook of Canine and Feline Urinalysis.* St. Louis, MO, Ralston Purina Co, 1981, pp 15–16, 21–34.
2. Fenner WR: *Quick Reference to Veterinary Medicine.* Philadelphia, JB Lippincott Co, 1982, pp 546–547.
3. Barsanti JA, Finco DR: Laboratory findings in urinary tract infections. *Vet Clin North Am [Small Anim Pract]* 9(4):731–734, 1979.
4. Lane DR: *Jones' Animal Nursing,* ed 3. Willowdale, Ontario, Pergamon of Canada, 1980, p 400.
5. McCurnin DM: *Clinical Textbook for Veterinary Technicians.* Philadelphia, WB Saunders Co, 1985, pp 178–179.
6. Pratt PW: *Medical Nursing for Animal Health Technicians.* Goleta, CA, American Veterinary Publications, 1985, pp 291–296.
7. Osborne CA, Lees GE, Polzin DJ, Kruger JM: Immediate relief of feline urethral obstruction. *Vet Clin North Am [Small Anim Pract]* 4(3):585–597, 1984.

URINE COLLECTION
IN CATS AND DOGS. PART II.
URINARY CATHETERIZATION*

Sharon Philip, AHT

Knutsford, British Columbia

Urine can be collected from veterinary patients through natural micturition, manual expression of the bladder, cystocentesis, or urinary catheterization. Of these methods, urinary catheterization is the most commonly used in dogs and is

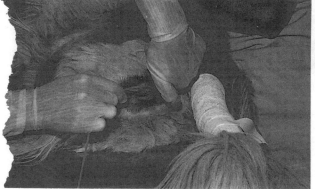

also used in cats. Urinary catheterization requires passing a catheter into the bladder through the

Originally published in Volume 11, Number 1, January/February 1990

TABLE I
Recommended Sizes and
Types of Urinary Catheters

Patient	Catheter	Size
Male or female cat	Tomcat	3.5 French[a]
	Jackson	3.5 French
Male dog		
Weighing up to 12 kg	Polypropylene or rubber	3.5–5 French
Weighing 12–35 kg	Polypropylene or rubber	8 French
Weighing more than 35 kg	Polypropylene or rubber	10–12 French
Female dog		
Weighing up to 5 kg	Polypropylene or rubber	5 French
Weighing 5–23 kg	Polypropylene or rubber	8 French
Weighing more than 23 kg	Polypropylene or rubber	10–14 French

[a]One French unit equals 0.33 mm.

urethra and then using a syringe to aspirate the urine. Because of the risk of iatrogenic trauma and infection, every precaution should be taken to ensure that the procedure is as gentle and aseptic as possible.

A urine specimen taken by urinary catheterization may be contaminated by the normal flora (primarily gram-positive staphylococci and streptococci and possibly some gram-negative organisms,[1,2] micrococci,[2] and mycoplasmas[1]) of the urethra as well as red blood cells and protein if any trauma occurred to the urethra. If culture and sensitivity studies or microscopic examination is required, contamination of the urine has to be taken into account; the protein and blood levels reflected by the chemistry strips may also have to be reinterpreted. Discarding the first portion of the collected urine specimen helps to reduce contamination.[1,2]

Indwelling catheters and repeated catheterization should be avoided because they increase the risk of bladder infection by the normal urethral flora present on the catheter. Cystocentesis may therefore be the preferred method of urine collection unless the animal is too large or obese for cystocentesis to be practical. Cystocentesis is particularly advisable when an animal is already predisposed to urinary tract infection. Such patients are particularly susceptible to iatrogenic infection as a result of urinary catheterization.

Types of Catheters

Catheters of various sizes, shapes, and materials are available (Table I). This article discusses the catheters most commonly used in small animals.

Polypropylene catheters are flexible, have a closed end, and are available in various diameters but only one length (Figure 1). They are the most commonly used catheters for male and female dogs. Polypropylene catheters can be sterilized in an autoclave and are therefore reusable. Care must always be taken to check the tip of such catheters for rough edges around the openings.

The metal female dog catheter is reusable but is available in only one size (Figure 1). This catheter is *not* highly recommended. Because it is rigid, it may damage the urethra or bladder.[1,3] In addition, insertion of a metal catheter is particularly uncomfortable for the patient if the catheter was not warmed before use.

Rubber catheters for male and female dogs are the least traumatic of the dog catheters. Rubber catheters are available in various sizes and can be reused several times. The rubber, however, cannot withstand repeated sterilization in an autoclave; and cold sterilization is not recommended because the rubber may absorb the chemicals. Because of their flexibility, rubber catheters are less traumatic but can be more difficult to insert.[3]

Tomcat catheters (Figure 2) are made of polypropylene. These catheters are available in one width, in two lengths, and with either an open or closed end. These catheters can be reused, but the tip must always be checked for roughness before use.

The Jackson cat catheter (Figure 2) is a soft plastic closed-end catheter with a small metal stylet. At the open end, the catheter can be sutured to the prepuce. Sutures are recommended if an indwelling catheter is used. The flexibility of the Jackson catheter makes it much less traumatic than the tomcat catheter. Because Jackson catheters are available in two diameters, they are particularly useful for young male cats. Jackson catheters are not reusable, how-

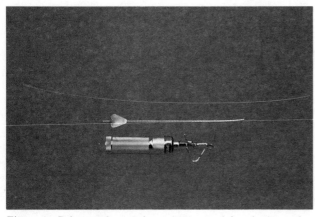

Figure 1—Polypropylene catheter (*top*), metal female dog catheter (*middle*), and vaginoscope (*bottom*).

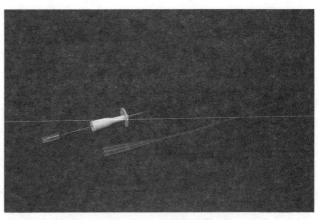

Figure 2—Jackson cat catheter (*top*) and tomcat catheter (*bottom*).

ever, and are more costly than tomcat catheters.

Foley catheters are indwelling catheters with an inflatable cuff at the tip. After insertion, the tip is inflated, thereby preventing the catheter from being pulled out of the bladder. Proper placement of this catheter is essential before the cuff is inflated. The cuff should *never* be inflated unless a steady stream of urine is flowing from the tube; otherwise, the cuff may be inflated while it is in the urethra.

Care of Urinary Catheters

Only sterile catheters in good condition should be used. Because trauma or infection may result from catheterization even if good equipment and excellent technique are used, nonsterile catheters or catheters in poor condition should never be used. The following procedure for the care of urinary catheters is used at the Department of Animal Health Technology at Cariboo College, Kamloops, British Columbia, Canada:

- The catheter is rinsed out immediately after use to prevent debris, blood, or protein from congealing in the tip.
- The tip of the catheter is checked for sharp edges, especially around the openings. If the catheter is damaged in any way, it is discarded.
- A large syringe is used to rinse the catheter with a mild soap solution. The catheter is then rinsed three or four times with water. Proper rinsing is essential to prevent residual soap from interfering with urinalysis.
- Another large syringe is used to blow any remaining water out of the catheter.
- The catheters are individually packaged and labeled.
- The catheters are sterilized in an autoclave or with ethylene oxide.

For the following reasons, chemical sterilization of urinary catheters is not recommended:

- Chemical solutions that effectively sterilize are irritating to mucous membranes. The catheter therefore cannot be used until it is rinsed. Rinsing contaminates the catheter unless sterile water is used.[1]
- Residual chemicals on the catheter may inhibit growth of bacteria in urine cultures and may affect urinalysis.[1]
- With chemical sterilization, the catheter cannot be passed through the wrapper; instead, the user must wear gloves, which is less convenient when catheterizing male dogs.

Catheterization of Male Dogs

Figure 3 depicts the anatomy of the lower urinary tract in male dogs. A male dog to be catheterized should be placed in lateral recumbency with the upper portion of the hindlimb pulled away from the site of operation.

The length of catheter to be inserted should be estimated as shown in Figure 4. This estimate helps reduce the bladder trauma associated with overinsertion of the catheter.[1,4]

If the dog has long hair, the hair at the tip of the prepuce should be trimmed (Figure 5). The prepuce should be gently cleansed with surgical scrub and rinsed well. A soap residue may cause the urine sample to appear cloudy, inhibit the growth of microorganisms in the specimen, or cause lysis of cells.[1]

A sterile catheter package is opened and the tip of the catheter exposed. Sterile lubricant (e.g., 2% lidocaine hydrochloride gel) is applied (Figure 6). The package is opened only enough to lubricate the tip of the catheter. The catheter is left in the package, thus allowing the operator to

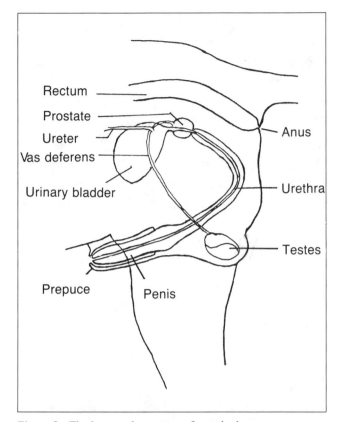

Figure 3—The lower urinary tract of a male dog.

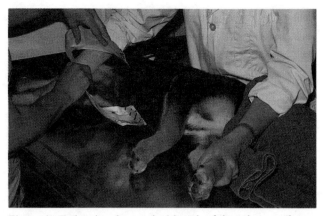

Figure 4—Estimating the required length of the urinary catheter.

pass the catheter directly from the package and obviating the need for gloves.

The operator's hands should then be scrubbed. The operator then puts on gloves (gloves are optional if the catheter is sterilized in an autoclave and therefore can be left in the package).

The prepuce is retracted to expose the penis (Figure 7). A small amount of mild antiseptic solution is applied to the penis.

While keeping the prepuce retracted at all times with one hand, the operator uses the other hand to pass the catheter into the urethra. As shown in Figure 8, the catheter is gradually withdrawn from the package as it is being inserted into the urethra.

The catheter should pass easily. If insertion is difficult or if the animal shows signs of discomfort, the operator should reevaluate the size of the catheter being used. When the catheter reaches the ischial arch, the operator may meet with some resistance in passage of the catheter. If the resistance cannot be easily overcome by gentle, steady pressure (the catheter must not be twisted), the appropriate size of catheter should again be reevaluated.

Once the catheter is in the bladder, urine should begin to flow into the package. The first few milliliters of urine should be discarded, and 6 to 12 ml should then be col-

lected in a sterile syringe by aspiration from the end of the catheter (Figure 9). If the catheter has been inserted as far as the mark that represents estimated required length but urine is not obtained, the syringe should be attached and the operator should try to aspirate urine. Digital pressure on the bladder is *not* recommended because it may cause the catheter to traumatize the bladder.[1,4]

Once the sample has been collected, the operator may wish to infuse the bladder with a sterile antiseptic solution. Such infusion, however, may cause complications. Infusing the solution may contaminate the bladder by flushing in bacteria that were picked up from the distal urethra while the catheter was being inserted.[5] Multidose stock solutions of antiseptic may over time become contaminated with resistant bacteria.[4,5]

Infused antiseptic solutions become diluted as urine is produced and may be of little benefit.[5] If the operator is concerned about possible contamination or if blood is found in the catheter after withdrawal, parenteral or enteral administration of antibiotics is probably more effective than infusion of antiseptic solutions into the bladder.[5]

Catheterization of Female Dogs

In catheterization of female dogs, the urethral orifice can be identified visually with the aid of a vaginoscope or the orifice can be identified by palpation. Figure 10 depicts the anatomy of the lower urinary tract in female dogs.

Visual Identification of the Urethral Orifice

If the urethral orifice is to be identified visually, the patient is restrained in a standing position with an assistant holding the dog's tail to one side. If the dog is large or the

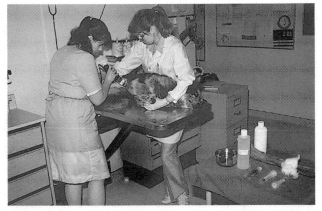

Figure 5—Long hair is trimmed from the tip of the prepuce of male dogs.

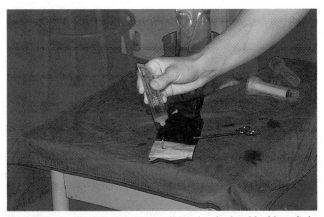

Figure 6—Sterile lubricant (e.g., lidocaine hydrochloride gel) is applied to the tip of the catheter.

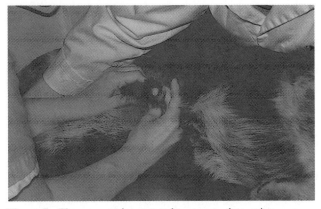

Figure 7—The prepuce is retracted to expose the penis.

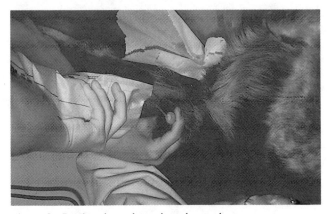

Figure 8—Passing the catheter into the urethra.

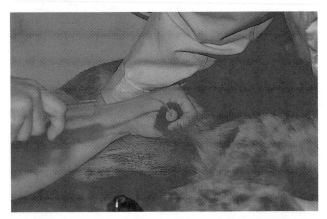

Figure 9—Collecting a urine sample in a sterile syringe.

assistant is of short stature, the dog can be catheterized in lateral recumbency.

The lips of the vulva and the surrounding hair are cleansed with antiseptic scrub, rinsed well, and sprayed with antiseptic solution. If the patient has long hair, the operator may need to trim some of the hair from the vulva to avoid contaminating the catheter as it is inserted.

The package of a sterile catheter of the appropriate size is opened, and the tip of the catheter is lubricated with 2% lidocaine hydrochloride gel. During catheterization of female dogs, the package is opened completely because it is easier to wear gloves than to pass the catheter through the packaging, as it may block the operator's vision.

The operator's hands should be washed. Sterile gloves should be put on. A sterile speculum with a light source is needed for this procedure. A vaginoscope (Figure 1), an otoscope with a large cannula, or a nasal speculum can be used. The instrument should be large enough to straighten out most of the folds of the vaginal wall; otherwise, it would be difficult to locate the urethral orifice among the folds. I have found that large female dogs are easier to catheterize by the tactile method because most specula are not long enough to reach the urethral orifice or wide enough to straighten out the vaginal folds in large dogs; the urethral orifice is consequently difficult to find in these patients. For catheterizing small female dogs, however, the visual method is preferred because the vagina of a small

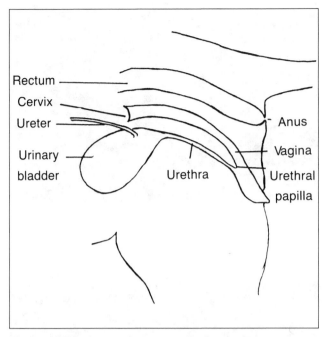

Figure 10—The lower urinary tract of a female dog.

Rectum
Cervix
Ureter
Urinary bladder
Urethra
Anus
Vagina
Urethral papilla

dog may be too small to tolerate digital palpation.

If the speculum has been stored in a cold-sterilization tray, the speculum should be rinsed with warm, preferably sterile water. If the speculum has been wrapped and has been sterilized in an autoclave, a small amount of 2% lidocaine hydrochloride gel should be placed on the tip of the speculum. After preparing the speculum, the operator should use one hand to insert the speculum into the vagina and direct the tip first dorsally, then cranially. This procedure avoids the clitoral fossa.

Once the operator has located the urethral orifice visually on the ventral floor of the vagina approximately 3 to 5 cm (1.5 to 2 inches) inside the vagina,[1,4] the operator should use the other hand to insert the catheter approximately 6 to 12 cm (3 to 6 inches) (Figure 11).

The speculum can now be removed; the operator should take care not to withdraw the catheter while removing the speculum. After allowing the first 2 to 3 ml of urine to flow from the catheter, the operator should attach a sterile syringe and collect 6 to 12 ml of urine (Figure 12). If no urine flows from the catheter but the operator is certain that the catheter has been placed correctly, the operator should try to aspirate urine into a syringe. As with male dogs, manual compression on the bladder to force the urine to flow is contraindicated because of the increased risk of iatrogenic trauma.

For the mentioned reasons, I do not routinely flush the bladder after collection of a urine specimen. Aseptic technique should be maintained; antibiotics are recommended only if there is evidence of trauma when the catheter is withdrawn or if there have been repeated attempts to catheterize the patient.

Tactile Identification of the Urethral Orifice

As mentioned, the tactile method is most successful in large canine breeds. It takes a little more practice initially but is less awkward than trying to manage a speculum and a catheter at the same time. The tactile method has limited usefulness in small breeds, however.

The patient should be restrained in a standing position with an assistant holding the tail to one side. It may be easier to restrain large patients in lateral recumbency.

The vulval area is cleansed as in the visual method. The preparation of the catheter is also the same as that done for the visual method.

The operator's hands must be washed. After putting on gloves, the operator should lubricate a finger with 2% lidocaine hydrochloride gel. The lubricated finger is inserted into the vagina dorsally and then cranially (the same way that a speculum is inserted) approximately 3 cm (1.5 inches) (Figures 13 and 14). The operator then gently palpates the vestibular floor for the urethral papilla (or tubercle). The urethral papilla feels like a soft, round mass 0.5 to 1 cm in diameter.[4] The operator can sometimes feel a depression (the urethral orifice) in the vaginal floor; the urethral papilla is just cranial to the depression.

The operator places a finger on top of the papilla and uses the other hand to pass the catheter beneath the papilla down into the bladder. If the operator can feel tissue between a finger and the catheter, the catheter has been correctly placed. If the operator can feel the catheter sliding under a finger, the catheter is going toward the cervix; the operator must pull the catheter back and redirect it. Once the catheter is in place, the procedure is the same as that used in the visual method.

Catheterization of Male Cats

Figure 15 depicts the anatomy of the lower urinary tract in male cats. For urinary catheterization of male cats, sedation or general anesthesia may be required depending on the nature of the cat and the experience of the operator. The cat is placed in dorsal recumbency with the hindlimbs pulled cranially.

The prepuce is gently cleansed with antiseptic scrub and rinsed well; antiseptic solution is then applied. If the pa-

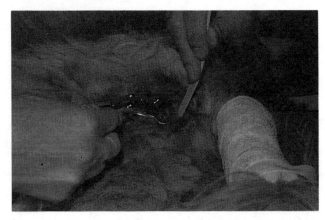

Figure 11—Visual catheterization of a female dog.

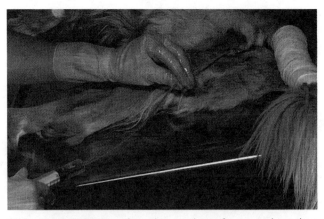

Figure 12—Collection of a urine specimen from a catheter in a female dog.

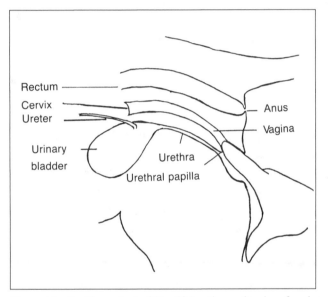

Figure 13—Tactile method of identifying the urethra in a female dog.

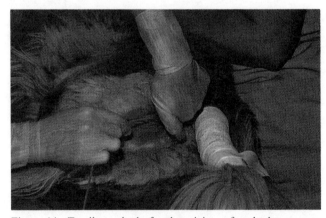

Figure 14—Tactile method of catheterizing a female dog.

tient has long hair, some trimming of the fur may be required; but wetting of the fur usually suffices.

The operator should open the package of a sterile catheter and lubricate the end of the catheter with 2% lidocaine hydrochloride gel if the patient is not anesthetized. For routine urine collection, a closed-end tomcat catheter (Figure 16) is preferred because it is less traumatic.[4]

The operator's hands should be washed, and the operator should put on sterile gloves. With one hand, the operator retracts the prepuce, exposes the penis, and gently puts traction on the penis in a caudal direction (Figure 17). Traction helps to straighten the penile flexure. The assistant then drops a small amount of antiseptic solution onto the penis.

With the free hand, the operator passes the catheter into the urethral orifice while keeping the catheter parallel to the spine (Figure 18). If resistance is met and the patient does not have a blocked urethra, the penis should be gently extended further in a caudal direction and steady, gentle pressure applied to the catheter. As in dogs, rotation of the catheter is not recommended.[3]

Once the catheter is in the bladder and urine is flowing, the urine sample is collected by the same method used in dogs. The first 1 to 2 ml is discarded, and 6 to 12 ml of urine is collected in a sterile syringe.

Catheterization of Female Cats

Sedation or general anesthesia may be required to perform urinary catheterization in a female cat. The patient is placed in lateral recumbency with the tail pulled to one side.

The vulva is gently cleansed with antiseptic scrub and rinsed well. Antiseptic solution is then applied. A small sterile speculum with a light source is required to identify the urethral orifice visually. The speculum is prepared in

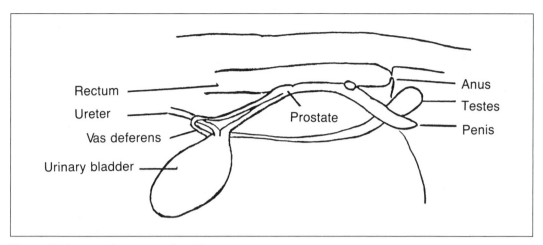

Figure 15—Lower urinary tract of a male cat.

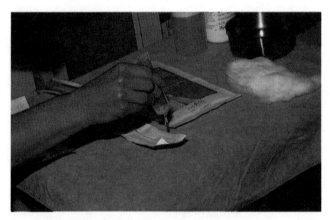

Figure 16—Lubricating the end of a tomcat catheter.

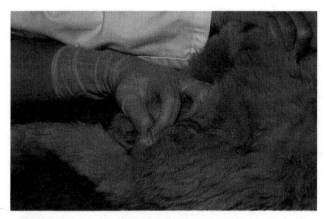

Figure 17—Retracting the prepuce of a male cat.

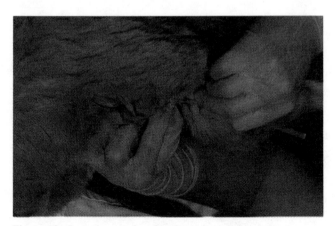

Figure 18—Inserting a urinary catheter in a male cat.

the same manner as that done for female dogs.

The package of a closed-end tomcat catheter is opened, and the tip of the catheter is lubricated with sterile gel. If the cat is not anesthetized, 2% lidocaine hydrochloride gel is used.

The operator's hands should be washed, and the operator should put on sterile gloves. With one hand, the operator places the speculum into the vagina and locates the urethral orifice on the vestibular floor. With the other hand, the operator passes the catheter into the bladder. The procedure for collecting the specimen is the same as that described for dogs and male cats.

■

REFERENCES

1. Osborne CA, Stevens JB: *Handbook of Canine and Feline Urinalysis.* St. Louis, MO, Ralston Purina Company, 1981, pp 15–16, 21–34.
2. Barsanti JA, Finco DR: Laboratory findings in urinary tract infections. *Vet Clin North Am [Small Anim Pract]* 9(4):731–734, 1979.
3. Pratt PW: *Medical Nursing for Animal Health Technicians.* Goleta, CA, American Veterinary Publications, 1985, pp 291–296.
4. Crow SE, Walshaw SO: *Manual of Clinical Procedures in the Dog and Cat.* Philadelphia, JB Lippincott Co, 1987, pp 110–124.
5. Kirk RW: *Current Veterinary Therapy VIII, Small Animal Practice.* Philadelphia, WB Saunders Co, 1983, pp 1097–1100.

■

BIBLIOGRAPHY

Evans HE, deLahunta A: *Miller's Guide to the Dissection of the Dog,* ed 2. Philadelphia, WB Saunders Co, 1980, p 164.

Fenner WR: *Quick Reference to Veterinary Medicine*. Philadelphia, JB Lippincott Co, 1982, pp 546–547.

Gilbert SG: *Pictorial Anatomy of the Cat*, ed 2. Toronto, Ontario, University of Toronto Press, 1979, pp 56, 58.

Lane DR: *Jones Animal Nursing*, ed 3. Willowdale, Ontario, Pergamon of Canada, 1980, p 400.

McCurnin DM: *Clinical Textbook for Veterinary Technicians*. Philadelphia, WB Saunders Co, 1985, pp 178–179.

Osborne CA, Lees GE, Polzin DJ, Kruger JM: Immediate relief of feline urethral obstruction. *Vet Clin North Am [Small Anim Pract]* 14(3):585–597, 1984.

The Technician's Role in the Management of Cats with Lower Urinary Tract Disease

David B. Joseph, AHT

Northridge, California

Feline lower urinary tract disease (which was formerly called feline urologic syndrome (FUS)) can be life threatening. This condition occurs when high levels of dietary magnesium in addition to other products in urine combine to produce

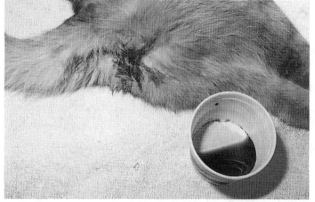

tiny struvite crystals that eventually form tiny sandlike stones and block the distal end of the urethra. Most clinical cases occur in male cats between one and six years of age. Veterinary technicians should become familiar with this disorder and its nursing care. With prompt medical treatment, this condition can be corrected; many affected cats recover completely.

Causes

The causes of feline lower urinary tract disease have not been clearly established, although numerous factors are being considered. Some of these factors include hygiene of the litterbox (e.g., soiled litter in a multicat household or the consistency of the litter), viruses, bacteria, dietary factors (e.g., high magnesium intake), and surgical factors (e.g., early castration). The predominance of urolithiasis in male cats has been attributed to the narrow width of the urethral lumen in comparison with that of females. Another factor that may induce lower urinary tract disease in cats is increased urine pH. As the pH rises above 6.8, struvite crystal formation becomes more frequent.

Recent studies have examined the possible role of excessive dietary magnesium levels. Three separate 12-month studies involved a total of 158 cats. The cats were then divided into three groups that were fed different rations containing different amounts of dietary magnesium. When dietary magnesium levels were greater than 0.75%, 55 of 72 cats became obstructed within nine months. When dietary magnesium levels were between 0.37% and 0.40%, 30 of 43 cats became obstructed. When dietary magnesium levels were less than 0.10%, none of the 43 cats became obstructed; however, urinary calculi were found in the bladders of these animals at necropsy.

Clinical Presentation

Cats with feline lower urinary tract disease are often presented to veterinary hospitals because of straining in the litterbox, some hematuria, pollakiuria (frequent attempts at urination), and licking of the penis. The most common owner complaint, however, is that the cat appears to be constipated.

As the disorder progresses, other clinical signs include vomiting, depression, signs of pain in the abdomen, and hypothermia. Often, cats are presented in lateral recumbency with bradypnea and bradycardia. These cases should be treated as emergencies.

Initial Management

The first step in the treatment of cats with lower urinary tract disease is to relieve the obstruction and reinstate elimination of urine. Physical restraint (i.e., wrapping the cat in a towel or blanket) in combination with a topical anesthetic usually allows the insertion of an indwelling urinary catheter into the urethra.

When the risk of damaging the urethra outweighs the risk of sedation, the cat should be anesthetized with an ultra–short-acting barbiturate, such as sodium thiamylal (which is excreted by the liver) in conjunction with a phenothiazine derivative (e.g., acepromazine maleate)—except in severe cases of depression.

If the cat is severely depressed and has severe bradycardia, a barbiturate may depress the cardiovascular system enough to cause cardiovascular collapse. In these cases, ketamine hydrochloride (2.2 to 4.4 mg/kg) can be used. The use of ketamine hydrochloride may be beneficial in these cases because ketamine increases the heart rate, thus helping to counteract bradycardia.

Cats that are obstructed and not depressed but have known renal compromise or azotemia should receive a reduced dose of ketamine hydrochloride because the kidneys excrete this agent in its active form. Normal doses could prolong the recovery of cats with renal insufficiency.

Epidural anesthesia can also be used but should only be performed by the veterinarian. An injection of 1 to 1.5 ml of 2% lidocaine hydrochloride can be made into the lumbosacral junction. This procedure provides regional perineal anesthesia.

The use of inhalation anesthetics (e.g., halothane or isoflurane) with or without the addition of nitrous oxide can provide a safe way to relax the cat before the insertion of an indwelling urinary catheter. If the animal is presented in lateral recumbency with severe dehydration and lethargy, a urinary catheter may be placed without anesthetic.

To prepare the cat for a urinary catheter, the cat should be placed in dorsal recumbency. The foreskin is retracted to expose the penis. A mild warm-water cleansing of the penis removes excessive dirt. With sterile technique, a 3.5 French open-end tomcat urinary catheter is lubricated with sterile lubricating jelly and gently inserted into the urethra. If the catheter cannot pass easily into the bladder, it may be necessary to use hydropropulsion. A 20-cc syringe with a small metal cannula is filled with 0.9% saline and gently inserted into the urethra. With gentle pressure, the cannula is moved in and out with the saline being directly applied into the urethra. The objective is to push struvite stones back into the bladder and allow placement of the urinary catheter.

If hydropropulsion does not clear the urethra and all other viable options except surgery have failed to alleviate the blockage and remove urine from the animal, cystocentesis should be performed. A 22-gauge 3.75-cm (1.5-inch) needle is attached to a three-way valve that is attached to a 20-cc syringe. The animal must be restrained and unable to move; otherwise the bladder may be lacerated. Under normal conditions, the bladder tissue is strong enough to withstand cystocentesis; but in cases of feline lower urinary tract disease, the bladder tissue may be friable.

If hydropropulsion was successful, urinary catheterization complete, and the blockage cleared, the urinary catheter can be placed and sutured to the prepuce. The next step is to flush the urinary bladder with lactated Ringer's solution or 0.9% saline. I have used a small sterile container with 250 ml of either solution to gently infuse 10 to 20 cc of fluid into the bladder and then withdraw the solution until it comes back clear. Some clinicians may elect to have the technician infuse a small amount of iodine solution in the flush solution as an antibacterial agent. After the bladder is completely flushed, the technician can then proceed to draw blood from the jugular vein for evaluation of the hemogram and serum biochemistries. Urinalysis and urine culture and sensitivity studies should be included. Voided urine can be collected for analysis after urine flow has been reestablished.

An indwelling intravenous catheter should also be placed in the cephalic vein. The fluid of choice is lactated Ringer's solution. Rehydration fluid volumes may be calculated by estimating clinical dehydration and then applying the following formula:

$$\text{Dehydration (\%)} \times \text{weight (kg)} \times 227 = \text{fluid replacement (ml)}$$

or

$$\text{Dehydration (\%)} \times \text{weight (lb)} \times 500 = \text{fluid replacement (ml)}$$

An additional 22 ml/kg (10 ml/lb) should be added to calculated volumes to replace insensible losses.

To ensure that renal shutdown has not occurred, a sterile urine collection system should be instituted as the best method of monitoring urine output. This collection system is made by taking an empty sterile intravenous fluid container and a sterile administration set and attaching the administration set to the indwelling urinary catheter using 1-inch tape and attaching the other end to the intravenous fluid bottle. It is important to remove the dial on the administration set because it could restrict the flow of urine; this error could be lethal. The collection system should be placed lower than the animal to allow gravity to pull the urine down into the bottle.

Use and Care of Indwelling Urinary Catheters

After the initial obstruction has been relieved and replacement fluid therapy has begun, the veterinary technician must provide proper care of the indwelling urinary catheter. Because hair is a major source of bacterial contamination, it is often best to shave the area around the penis before the urinary catheter is inserted. Not only does shaving help prevent contamination of the urinary catheter (the bacteria may migrate up the catheter and into the bladder), it helps prevent urine scalding of the patient. Parenteral ampicillin reduces the frequency and severity of catheter-induced urinary tract infections. The length of time that the catheter should remain in place depends on the individual patient, but the catheters should be used for as short a time as possible. The usual duration of catheter use is 24 to 72 hours.

The technician must monitor the patency of the catheter and the reaction of surrounding tissue. The technician must also be alert for contamination of the catheter by fecal material.

To prevent the cat from removing the catheter or destroying the urine collection system, an Elizabethan collar should be placed around the cat's neck. Some clinicians elect not to institute a closed urine collection system. In such cases, the cat should be placed in a cage that has a grate or rack flooring so that urine can fall freely to the bottom of the cage.

Emergency Treatment

Urinary obstruction for 24 hours or longer constitutes an emergency. Most cats that have had urinary blockage longer than 24 hours have the following clinical signs: vomiting, metabolic acidosis, severe dehydration, cardiac arrhythmia, elevated serum urea nitrogen and creatinine, and hyperkalemia. Some cats are comatose and unresponsive to painful stimuli on presentation.

The following steps are taken in emergency treatment of cats with urinary obstruction:

- Do not use intravenous barbiturates; avoid use of ketamine hydrochloride in cats with severe acidosis or azotemia.
- Use inhalation anesthesia if possible (e.g., a combination of nitrous oxide, oxygen, and halothane or a combination of oxygen and isoflurane). Be ready to intubate the cat.
- If severe uremia and acidosis are present, begin fluid therapy before dislodging the blockage and passing a urinary catheter.

• Support the animal's body temperature to avoid hypothermia.

When severe hyperkalemia is life threatening, the administration of insulin and dextrose helps drive extracellular potassium back into cells. Intravenous insulin (0.5 U/kg) is followed by two grams of dextrose per unit of insulin. One quarter of the dextrose dose is administered over a five-minute period; and the remainder is incorporated into the intravenous fluids, thus making a 2.5% dextrose solution.

Metabolic acidosis can be fatal if not treated in time. If hyperkalemia does not resolve after fluid therapy has begun, sodium bicarbonate should be administered. The amount of sodium bicarbonate to give to a patient is determined by the following formula:

$$\text{Bicarbonate dose (mEq/L)} = \text{base deficit (mEq/L)} \times \tfrac{1}{3} \text{ of body weight (kg)}$$

When the proper dose of sodium bicarbonate has been determined, one quarter of the dose is given in an intravenous bolus. The remainder is then incorporated into the intravenous fluids. Rarely does bicarbonate therapy have to be repeated.

Maintenance Therapy

After the urinary catheter has been removed, the cat should be hospitalized an additional 24 hours to check the muscle tone of the bladder. Many cats that undergo treatment for lower urinary tract disease lose bladder tone and the ability to urinate voluntarily. The technician must ensure that the cat is able to eliminate and must report these findings to the veterinarian. If the cat is unable to urinate by itself, gentle manual compression of the bladder will help relieve accumulated urine and allow the overstretched bladder muscles to return to normal size. To perform manual compression of the bladder, the technician locates the bladder in the caudal abdomen and applies gentle but steady digital pressure until a stream of urine is obtained. If digital pressure alone is insufficient to resolve bladder atony, pharmacologic agents are then used to help the bladder regain tone.

Several drugs are available to veterinarians to help improve contractions of the bladder muscle and enable the cat to return to a normal urination pattern; technicians should become familiar with these drugs and their potential side effects. Before any drug therapy is instituted, a complete data base (consisting of serum and biochemical profile, hemogram, urinalysis, and electrocardiography) should be available to the veterinarian for review.

Bethanechol chloride is a cholinergic agent used to stimulate and enhance bladder contractions that aid in the return to normal urination. Bethanechol chloride is given orally (5 to 25 mg every eight hours). Side effects of this agent include gastrointestinal distress (i.e., vomiting, diarrhea, cramping, and anorexia), hypersalivation, and cardiac abnormalities (with overdose). This agent is best given when the patient's stomach is empty.

Isometheptene is used to relax hypertonic or spastic smooth muscle; this condition frequently occurs in cats with lower urinary tract disease. Isometheptene is given orally at a dose of 65 mg twice a day. Side effects of this agent are rare but include overstimulation of the pilomotor reflex (fright reaction) and hypertension.

Phenoxybenzamine is an α-adrenergic blocker that is given when cats cannot empty the urinary bladder and affects the detrusor sphincter. Phenoxybenzamine hydrochloride is given orally (2.5 to 7.5 mg once a day for five days). Side effects of phenoxybenzamine hydrochloride include hypotension, miosis (contraction of the pupil), tachycardia, and nasal congestion. Phenoxybenzamine hydrochloride must be used with caution in cats that have preexisting cardiovascular disease.

Urine culture and sensitivity testing are used in selecting antibiotics. Antimicrobial therapy should continue for up to four weeks.

Dietary Management

Proper nutritional management of cats with lower urinary tract disease is important to a full recovery. Technicians can help clients understand that a special diet is needed to prevent recurrence.

The initial step is to change the diet to a product that is formulated to facilitate the dissolution of struvite crystals in urine (e.g., Prescription Diet® Feline s/d®—Hill's Pet Products). Many cats readily accept this diet, but some may not. To enhance palatability, the product can be gently warmed to room temperature. The diet is usually initiated in the hospital after parenteral support has been discontinued. Technicians should also instruct clients that no other treats, vitamins, or feedings of the previous diet should be used during dissolution therapy, which may last as long as two to three months. The dissolution diet can be used for long-term maintenance; however, its high sodium content may lead to other complications, such as congestive heart failure.

Client Education

After all clinical evidence of crystalluria has been resolved, the cat should be fed a maintenance diet that is formulated to prevent the recurrence of feline lower urinary tract disease (e.g., Prescription Diet® Feline c/d®—Hill's Pet Products). Because this diet is complete, no supplementation is needed.

Clients can help prevent feline lower urinary tract disease. The initial presentation of the kitten to a veterinary hospital for vaccinations is the ideal time to begin informing clients about this disease.

Cat owners should be told about the various available diets and instructed in the proper way to interpret food labels so that they can select a low-magnesium diet. Cat owners should also be told that cats may show little interest in a new food. If warming the food to room temperature does not seem to improve palatability, I recommend adding a small amount of garlic powder to the food. If the cat does not readily accept a new diet, a gradual change is recommended. The client should mix a little of the new diet with the old diet, gradually replacing the old diet with the new over one to two weeks.

Some clients do not purchase the special diets because of their high cost. A less expensive management option involves the use of urinary acidifiers. Two of the most common types of urinary acidifier used in veterinary medicine are DL-methionine and ammonium chloride. As with any therapeutic agent, clients should be instructed in the proper use of urinary acidifiers.

A low-magnesium diet must be used in conjunction with the acidifier. The proper dose of acidifier must be used, and the product must be given every time the cat eats. Urinary acidifiers may be unpalatable and cause vomiting in some cats. This side effect occurs more often with ammonium chloride than with DL-methionine. Kittens must not be permitted to consume an adult's ration to which a urinary acidifier has been added. Urinary acidifiers are also contraindicated in cases of urate calculi, metabolic acidosis, or hepatic failure. Although a special maintenance diet is more convenient for some clients, many cats have successfully been maintained with urinary acidifiers and a low-magnesium ration.

Cleanliness of the litterbox at home is also important because some cats refuse to eliminate in a dirty litterbox. If water consumption is too low, a small amount of salt may be added to the diet to increase water consumption.

Once the cat has recovered from the initial episode of lower urinary tract disease and is ready to be discharged, the technician should explain to the client the proper method of administering medication. The technician should allow the client to administer the first dose of medi-

TABLE I
Laboratory Values for a Cat with Lower Urinary Tract Disease

Parameter	Patient's Values[a]	Normal Values
Blood urea nitrogen (mg/dl)	245	15–35
Serum creatinine (mg/dl)	11.8	1.0–2.0
Serum phosphorus (mg/dl)	15.5	3.0–5.0
Serum potassium (mEq/L)	8.8	4.3–5.2
White blood cell count ($\times 10^3$ cells/μl)	25.0	5.5–19.5

[a]These values were measured at presentation. When the tests were repeated one week later, the results were normal.

cation to the animal while the animal is in the examination room; this practice helps build the client's confidence in administering medication. The client should also be instructed that all medication should be finished unless the veterinarian directs otherwise. Clients should be encouraged to call the hospital if questions arise or if there seems to be no further improvement in the cat's condition. Clients should also be informed that the condition may recur and that surgical intervention may be necessary.

Clinical Case

A seven-year-old castrated male cat was presented to a veterinary clinic because of straining in the litterbox and some hematuria (blood in the urine) during the previous two days. The patient's body temperature was 37.5°C (99.5°F), and abdominal palpation revealed that the urinary bladder was large and hard. All other findings were within normal limits. The diagnosis of feline lower urinary tract disease was made.

An indwelling intravenous catheter was placed in the cephalic vein. Blood was drawn from the jugular vein for evaluation of the animal's hemogram and serum biochemistries. An intravenous drip of 0.9% saline was started. The cat was anesthetized with an intravenous injection of ketamine hydrochloride and diazepam so that the obstruction could be relieved and an indwelling urinary catheter could be placed and sutured. An intramuscular injection of prednisone (10 mg) was given to help alleviate urethral swelling, and ampicillin (100 mg) was given to prevent infection. An Elizabethan collar was not applied, and the cat dislodged the catheter the day after it was inserted.

Laboratory findings (Table I) supported a diagnosis of feline lower urinary tract disease. After a few days of hospitalization and treatment with injectable ampicillin, the cat was discharged to the owners with a prescription for antibiotics and instructions for a dietary change. During the follow-up examination one week later, all findings were within normal limits. At the time of this report, the cat is healthy.

Summary

Feline lower urinary tract disease can be managed well with dietary and antimicrobial therapy, although the causes of the condition are still incompletely understood. Veterinary technicians must understand the importance of proper medical, dietary, and antimicrobial therapy. If diagnosed early and treated aggressively, feline lower urinary tract disease is curable; the cat can lead a normal life.

Acknowledgments

The author wishes to thank Kristy Menke, General Manager, Porter Pet Hospital, for the case history and Dr. Mike Gerardo of Rancho Sequoia Veterinary Hospital.

■

BIBLIOGRAPHY

Ettinger SJ: Feline urolithiasis syndrome, in *Textbook of Veterinary Internal Medicine*. Philadelphia, WB Saunders Co, 1975, pp 516–520.

Finco DR: Feline urologic syndrome: Management of the critically ill patient, in *Current Veterinary Therapy. VII*. Philadelphia, WB Saunders Co, 1980, pp 1188–1190.

Lees GE, Osborne CA: Feline urologic syndrome: Removal of urethral obstructions and the use of indwelling urethral catheters, in *Current Veterinary Therapy. VII*. Philadelphia, WB Saunders Co, 1980, pp 1191–1196.

Lewis LD, Morris ML: Diet as a causative factor of feline urolithiasis, in *The Veterinary Clinics of North America, Disorders of the Feline Lower Urinary Tract*. Philadelphia, WB Saunders Co, 1984, pp 415–420.

Lewis LD, Morris ML: Feline urolithiasis syndrome, in *Small Animal Clinical Nutrition*. Topeka, KS, Mark Morris Associates, 1987, pp 9-1–9-30.

Plumb DC (ed): *Veterinary Pharmacy Formulary*, ed 2. O'Fallon, IL, Veterinary Software Publishing, 1989.

Management of Fecal Impaction in Geriatric Cats

Johnny D. Hoskins, DVM, PhD

Diplomate, ACVIM

Department of Veterinary
 Clinical Sciences

School of Veterinary Medicine

Louisiana State University

Baton Rouge, Louisiana

Fecal impaction is an extremely common disorder in middle- to older-aged domestic cats. It is synonymous with constipation, as the colon is the primary target organ involved.[1] Constipation is a condition in which bowel movements are

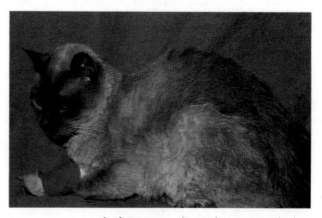

infrequent or incomplete. Fecal impaction therefore should be considered likely in any

Originally published in Volume 11, Number 8, September 1990

TABLE I
Causes of Fecal Impaction in Geriatric Cats

Category	Cause
Food and liquids	Excessive nondigestible bulk or fiber, hair impaction, foreign material, dehydration
Drugs	Agents that add to stool density (e.g., sucralfate, barium sulfate, antacids containing aluminum, calcium preparations); agents that alter colonic motility (e.g., narcotics, anticholingerics, oral iron preparations, vincristine, antihistamines, phenothiazines, diuretics, chronic laxative abuse)
Neurologic problem	Ileus, paraplegia, neurologic disorder, spinal cord or sacral nerve disease, central nervous system disease, lead intoxication, dysautonomia, pseudoobstruction, hypokalemia, intervertebral disk disease
Traumatic insult	Pelvic or spinal fracture, hematoma or contusion, laceration
Metabolic disease	Hyperthyroidism, hyperparathyroidism, pseudohyperparathyroidism, chronic renal failure, cancer
Perineal or rectal pain	Septic or nonseptic inflammation, lodged foreign object, pelvic fracture, rectal prolapse, perianal abscessation or fistula, rectal or anal growth or stricture, anal sac impaction, abscess, or infection
Colonic, rectal, or anal obstruction	Neoplasia or granulomatous inflammation, misaligned healed pelvic fracture, rectal prolapse, pseudocoprostasis, extracolonic compression, cystic uterus masculinus, sublumbar lymphadenopathy, perineal hernia
Behavioral	Elimination problems (refusal to defecate, no available litter boxes), territorial fighting, change of environment, situational depression
Miscellaneous	Idiopathic megacolon, inability to ambulate or squat, persistent inactivity, irritable bowel syndrome

cat presented with vague history and physical findings or in cats with infrequent or incomplete passage of stool. In most cases, the diagnosis is straightforward; but several complications often occur. Long-term, conservative medical management can be initiated after stabilization and rehydration of a cat presented in a decompensated state. Because treatment of fecal impaction can be frustrating, prevention is a better alternative in the management of geriatric cats.

Causes of Fecal Impaction

Fecal impaction is usually the result of a number of interacting pathophysiologic factors. Various causes that can contribute to fecal impaction in geriatric cats are listed in Table I.

The most common cause of infrequent or incomplete defecation in middle-aged cats is a mixture of feces and nondigestible hair or bones. In geriatric cats, lack of mobility plays an important part in causing fecal impaction. The ability to ambulate and exercise promotes colonic motility. The problem is magnified when daily routines are disturbed, which can occur during boarding or hospitalization. Geriatric cats are also subject to serious underlying disease, including cancer of the colon, hepatic disease, chronic renal disease, hyperthyroidism, electrolyte imbalance, and congestive heart failure; all of these often contribute to constipation.[2–4]

In addition, the use of calcium preparations and antacids containing aluminum in the management of a geriatric cat with chronic renal failure contributes to the risk of impaction.[5] Not only does renal failure increase the likelihood of impaction, but malnutrition and the use of immunosuppressive agents increase the incidence of subsequent complications.

Clinical Findings

The presentation of a geriatric cat with fecal impaction can be subtle and nonspecific. Impaction should be considered when evaluating cats presented with clinical deterioration, especially if the frequency or consistency of bowel movements has changed. Continual passage of some stool does not necessarily rule out impaction. If the frequency of bowel movements is fewer than one every other day, impaction should be included in the differential diagnosis.

Thorough abdominal palpation, a procedure that is well tolerated by cats, can detect most cases of fecal impaction. Abdominal palpation typically reveals fecal masses that fill the entire length of the colon; but fecal masses can occur only as a proximal or high impaction, which is a type of impaction that usually suggests neoplasia or stricture of the colon. In addition, impacted feces can be of any consistency, ranging from soft to hard, and can take many forms, such as a single mass or multiple pellets.

Cats presented with fecal impaction are generally dehydrated. They may assume a crouching, hunched attitude indicative of abdominal pain; and obvious abdominal distention is occasionally observed. Such signs as anorexia, depression, lethargy, nausea, vomiting, and abdominal pain are typical of impaction[6,7]; however, signs of other internal organ failure can also be present.

In geriatric cats, paradoxical diarrhea and fecal incontinence may be among the most common presenting signs.[6,7] Regardless of the cause of fecal retention, the colon's normal absorption of electrolytes and water leads to hardening of the feces; and the normal peristaltic activity of the colon causes the packing of feces into a discrete mass or masses. Because of the limited distensibility of the anal canal and marked distensibility of the rectum, a mass of fecal material can become too large to pass. The result can be a ball-valve effect that allows seepage of liquid stool around the obstructing mass of harder feces during frequent attempts at defecation. In addition, urinary problems associated with frequency, retention, and overflow incontinence can be caused by the mechanical effects of fecal impaction. In geriatric cats, urinary and fecal problems occurring together can imply a shared neurologic basis. Rectal prolapse can also result from severe straining associated with the impaction.

Laboratory and Radiographic Findings

Laboratory abnormalities associated with fecal impaction are nonspecific. Leukocytosis can occur; and electrolyte abnormalities, such as hyponatremia or hypokalemia, can be associated with impaction. Stool that is positive for blood might reflect mucosal irritation from the impaction; however, the same finding can also be a sign of an underlying neoplasm of the colon.

When fecal impaction is suspected but abdominal palpation is negative, noncontrast abdominal radiographs should be taken, observing for accumulation of feces or signs of obstruction, such as colonic dilatation and unusual air-fluid levels in the small intestine. On plain radiographs, fecal masses typically have a bubbly or speckled appearance and are generally visible.

Complications of Fecal Impaction

The most serious complication of fecal impaction is incontinence. The continuous seepage of moist bacteria-laden mucus and fecal material fosters the development of perineal irritation and ulceration. Concomitant infections of the urinary tract can also be caused by this contamination because of the direct passage of bacteria from the perineum into the urinary bladder.

Obstruction of the colon or rectum also commonly occurs with fecal impaction. The effects of pressure and ischemic necrosis on the wall of the colon can produce fecal mass–induced ulcerations that generally are clinically silent unless a complication follows. Occult bleeding of ulcers can occur, but massive bleeding is not common. Mass-induced ulcerations rarely perforate. Clinical findings suggesting perforation include a history of fecal impaction coupled with signs of localized or generalized peritonitis and radiographic evidence of free peritoneal air or contrast medium outside the confines of the intestinal lumen.

Less common complications that can be attributed to fecal impaction in geriatric cats include autonomic dysreflexia, pneumothorax from straining, hepatic encephalopathy, rectal prolapse, hypoxia, and profound shock from massive loss of fluid into the intestinal lumen.

Prevention of Fecal Impaction

Prevention is the preferred approach to managing fecal impaction. Such provisions as adequate dietary fiber, regular exercise, treatment of underlying disease, regular grooming, minimal changes in environment, and limited medication often prevent fecal impaction. Most commercial cat foods are low in dietary fiber, with the average commercial product containing 2.0% to 2.7% of crude fiber on a dry-matter basis. Because more dietary fiber is recommended for the successful management of recurrent fecal impaction,[8] clients should be advised to replace the typical commercial cat food with a product that contains more fiber (e.g., Prescription Diet® Feline r/d® or w/d®— Hill's Pet Products).

Other simple measures to follow include sufficient time for the gastrocolic reflex to operate after the cat has eaten, easy access to outdoor toilet facilities, and availability of litter boxes conducive for defecation.

The regular use of laxatives in geriatric cats with recurrent constipation is sometimes necessary but carries risk. In general, bulk-forming laxatives are the safest and most effective agents in the prevention of impaction.[6,7] Adequate hydration and electrolyte balance must be ensured. In all instances, the goal should be to have the cat pass soft, formed feces and to defecate regularly—at least daily or every other day. Commercial veterinary laxatives containing petrolatum as the active ingredient are useful for preventing impaction caused by hair balls.

Treatment of Fecal Impaction

The treatment of fecal impaction consists of gentle removal of impacted fecal material and, if possible, removal of the underlying cause.[6,7] A cat with mild to moderate fecal impaction can generally be treated with oral laxatives and frequent, small-volume enemas. A cat with more severe fecal impaction is usually dehydrated and requires fluid replacement therapy to resolve the dehydration and electrolyte abnormalities before correction of the impaction can be attempted. Manual fragmentation and removal of a fecal mass or masses should be accomplished as slowly and gently as possible. It is less traumatic for a geriatric cat if the fecal material is softened and removed after two or three days than if the entire impaction is removed quickly.[6,7]

In cats with mild to moderate fecal impaction and after fluid replacement therapy has been accomplished, oral administration (about 10 to 20 ml/kg of body weight every 12 hours) of an isosmotic solution of poorly adsorbable polyethylene glycol containing electrolyte solution (Colyte®—Reed & Carnrick; GoLytely®—Braintree Laboratories) can be used for completing the removal of residual feces.[9,10]

Laxatives

Because the effects of laxatives are mild, they usually eliminate formed feces. Some common laxative agents are presented in Table II. Laxatives that contain docusate sodium and docusate calcium act as detergents to alter surface tension of liquids and promote emulsification and softening of the feces by facilitating the mixture of water and fat. The patient must be well hydrated, however, before agents containing these substances are administered because they decrease jejunal absorption and promote colonic secretion.[6,7] Furthermore, these laxatives should not be administered in conjunction with mineral oil because they aid in absorption of the mineral oil.

Mineral oil (liquid petrolatum) and white petrolatum are nondigestible and poorly absorbed laxatives. They soften feces by coating them to prevent colonic absorption of fecal water and promote easy evacuation. A small amount of oil absorption does occur, but the primary danger of giving mineral oil is laryngotracheal aspiration resulting from its lack of taste.[6,7] Bulk-forming laxatives, such as psyllium, canned pumpkin, and coarse bran, increase the frequency of evacuation of the proximal colon via stimulation produced by added bulk or volume. They soften feces because of the water retention that occurs. Natural psyllium products contain coarse bran; therefore, clients should be advised to administer these products with moistened food to ensure a high degree of water intake.

Another useful laxative is bisacodyl; this agent exerts its action on colonic mucosa and intramural nerve plexuses. Stimulation is believed to be segmental and axonal, producing contraction of the entire colon independent of its resting tone.[6,7] It should be used only in well-hydrated cats and is contraindicated when intestinal obstruction is present.

Lactulose (a synthetic disaccharide of galactose and fructose) and lactose (available as household milk) also have laxative effects. Following oral administration, they are metabolized to organic acids by intestinal bacteria and promote an osmotic catharsis of feces. The dose should be individualized on the basis of stool consistency and titrated until a semiformed stool is obtained (two to three soft bowel movements per day).[11] An overdose of lactulose can, however, induce intestinal cramping, profuse diarrhea, flatulence, dehydration, and acidosis. Cats, in general, resent the taste of lactulose but generally like milk.

Enemas

Enemas act by softening feces in the distal colon and thereby stimulate colonic motility and the urge to defecate. The enema fluid should be room temperature or tepid when used. Tap water, normal saline solution, and sodium biphosphate solution add bulk; and petrolatum oils soften, lubricate, and promote the evacuation of hardened fecal material.[7] Soap, hydrogen peroxide, and hot-water enemas should never be used because they irritate the colonic mucosa and can cause bleeding.

For debilitated cats, normal saline solution and tap water (about 5 ml/kg of body weight) are generally preferred. In general, better results with a normal saline solution or a tap-water enema are obtained if the enema is repeated several times using small volumes.[7] Small volumes are retained for longer periods, therefore allowing time for the

TABLE II
Therapeutic Products for Management of Fecal Impaction in Cats

Therapeutic Agent	Dose Regimen	Comments
Bisacodyl	1 tablet (5 mg) daily given orally	Available in 5- and 10-mg tablets and 5-mg suppository; takes 6–12 hr to take effect; animal should be well hydrated and feces softened before its use
Bran (coarse)	1–3 tbsp mixed in 400 g of canned food daily or every 12 hr	Available in powder form; takes 12 to 24 hours to take effect
Bran cereals	3–5 tbsp mixed in food daily	Available as breakfast cereals
Canned pumpkin	1–4 tbsp mixed in food daily	Available as pie filling
Docusate sodium	1 capsule (50 mg) daily given orally	Available in 50- and 100-mg capsules, 1% liquid, 4 mg/ml syrup; takes 12–72 hr to take effect; animal should be well hydrated before its use; do not use with mineral oil
Docusate calcium	1–2 tablets (50 mg) daily given orally	Available in 50- and 240-mg tablets; similar activity and precautions as for docusate sodium
Lactose	Add to diet to effect	Available in household milk
Lactulose	0.25–1 ml daily or every 12 hr orally to start, then adjust dose to stool consistency and 2–3 bowel movements per day	Overdose can cause diarrhea, flatulence, intestinal cramping, dehydration, acidosis
Mineral oil	5–20 ml every 12 hr given orally or rectally	Available in liquid form; use with caution orally (causes lipoid aspiration pneumonia); should be given only between meals; takes 6–12 hr to take effect
Psyllium (natural)	1–3 tsp mixed with food daily or every 12 hr	Available in powder form; takes 12–24 hr to take effect
White petrolatum	1–5 ml daily given orally, then 2–3 days/wk	Available in paste form; should be given only between meals; takes 12–24 hr to take effect

impaction to soften and fragment. Mineral oil (5 to 20 ml) can be instilled directly into the colon and rectum if the feces are extremely hard. Hexachlorophene-based soaps should not be used, as they can cause central nervous system damage.[7] Although sodium phosphate retention enemas (e.g., Fleet Enema®—C. B. Fleet) are convenient preparations for the relief of fecal impaction, their use is generally contraindicated because they can cause potentially fatal hyperphosphatemia, hypernatremia, hyperosmolality, hypocalcemia, and acidosis.[12,13]

Surgery

If medical management with laxatives and/or enemas fails, surgery may be necessary. The goals of surgery are removal of impacted feces and correction of the underlying cause. For severe, recurrent constipation or megacolon that is nonresponsive to conservative medical management, subtotal colectomy is considered to be a viable option.[14]

Summary

The management of fecal impaction in geriatric cats is often complicated by normal age-related changes in body systems and by spontaneous concurrent disease or traumatic insult. Thorough evaluation of the cat's history, clinical signs, and laboratory and radiographic findings can demonstrate complicating factors and permit successful treatment of fecal impactions. The preferred management approach, however, is prevention. In geriatric cats, provision of adequate dietary fiber and regular exercise can assist in prevention of fecal impaction.

■

REFERENCES

1. Burrows CF: Disorders of gastrointestinal motility: More than you think. *Proc Am Coll Vet Intern Med* 6:573–575, 1988.
2. Bell FW, Osborne CA: Treatment of hypokalemia, in Kirk RW (ed): *Current Veterinary Therapy. IX.* Philadelphia, WB Saunders Co, 1986, pp 101–107.
3. Ross LA: Healthy geriatric cats. *Compend Contin Educ Pract Vet* 11(9):1041–1046, 1989.

4. Osborne CA, Abdullahi S, Polzin DJ, et al: Manifestations of feline renal failure. *Proc World Small Anim Cong*:55, 1985.
5. Allen TA: Management of advanced chronic renal failure, in Kirk RW, Bonagura JD (eds): *Current Veterinary Therapy. X.* Philadelphia, WB Saunders Co, 1989, pp 1195–1198.
6. Burrows CF: Medical diseases of the colon, in Jones BD, Liska WD (eds): *Canine and Feline Gastroenterology.* Philadelphia, WB Saunders Co, 1986, pp 221–256.
7. Burrows CF: Constipation, in Kirk RW (ed): *Current Veterinary Therapy. IX.* Philadelphia, WB Saunders Co, 1986, pp 904–908.
8. Burrows CF, Kronfeld DS, Banta CA, et al: Effects of fiber on digestibility and transit time in dogs. *J Nutr* 112:1726–1732, 1982.
9. Richter KP, Cleveland MvB: Comparison of an orally administered gastrointestinal lavage solution with traditional enema administration as preparation for colonoscopy in dogs. *JAVMA* 95:1727–1731, 1989.
10. Burrows CF: Evaluation of a colonic lavage solution to prepare the colon of the dog for colonoscopy. *JAVMA* 195:1719–1721, 1989.
11. Center SA: Feline liver disorders and their management. *Compend Contin Educ Pract Vet* 8(12):889–903, 1986.
12. Atkins CE, Tyler R, Greenlee P: Clinical, biochemical, acid-base, and electrolyte abnormalities in cats after hypertonic sodium phosphate enema administration. *Am J Vet Res* 46:980–988, 1985.
13. Jorgenson LS, Center SA, Randolph JF, et al: Electrolyte abnormalities induced by hypertonic phosphate enemas in two cats. *JAVMA* 187:1367–1368, 1985.
14. Bright RM, Burrows CF, Goring R, et al: Subtotal colectomy for treatment of acquired megacolon in the dog and cat. *JAVMA* 188:1412–1416, 1986.

Pain Management

CRITICAL CARE COMPANION ANIMAL is a regular feature of *Veterinary Technician®*. This month's feature was written especially for *Veterinary Technician* readers by Johnny D. Hoskins, DVM, PhD, Department of Veterinary Clinical Sciences, School of Veterinary Medicine, Louisiana State University, Baton Rouge, Louisiana. Dr. Hoskins is a Diplomate of the American College of Veterinary Internal Medicine.

Pain is defined as an unpleasant sensory and emotional experience associated with actual or potential tissue damage.[1] The various causes and effects of pain in animals remain poorly understood. Neuroanatomy, physiology, and behavioral information indicate that pain perception in humans and animals is remarkably similar.[2,3]

The lowest stimulus perceived to be painful or that results in a painful response is known as the pain detection threshold. Studies have indicated that humans and animals begin to identify noxious stimulation at approximately the same intensity.[3,4] Therefore, veterinarians and technicians should use their understanding of human pain during assessment of an animal in pain or when anticipating a painful response in a patient after noxious stimulation. Very often, the veterinarian's or technician's assessment of pain intensity resulting from noxious stimulation is based solely on human pain perception standards. Veterinary professionals must also be aware of the possibility of unexpressed pain. Although an animal may be exhibiting stoic behavior, it is not prudent to disregard pain management if tissue injury has occurred.[3]

Signs of Pain in Dogs and Cats

The signs of pain in dogs or cats vary.[5] The animal may vocalize (i.e., moan, cry, or whimper), attempt escape, self-mutilate the affected area, or become aggressive when a painful area is approached or manipulated. Weight-bearing lameness, unusual body posture, restlessness (pacing or continuously getting up and down), and prolonged recumbency may indicate pain. The animal also may move slowly and stiffly in conjunction with diminished activity.

Animals with abdominal pain tend to tighten their abdominal muscles; animals with thoracic pain tend to breathe shallowly and abduct their elbows. Other responses to pain include tachypnea (or panting), tachycardia, cardiac arrhythmia, mydriasis, hypersalivation, hyperglycemia, and pale mucous membranes.[5] Drug therapy with opioid and nonopioid analgesics is the principal means of successful pain management in most dogs and cats.

Drug Therapy in Pain Management
Opioid Analgesics

Opioid analgesics act by binding opiate receptors and thus activate central nervous system endogenous pain suppression systems.[4] After binding with receptors, opioid analgesics induce a conformational change in the receptors and an analgesic effect results. The ability of opioid analgesics to produce this effect has little relationship to the potency of the opioid or affinity for the receptor.[6] Opioid analgesics commonly used for pain management include morphine sulfate, oxymorphone hydrochloride, fentanyl citrate, meperidine hydrochloride, and butorphanol tartrate.

Nonopioid Analgesics

Nonopioid analgesics include nonsteroidal antiinflammatory drugs and acetaminophen. Nonsteroidal antiinflammatory drugs diminish pain and suppress the inflammatory response. Thus, they are helpful in relieving pain of low to moderate intensity[7] but are of little benefit in managing severe pain or postoperative pain in dogs and cats (especially during the first 48 hours after surgery).[6] Opioid analgesics and nonsteroidal antiinflammatory drugs may act synergistically and potentiate pain relief.[7] Nonopioid analgesics are believed to act in tissue at the pain receptor level by impairing the impulse generation or conduction that results in pain perception.[7]

Nonsteroidal antiinflammatory drugs that have been commonly used in dogs and cats include aspirin, ibuprofen, flunixin meglumine, naproxen, meclofenamic acid, and phenylbutazone. These drugs are readily absorbed from the gastrointestinal tract, metabolized by the liver, and excreted in urine. The side effects of most nonsteroidal antiinflammatory drugs are many and common, including gastric and intestinal ulceration, hemorrhage, and/or perforation; impaired platelet aggregation; renal failure secondary to preexisting renal disease; hypersensitivity; and occasional blood dyscrasias.[7,8] Nonsteroidal antiinflammatory drugs that are less likely to produce undesirable gastrointestinal and renal side effects are aspirin, phenylbutazone, and meclofenamic acid.[8]

Ibuprofen, of all nonopioid analgesics, causes the most extreme side effects in dogs and cats. Since 1974, ibuprofen has been available in the United States as a prescription antiinflammatory and pain management drug for humans.[9] In 1984, ibuprofen was approved for nonprescription use in humans. Since that time, poisoning of dogs and cats with ibuprofen has increased at an alarming rate.

Many advertisements for ibuprofen products claim that they are more effective than other nonsteroidal antiinflammatory drugs, such as aspirin. Clients may therefore be led to believe that if the product is better for them, then it must also be better for their pets, especially those with pain resulting from degenerative joint disease (arthritis) or other painful chronic ailments. Ibuprofen can currently be purchased as plain and film-coated tablets, caplets, and suspension in more than 24 over-the-counter proprietary products and many generic products.

Ibuprofen controls pain by inhibiting cyclooxygenase, a major enzyme in the arachidonic pathway leading to prostaglandin synthesis[10] (prostaglandins are important local mediators of inflammation and pain). Therapeutic doses of ibuprofen cause overt bleeding through inhibition of platelet aggregation, although impaired platelet function is generally reversible within 24 hours after discontinuation of the drug. Ibuprofen does not affect whole blood clotting or prothrombin times.

Ibuprofen is extremely toxic when administered to dogs and cats at the same doses given to humans.[10,11] Ibuprofen should never be administered to cats and, when administered to dogs, should be given at much lower doses than for humans (usually not to exceed 2 to 3 mg/kg body weight orally twice a day). Signs of ibuprofen toxicity noted in dogs, in order of frequency, include vomiting, depression or stupor, diarrhea, anorexia, incoordination, bloody stool (fresh blood or melena), increased urination, and excessive thirst. Ibuprofen also causes altered renal function and profuse bleeding from the gastrointestinal tract. Ibuprofen should not be administered to pregnant or lactating dams and preferably not to puppies. In cats, internal bleeding does not occur as often as it does in dogs but rapid breathing and panting are seen more frequently.

Therapy for dogs and cats presented for recent ibuprofen toxicity begins with inducement of vomiting (if ingestion occurred within two hours of presentation), oral administration of activated charcoal (at least two or three doses, six hours apart), and intravenous administration of fluids to enhance perfusion of the kidneys and other body organs. For signs of toxicity in the gastrointestinal system, ulcer-coating agents (i.e., sucralfate) to protect the mucosa and histamine H_2 receptor blocking agents, such as cimetidine and ranitidine, to decrease the gastric acid secretion are administered. The ulcer-coating agents and the histamine H_2 receptor blocking agents do not directly reverse the effects of ibuprofen on the gastrointestinal tract but do provide supportive therapy. The bleeding is occasionally so severe that transfusion of freshly collected whole blood is warranted. Ibuprofen toxicity can usually be reversed with supportive therapy in three to five days. In one case in my experience, however, it took three weeks and six transfusions of whole blood to save a dog that had been given an overdose of ibuprofen.

Considering the relative risk of ibuprofen toxicity, clients should be warned not to give ibuprofen to their pets unless done so under the direct supervision of a veterinarian. In most cases, aspirin is still a much safer alternative. When ibuprofen is being given, periodic evaluation for clinical improvement, monitoring for compli-

cations, and attempts at dose reduction should be part of the treatment plan.

Acetaminophen inhibits prostaglandin synthesis in the central nervous system. Although acetaminophen does not induce impaired platelet function or gastrointestinal tract ulceration, acetaminophen can produce hepatotoxicity that can be detrimental to animals. Acetaminophen is contraindicated in cats.

Guidelines for Pain Management

Successful management of pain in dogs and cats involves several distinct components.[12] Because pain is a sign of underlying disease or tissue injury, recognition and treatment of the source of pain is important. Thereafter, pain management may involve the use of appropriate analgesic drugs. In general, short-term use of opioid analgesics is the most beneficial therapy for animals with acute pain resulting from surgery.

Animals with chronic pain, such as that caused by degenerative joint disease, often experience at least partial amelioration of pain during treatment with one of the nonsteroidal antiinflammatory drugs. In general, the most effective therapeutic approach in animals with chronic pain is to begin with aspirin and then advance to other drugs if the pain is not relieved.[12] Veterinarians and technicians must remember that such side effects as renal toxicity and gastrointestinal ulceration result from the more potent nonsteroidal antiinflammatory drugs.

Pain management in cats should follow the basic parameters set for dogs with a few exceptions. Aspirin, administered no more than every three days, is the nonsteroidal antiinflammatory drug of choice. Opioid analgesics are effective in managing pain after surgery in cats as well as in dogs. Cats experience excitatory effects of opioid analgesics if inappropriately high doses are given. Doses of opioid analgesics given to cats should be lower than doses given to dogs.[12]

REFERENCES

1. Schecter NL: An approach to the child with

pain. *Patient Care* 30:116–133, 1988.

2. Kitchell RL: Problems in defining pain and peripheral mechanisms of pain. *JAVMA* 191:1195–1199, 1987.
3. Crane SW: Perioperative analgesia: A surgeon's perspective. *JAVMA* 191:1254–1257, 1987.
4. Sawyer DC: Understanding animal pain and suffering. *Proc 55th Annu AAHA Vet Tech Prog*:1–6, 1988.
5. Johnson JM: The veterinarian's responsibility: Assessing and managing acute pain in dogs and cats. Part I. *Compend Contin Educ Pract Vet* 13(5):804–809, 1991.
6. Benson GJ: The recognition and alleviation of animal pain and suffering: Opioid analgesics. *Proc 55th Annu AAHA Vet Tech Prog*:7–17, 1988.

7. Jenkins WL: Pharmacologic aspects of analgesic drugs in animals: A review. *JAVMA* 191:1231–1240, 1987.
8. Haskins SC: Use of analgesics postoperatively and in a small animal intensive care setting. *JAVMA* 191:1266–1268, 1987.
9. Simon LS, Mills JA: Nonsteroidal antiinflammatory drugs: New nonsteroidal antiinflammatory drugs. *N Engl J Med* 302:1237–1243, 1980.
10. Scherkl R, Frey HH: Pharmacokinetics of ibuprofen in the dog. *J Vet Pharmacol Ther* 10:261–265, 1987.
11. Adams SS, Bough RG, Cliffe EE, et al: Absorption, distribution, and toxicity of ibuprofen. *Toxicol Appl Pharmacol* 15:310–322, 1969.
12. Sackman JE: Pain. Part II. Control of pain in animals. *Compend Contin Educ Pract Vet* 13(1):181–193, 1991.

UPDATE

The following table lists analgesic agents used in dogs and cats.

Analgesic Agents for Use in Small Animals

Drug	Dosage Dog	Dosage Cat
Mild Analgesic Agents		
Acetaminophen	10–15 mg/kg tid-qid; PO	None (toxic)
Aspirin	10 mg/kg bid-tid; PO	10 mg/kg every 48 hours; PO
Flunixin meglumine	0.5–1.0 mg/kg sid; IV for 1–3 days	None
Phenylbutazone	10 mg/kg bid-tid; PO, IV	None
Narcotic Analgesic Agents		
Codeine	2 mg/kg qid; PO, SC	None
Meperidine	2–5 mg/kg every 2–4 hours; IM	Same as for dog
Methadone	0.11–0.55 mg/kg every 4 hours; IM	None
Morphine	0.25–1.25 mg/kg every 3–6 hours; IM, IV, SC	0.05 mg/kg every 3–6 hours; IM, SC
Oxymorphone	0.05–0.2 mg/kg every 3 hours; IM, IV, SC	0.01 mg/kg every 3 hours; IM, IV, SC
Narcotic Antagonists		
Butorphanol	0.1–0.2 mg/kg every 2–4 hours; IV *or* 0.2–0.4 mg/kg every 2–4 hours; IM, SC	Same as for dog
Nalorphine	1 mg/kg; IM, IV, SC	Same as for dog
Naloxone	0.01–0.04 mg/kg; IM, IV, SC	Same as for dog
Pentazocine	1.5–3.0 mg/kg every 2–3 hours; IM, IV	0.75–1.5 mg/kg every 2–4 hours; IV

Management of the Cancer Patient*

Elsa Beck, DVM
Joan Sheetz, AHT

Comparative Oncology Unit
College of Veterinary Medicine
Colorado State University
Fort Collins, Colorado

Cancer is not a topic most people enjoy. It cannot be ignored, however, and undoubtedly may touch each of us at some point in our lives. Current statistics show that one of four people in the United States will develop some form of cancer and one of six will die from it.[1]

This article discusses the various cancer treatment options available in veterinary medicine, the diagnostic procedures, and some management techniques.

Why treat animals with cancer? There are several good reasons. First, cancer is the leading cause of death. In one study of autopsied dogs, 23% of all deaths were attributed to cancer. Moreover, when dogs older than 10 years of age were considered, almost one half (45%) of all deaths were cancer related[2]; the number of older pets is constantly increasing because the life span of domestic animals is greater as a result of better preventive health care, better nutrition, enforced leash laws, and earlier diagnosis of disease. Because of all these factors, the number of cancer cases seen in veterinary practices will continue to increase.

Another reason to treat a pet with cancer is that most forms of cancer are treatable; cancer therapy can provide additional years of happy, pain-free life. Many cancers can be cured totally by surgery, while others can be cured or controlled with radiation therapy. Although chemotherapy provides a complete cure in only one type of cancer, other types can be controlled with drugs. Immunotherapy attempts to overcome cancer by stimulating the body's natural immune system. Newer types of therapy under development are hyperthermia to elevate the temperature of the affected area and cryotherapy to freeze the affected area. Combinations of these treatment modalities are often successful when a single measure has failed.

Another reason to treat pet cancer is that recent sociologic studies show that 50% of pet owners consider their pets to be equivalent to a human member of the family.[3] Often a pet has been with its owner(s) longer than the children have been, or the pet has served as a child substitute for a childless couple. For many single adults, a pet assumes the position of a companion, friend, and confidant. Furthermore, studies have shown that pets make significant contributions to the emotional and psychological well-being of the elderly, disabled, or emotionally disturbed or extremely shy children. "Animals can provide a boundless measure of acceptance, adoration, attention, forgiveness and unconditional love. Animals also contribute to their owner's concept of self-worth and sense of being needed."[4] Thus, each animal is very special to its owner; and a positive, sympathetic attitude toward the diagnosis and treatment of a pet can comfort and reassure the client.

Because cancer is so prevalent in both human and veterinary medicine, the owners of pets with cancer often are closely associated with human cancer patients. Clinical histories often reveal that an owner or owner's spouse, mother, sister, or brother is undergoing, or has undergone, some type of cancer treatment. A callous word, premature advice to euthanatize, or insinuations

*This article was supported in part by PHS Grant #1 PO1-CA 29582 awarded by the National Cancer Institute, Department of Health and Human Services.

that therapy is useless therefore may be insulting or upsetting to the owner. On the other hand, a positive attitude concerning therapy may encourage the client to accept a relative's cancer more easily.

Another motivation to treat pets with cancer involves the comparative research being conducted on various aspects of human and animal cancers. Animals share the same environment as their owners and thus are exposed to the same potential carcinogens.[5] In addition, the results of cancer therapy in animals can yield information that is valuable in improving treatment modalities for human cancer. For research purposes, the effectiveness of therapy is easier to evaluate in animals because they have shorter life spans and most cancers progress more rapidly in animals. In the treatment of human cancer, legal and moral constraints restrict experimentation with new forms of therapy or even minor modification of existing treatment regimens. Consequently, even though modification of a specific cancer treatment shows strong experimental evidence of being more effective and having fewer complications,

it may not be implemented in human medicine for years because it is considered unproven.

What is cancer and what causes it? The answer is not totally clear. Cancer, tumor, and neoplasia are all terms that refer to the uncontrolled growth of cells in the body. The normal control mechanisms that function to regulate the rate and amount of growth have failed. The reasons for this failure are not known entirely. Certain chemicals and viruses have been shown to cause cancer. Hormonal, genetic, environmental, nutritional, and congenital factors also have been associated with a higher incidence of cancer.[6]

Nomenclature

Cancer can be either benign or malignant. Benign tumors tend to have well-defined borders, grow slowly, and increase in size only in a local area. They generally will not impair the life of an animal and may not require treatment. Benign tumors are sometimes removed surgically if they are unsightly, subject to being injured (e.g., a sebaceous adenoma that is traumatized

TABLE I
Cell Type and Nomenclature of Common Tumors

Cell Type	Benign Tumor	Malignant Tumor
Epithelial tissue		
Stratified squamous cells	Papilloma	Squamous cell carcinoma
Liver cells	Hepatoma	Hepatocellular carcinoma
Bile duct	Bile duct adenoma	Bile duct carcinoma
Bladder	Papilloma	Transitional cell carcinoma
Kidney	Renal tubular adenoma	Renal cell carcinoma
Respiratory epithelium	Bronchial tubular adenoma	Bronchogenic carcinoma
Glands or ductal tissue	Adenoma	Adenocarcinoma
Sebaceous gland	Sebaceous gland adenoma	Sebaceous gland adenocarcinoma
Sweat gland	Sweat gland adenoma	Spiradenocarcinoma
Perianal gland	Perianal adenoma	Perianal adenocarcinoma
Ovary	Cystadenoma	Cystadenocarcinoma
	Teratoma	Granulosa cell tumor
Testis	Seminoma	Malignant seminoma
	Tubular adenoma	Malignant Sertoli cell tumor
	Interstitial cell adenoma	Interstitial cell carcinoma
Periodontal tissue	Epulis	Adamantinoma
Mesenchymal tissue		
Bone	Osteoma	Osteosarcoma
Cartilage	Chondroma	Chondrosarcoma
Fibrous connective tissue	Fibroma	Fibrosarcoma
Fat tissue	Lipoma	Liposarcoma
Joint capsule	Synovioma	Synovial cell sarcoma
Smooth muscle	Leiomyoma	Leiomyosarcoma
Striated muscle	Rhabdomyoma	Rhabdomyosarcoma
Mast cells	Mastocytoma	Mast cell sarcoma
Blood vessels	Hemangioma	Hemangiosarcoma
Pericyte	Hemangiopericytoma	Malignant hemangiopericytoma
Lymph vessel	Lymphangioma	Lymphangiosarcoma
Lymphoid tissue	None	Lymphosarcoma, lymphoma
Blood lymphocytes	Lymphocytosis	Lymphocytic leukemia
Blood neutrophils	Leukocytosis	Granulocytic leukemia
Blood monocytes	Monocytosis	Monocytic leukemia
Plasma cell	Plasmacytosis	Multiple myeloma

repeatedly during grooming), or mechanically interfere with normal movement (e.g., a large axillary lipoma that interferes with movement or an epulis on the gums that interferes with eating).

By contrast, malignant tumors tend to grow rapidly, invade into local normal tissue, and spread to distant locations through blood and lymphatic vessels. This spread to distant organs is referred to as *metastasis* and is often the life-limiting factor. Malignant tumors can be cured if they are controlled early enough to prevent local invasion or metastasis.

The nomenclature adopted to distinguish the types of tumors is straightforward. The prefix denotes the cell of origin, for example, the prefix *lipo-* means fat cells. The names of benign tumor cells usually are a combination of this prefix and the designation *-oma*; for example, *lipoma* is a benign tumor of the fat cells. In naming malignant tumors, the term *sarcoma* or *carcinoma* usually is added to the prefix. Thus, *lipo-* is the prefix for fat tissue, a benign fatty tumor is a *lipoma*, and a malignant fatty tumor is a *liposarcoma*. A benign tumor of glandular tissue is an *adenoma*, with *adenocarcinoma* denoting malignancy. Of course, there are always variations and exceptions. Normal skin cells are called *squamous cells*, a benign proliferation is a *papilloma*, while the malignant tumor is *squamous cell carcinoma*. Likewise, a benign tumor of plasma cells is *plasmacytosis*, with malignancy of these cells called *multiple myeloma*; while the sarcomas of blood cells are called *leukemias*. Table I shows the name and cell of origin of several common tumors.

Malignant tumors therefore are divided into two basic groups: carcinomas and sarcomas. The carcinomas arise from epithelial cells. They include tumors of the skin; associated glands; and cells that line the inside of the lungs, kidneys, liver, bile duct, and urinary tract. Sarcomas develop from mesenchymal (or supportive) tissue and include tumors of the bone, cartilage, joints, muscles, other connective tissues, blood and lymph vessels, white blood cells, red blood cells, and bone marrow cells.

The cell type of origin is determined by observing the tumor cells under a microscope; in a few cases, the cell type can be determined by cytologic evaluation of a fine-needle aspirate. Most tumors, however, should be diagnosed on the basis of the results of a biopsy and tissue histopathology. Submitting a biopsy for study is the most important step in diagnosing, prognosing, and instituting appropriate treatment for any mass or lump suspected of being cancer. Biopsies of skin tumors and needle aspirates of lymph nodes can be done on an animal while it is awake; however, before any animal undergoes a surgical biopsy or exploration for a mass, it should have a thorough health history, physical examination, and basic laboratory screening tests.

Diagnosis of Cancer
History

The general history of a patient with cancer should cover all areas of the animal's past and present health as well as specific questions concerning the suspected cancer. An adequate history should note when the clinical signs of cancer were first observed by the owner and how the appearance of the growth or other signs have changed. The behavior of the tumor provides valuable insight into the nature of the disease process; slow gradual growth tends to imply a more benign process, whereas recent rapid growth is more compatible with an infection of the tumor or a malignant process.

Physical Examination

The physical examination should evaluate the entire health status of the animal as well as focus on the suspected tumor. Eyes, ears, nose, throat, heart, lungs,

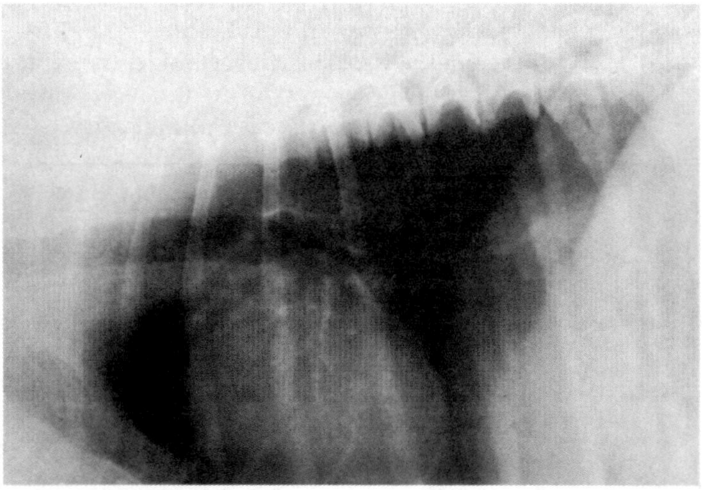

Figure 1A

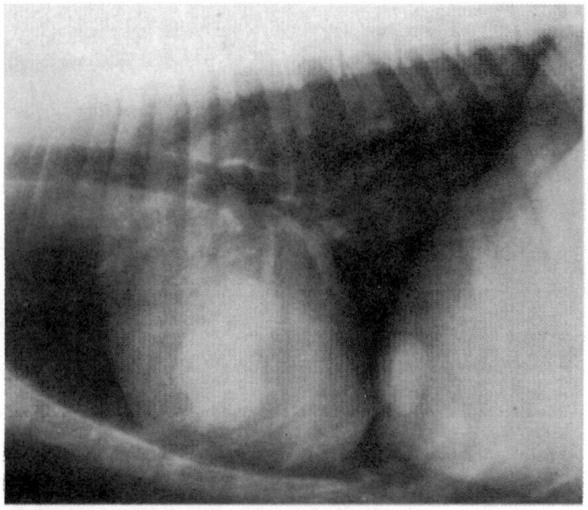

Figure 1B

Figure 1—(**A**) This right lateral view of a dog's thorax does not show any detectable metastasis. (**B**) The left lateral view (which has been turned to match the right lateral view) of the same dog shows definite metastases, which were not discernible on the right lateral view.

abdominal organs, urogenital tract, and skin should be evaluated first. Next, an exhaustive search of the animal should be done to identify any lumps and bumps undetected by the owner. Evaluating the size and comparing the bilateral symmetry of all lymph nodes are essential to judge regional spread of the tumor. Special attention should be directed to the lymph nodes, which drain fluid from the affected area. Any suspiciously enlarged lymph nodes should be aspirated and examined for cancerous cells.

Finally, attention must be directed to the mass itself. When possible, a record should be made of the height, width, depth, and location of the mass. Each mass should be described according to its relationship to the skin or deeper body structures, such as muscle or bone, or whether it is freely movable in the subcutaneous tissue. Any pigmentation, alopecia, or ulceration should also be recorded. These records can then be used to monitor changes in the size or behavior of the tumor(s).

Laboratory Tests

Basic laboratory screening tests are important, especially in any animal that is middle aged or older or if abnormalities are suspected during the physical examination. Ideally, laboratory tests should include a differential white blood cell count; packed cell volume; total protein; urinalysis; and such serum chemistries as glucose, blood urea nitrogen, and liver enzymes. A complete serum chemistry screen is appropriate in many cases. Further laboratory work might include a feline leukemia virus assay, bone marrow examination, electrocardiogram, or blood coagulation tests. Laboratory abnormalities may indicate internal tumor involvement or change the way the biopsy is performed or the cancer treated.

Radiography

Animals suspected of having cancer should be evaluated for lung metastasis. Chest radiographs should include two lateral views (both right and left sides down) and either a ventrodorsal or dorsoventral view. Metastatic lesions in the lungs may be visible only when the affected side of the lung is positioned upward. Minimal lung metastasis may be detectable only on the upward side because a fully inflated lung is necessary to supply the air contrast necessary for visualization. The downward side of the lung is compressed and partially deflated by the weight of the animal. Therefore, it contains little air to contrast with the mass (Figure 1). A radiograph of a mass located near a bone, such as the leg or jaw, should also be taken to determine whether there is any bony involvement.

Biopsy

After the general health of the animal and extent of disease have been determined, the patient is ready for biopsy. The biopsy site should be surgically clipped and prepped. Many methods of biopsy have been developed, including the use of hole punches, cutting needle instruments, and scalpel blades. A representative sample removed from the mass is referred to as an *incisional biopsy*, while complete removal of the mass is an *excisional biopsy*. The best samples are cleanly and sharply removed with little crushing or damage from heat and/or cold.

Biopsy tissue should be fixed in a 10% buffered formalin solution. Ideally, there should be 10 times more formalin than volume of biopsy for the first 24 hours (Figure 2). Large biopsies should be cut in slices until they are no thicker than 1 cm (Figure 3). Tissue that floats should be submerged using paper towels, gauze, or tongue depressors. After the initial 24 hours, the tissue can be packaged for shipment in smaller amounts of formalin (Figure 4). Plastic sample jars or two double-thickness plastic bags should be labeled clearly using a permanent-ink pen. Care should be taken not to use breakable shipping material, such as glass, or thin plastic sacks. Plenty of padding should be provided to prevent leakage. A sheet with the hospital's name and address and the name of the referring veterinarian should be included. A complete history, description, and location of the tumor should be given along with the species, age, breed, and sex of the animal. The interpretation of biopsies is not an exact science and often relies on the clinical behavior of the tumor.

The Decision to Treat

After a diagnosis is made, the veterinarian should discuss with the owner the characteristic behavior of the specific tumor and the treatment options. Patient age should rarely be used as a deterrent to treatment; age is not a disease, and the animal may survive for many years if it has no other life-limiting conditions. Even if the cancer is not curable, the quality of the pet's remaining life is important. Frequently owners feel guilty, cruel, and/or selfish for treating pets with cancer; however, animals undergoing cancer treatment often live longer with considerably less suffering than animals being treated for kidney or heart failure.

Owners and veterinarians must consider the general health of the animal as well as the tumor type when deciding whether to initiate treatment and when selecting the best treatment. The cost of cancer therapy must also be considered. In addition, some animals may have physical conditions that preclude anesthesia for surgical treatment or radiation therapy. These cases are best managed by chemotherapy if an effective drug is available.

Many owners may not have the resources to finance the most aggressive, up-to-date therapy available; euthanasia may be the only viable option in these cases. Owners electing euthanasia should never be made to feel guilty. Likewise, owners electing to treat the cancer also should never be made to feel guilty. The owner should be reassured that the decision to treat or euthanatize is helping, not torturing, the animal.

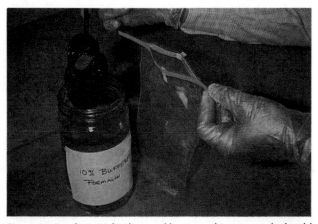

Figure 2—For the initial 24 hours of fixation, a biopsy sample should be submerged in formalin solution that is 10 times the volume of the sample.

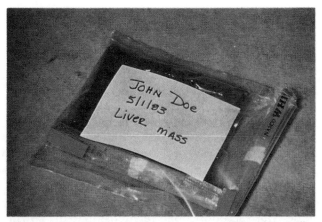

Figure 4—After fixation, the biopsy can be repackaged in a smaller volume of formalin. An unbreakable, clearly labeled container should be used to ship samples to the laboratory.

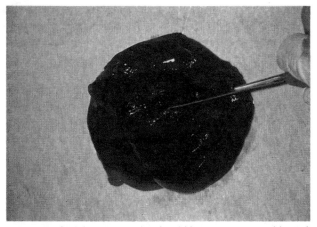

Figure 3—Thick biopsy samples should be cut in 1-cm widths with one edge left intact for continuity. This technique allows the fixative to penetrate adequately and preserve the tissue.

If the extent of disease is so obviously widespread that no form of therapy will provide relief, the owner should be gently but firmly counseled regarding the extent of disease, suffering of the pet, and lack of available treatment. Most owners will elect euthanasia if convinced that their pet is suffering and treatment will not resolve the suffering; however, if a pet is expected to be free of pain or discomfort for several months, the owner should be encouraged to enjoy this remaining time with the pet.

Treatment Options

Treatment should begin as soon after diagnosis as possible. The earlier the treatment is begun, the greater the chance for success. The most aggressive therapy that is appropriate should always be used initially because the first attempt at control has a better chance for success; recurrences of a tumor could be avoided if treated aggressively the first time, and the possibility of metastasis or untreatable local spread increases with each recurrence.

Surgery

The treatment of cancer has traditionally taken the form of surgery, radiation therapy, or chemotherapy. If the nature of the tumor allows complete removal, surgery is the easiest, quickest, and least expensive form of therapy and may provide a complete cure. If the cancer invades vital structures or is too large to remove surgically without destroying normal function, radiation therapy is the advisable option.

Radiation Therapy

Radiation therapy, which is available at a number of veterinary facilities (Figure 5), is the recommended treatment for several tumor types. Localized lymphosarcoma, hemangiopericytoma, oral squamous cell carcinoma, or dental tumors can be controlled successfully by radiation therapy. Many other types of cancers are now being evaluated for their radioresponsiveness.

One advantage of radiation therapy is the preservation of normal cosmetic and functional structure. The side effects of radiation are limited to the area receiving the dose of radiation. Almost no systemic effects (e.g., nausea, vomiting, or diarrhea) have been observed in animals. The localized changes to hair color, alopecia, and thinning of the haircoat (Figure 6) are generally well tolerated (the hair often becomes finer in consistency and a few shades lighter or darker). The skin in the radiation field tends to become more fragile and slower to heal than normal skin. In very severe skin reactions, the surface cells of the skin may die and leave superficial ulcers. Usually, these erosions heal within two to three weeks. Rarely, the reaction may be severe enough to cause necrosis or death of the tissue. Cosmetic surgery then may be necessary.

Radiation therapy is usually given in small increments of a cumulative dose. At Colorado State University, therapy is divided into 10 or 12 doses of 400 rads (4 Gy) each, given three days a week for a three- to four-week course. This division of the dose helps protect normal tissue by giving it an opportunity to repair from radia-

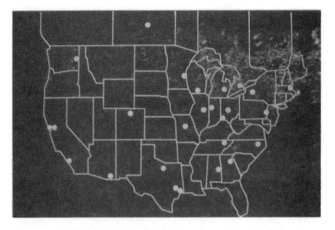

Figure 5—Locations in North America where radiation therapy currently is available for animals.

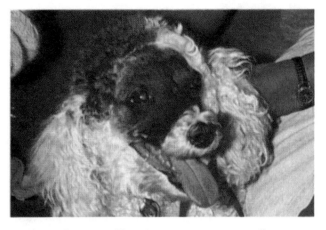

Figure 6—Alopecia and hyperpigmentation are typically apparent one month after radiation therapy.

tion damage between successive doses. This approach also provides a higher percentage of tumor cell kill because tumor cells generally do not repair as effectively as normal tissue does.

Each dose of radiation requires heavy sedation or brief anesthesia to ensure that the animal does not move and that only the targeted tissue receives the radiation. Repeated anesthesia rarely produces problems, even though the majority of animals undergoing radiation therapy are older than 10 years of age; at Colorado State University, only three of more than 1000 patients anesthetized for radiotherapy (over 10,000 anesthetic procedures) have been lost because of anesthetic-related incidents. Radiation therapy therefore is a valuable treatment option that should always be offered to a client; many clients are willing to send their pets long distances to radiation treatment centers.

Chemotherapy

Chemotherapy is the recommended option once the cancer becomes widely disseminated or involves internal organs that are not treatable by radiation or surgery. In human medicine, chemotherapy has been used successfully to control many tumors; however, veterinary medicine is in the early testing stages for using this treatment. Chemotherapy for animals has traditionally been less aggressive and less toxic than that used to treat cancer in humans, but this treatment also has been less effective in animals. Chemotherapy will cure transmissible venereal tumors and help control lymphosarcoma, mast cell tumors, multiple myeloma, and ulcerated perianal adenomas. Thyroid adenocarcinomas as well as pituitary adenomas and thyroid adenomas (benign tumors that produce active hormones and thus require treatment) may also be helped by chemotherapy. The benefits of chemotherapy range from complete cure for transmissible venereal tumors, to increased tumor-free time, to partial tumor regression, to alleviation of associated clinical signs, to slower progression of disease.

Each drug or group of drugs has its own indications,

dose, and side effects. Drug reactions can generally be divided into gastrointestinal upsets, specific organ toxicities, or bone marrow suppression. Mild vomiting and diarrhea are associated with several chemotherapeutic agents. Some drugs have toxicities restricted to a specific organ, such as myocardial toxicity with doxorubicin, inflammatory cystitis with cyclophosphamide, or neurotoxicity with vincristine. The dose-limiting factor for most drugs, however, is bone marrow suppression. Decreased production of cells by the bone marrow can result in anemia, clotting abnormalities from low platelet counts, or increased susceptibility to infection because of a low number of white blood cells. Combinations of chemotherapy, radiation therapy, and surgery often provide longer or more complete control than any given form of therapy used alone.

Nursing Support

The importance of careful, conscientious, and skillful veterinary nursing care during treatment cannot be overemphasized. Cancer patients, especially older patients, have poor immune function and are more susceptible to infection. It is crucial to minimize the risk of sepsis by practicing good hygiene, especially when preparing injection and blood-sampling sites. Keeping the patient comfortable and clean may be less glamorous than some other aspects of veterinary medicine, but it is very important.

Treatment of cancer often necessitates longer periods of hospitalization than is routinely required. It is easy for an animal to become depressed, stop eating, lose weight, and gradually debilitate while away from home. Empathy and concern for the patient can be expressed by gentleness, affection, and special attention to the animal's food and housing. A cold metal cage with a chunk of dog food in a bowl will be much more stressful than a warm towel, loving pats, and food in bite-sized morsels. Cats seem to find considerable security when placed in a small box faced away from the cage door. All patients must be sent home clean; the smell of urine or blood on the haircoat can make a lasting impression, and the animal's attitude and the degree of care it receives usually are readily apparent to the owner.

Client Education

Owner communication is very important. The client should understand what tests and treatments will be done on a pet and the possible side effects. Often, instructions given verbally to an owner who is in a state of emotional upset are forgotten quickly. Preprinted handouts outlining common side effects of a cancer therapy are helpful to send home with the client. As an alternative, especially when giving specific information to the client, the technician can write out all home-care instructions, giving any side effects that may accompany treatment. Owners feel more involved and reassured if they at least know the name of the cancer, the drugs or treatments that can be used, and the potential side effects.

Owners should be encouraged to call if they have any questions or problems. Clients often feel that the technician is more accessible than the veterinarian for answering questions because they hesitate interrupting the veterinarian from handling other cases. The technician should emphasize that no questions are stupid. Many times reassurance is all that is necessary. The technician can initiate the question-answer therapy by making periodic telephone calls that allow the owner to discuss issues that have been of concern. This approach increases the client's trust and faith in the technician's concern for the pet. This telephone technique also helps the owner feel more confident the next time the pet requires treatment or hospitalization.

Client Relationship

At some point, regardless of whether an animal has cancer, the subject of euthanasia frequently must be explored. The veterinary technician therefore must be prepared to relate with the client about this issue. Many owners feel terrible bereavement and guilt and cannot openly face this decision. The quality of each animal's life, however, is very important and the client must be supported in making a decision to euthanatize a pet. The degree of emotional attachment between an owner and a pet is often considerable. A pet that has been with a family for 14 years is not simply a dog or a cat but a friend and integral member of the family. The owner's grief should be acknowledged and understood, not avoided. The special relationship between the client and pet should be affirmed and supported by the technician, who should freely empathize with the owner. The owner should be assured that the veterinary staff has done all that was humanly possible to help the pet and that a decision to put the animal to sleep is both timely and fair. A carefully worded letter expressing condolences and sympathy is greatly appreciated.

"Cancer, unlike politics and religion, is not a topic of controversy. No one is for it. Cancer is not another word for death. Neither is it a single disease for which there is one cure. Instead, it takes many forms, and each form responds differently to treatment."[7] The efforts made by veterinary technicians on behalf of a cancer patient are often the most appreciated and rewarding aspects of their careers, rendering considerable personal satisfaction.

REFERENCES

1. Rubin P: Statement of the clinical oncologic problem, in Rubin P (ed): *Clinical Oncology*. American Cancer Society, 1983, pp 1-19.
2. Bronson FT: Variation in age at death of dogs of different sexes and breeds. *Am J Vet Res* 43:2057-2059, 1982.
3. Walshaw SO: Perspectives on pets and people. *Kal-Kan Forum* 2(5):4-14, 1983.
4. Busted L: *Animals, Aging and the Aged.* University of Minnesota Press, Minneapolis, 1983, p 23.
5. Hayes HM: The comparative epidemiology of selected neoplasms between dogs, cats, and humans: A review. *Eur J Cancer* 14:1299-1308, 1981.
6. Rensberger B: Cancer: The new synthesis—Cause, cure and prevention. *Science* September:38-39, 1984.
7. Mooney S: *A Snowflake in My Hand.* New York, Delacourt Press/Eleanor Friede, 1983, p 12.

Care of Neonatal Puppies and Kittens

Cheri A. Johnson, DVM, MS
Janet A. Grace, LVT
Veterinary Clinical Center
Michigan State University
East Lansing, Michigan

Although the vast majority of pregnancies and parturitions occur without complications, the first two weeks of life are the most precarious for puppies and kittens. Nearly all preweaning deaths occur during this period. The number of deaths is highest during the first three days. This vulnerability of puppies and kittens is influenced almost exclusively by the environment into which they are born and by the dam. Thus, the two most important aspects of neonatal care are provisions for an optimal environment and for optimal maternal health.

Environment

A clean, warm, dry site should be provided for parturition and the preweaning rearing of the young. A whelping or queening box is essential for optimal survival of the neonates. The box should be large enough for the dam to lie comfortably away from the litter if she desires but small enough so that the newborns are within easy reach. The sides should be high enough to prevent the young from wandering away but low enough for the dam to be able to come and go without difficulty.

Wood or plastic usually makes the best boxes. Wood should be sealed with nontoxic paint or sealer. A child's wading pool is an ideal whelping box, especially for larger canine breeds (Figure 1). Such pools are easy to clean and disposable when the puppies reach weaning age. Sturdy cardboard is acceptable for queening boxes, but such boxes must be replaced if they become wet. The box should be lined with clean, dry, soft, removable material, such as mattress pads, clean cloth, or newspaper. There must be no holes or loose strings to entangle the neonates. The fact that placental blood and normal postpartum vaginal discharge will stain fabric might influence the choice of lining material. Newsprint can soil light-colored fur. Straw, hay, and sawdust should not be used because they are too coarse and dusty.

The box should be placed where the owner wishes the birth and early rearing of the young to take place. The dam is introduced to this location and to the box a few weeks before her due date so that she is familiar and comfortable with them. She may become frustrated and frightened if forced to deliver her litter in unfamiliar surroundings.

A room (ambient) temperature of 80° to 85° F is recommended. This might be too warm for many dams, however. If there is doubt about the temperature, half of the box can be heated; the dam and the litter then can choose. Electric heating pads or electric blankets become too hot and may cause burns. Circulating water blankets or hot-water bottles are preferred. Heat lamps must be used with caution because they can be very hot and can cause burns. Neonatal puppies and kittens might be unable to move away from a heat source that is too hot. Drafts and dampness can chill neonates even when room temperature is adequate. Until a puppy or kitten is old enough to maintain its own body temperature, it requires a warm, dry, draft-free environment. Cardboard boxes housing neonates should never be placed on concrete; this can draw a considerable amount of heat from newborn puppies or kittens.

Newborns and the Dam

Any factor that influences the dam's health, labor, or delivery will affect the health of newborn puppies and kittens. Medications should not be given to a pregnant or lactating female without consulting the veterinarian. This includes such seemingly innocuous items as flea collars and medicated shampoos. It is reasonable to assume that whatever is in or on the dam will ultimately be in or on the

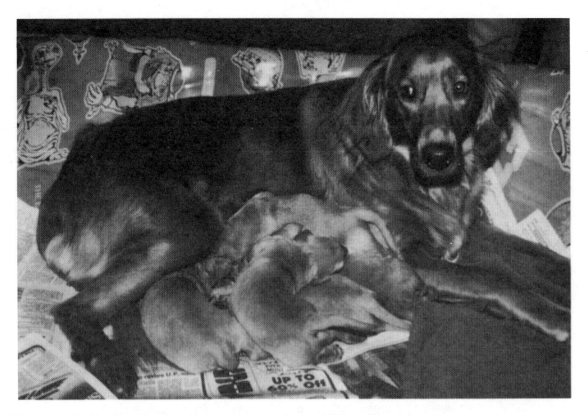

Figure 1—A bitch and her litter in a whelping box made from a child's wading pool.

neonate.

Neonatal losses increase when labor and delivery are prolonged. Labor can be prolonged if the dam is frightened, insecure, distracted, or upset. The dam must have private, familiar surroundings for parturition to proceed normally. Ideally, dams should be healthy, in excellent condition, and one to six years old. Females that are overweight, in poor condition, or older than six are likely to have smaller litters with lower birth weights, longer labor, and greater neonatal losses.

The technician or owner that is present during parturition should provide reassurance not interference. Anxiety will lessen milk flow, prolong labor, and increase the chances that the dam will injure the neonates or the observer. As soon as a puppy or kitten is delivered, the dam will lick the fetal membranes away from the newborn's face. She then proceeds to clean and dry its entire body. This cleaning is vital to bonding and recognition between the dam and the neonate. The newborn will be unable to breathe if the fetal membranes are not cleared away from its nose and mouth; if the mother fails to do this promptly, technician or owner assistance is necessary. The dam should be encouraged to do the rest of the cleaning, however. She will chew through the umbilical cord and eat the placenta; this is normal behavior. The remnant of the umbilical cord will dry up and fall off in two to three days. Frequent licking of newborns' abdominal and perineal areas is normal behavior for the dam. This is necessary to induce urination and defecation for the first two weeks of life.

Newborn puppies and kittens are unable to regulate their body temperature until they are two weeks old. They are completely dependent on their environment, especially their mother, to keep warm. Neonates maintain warmth primarily by snuggling against the dam and each other. Clipping the hair on bitches with very heavy coats, such as Siberian huskies, might enable them to recognize cool temperatures better and to be more willing to snuggle with the puppies. Clipping the hair from the mammary glands also will make it easier for the young to find the nipples.

Newborn animals have limited energy reserves and depend on nursing. There is no substitute for mother's milk, which provides all the nutrition needed. It is also the most important source of immunoglobulin (antibody). In dogs and cats, very little antibody crosses the placenta. Immunoglobulins are produced by the dam and passed to the neonates in the first milk, called *colostrum*. The immunoglobulins in colostrum protect neonates from infection until they are mature enough to produce their own antibodies.

Newborn puppies and kittens usually begin to nurse soon after birth. They should do so within the first two to three hours of life. Dams that are nervous or insecure might not nurse their young effectively. Because milk production requires energy, the dam's food and water provisions should be increased two to four times normal. More food and water are required than during pregnancy. Ideally, food is available at all times so that the dam can eat as much as she needs. If this is impossible, she should be fed at least three to four times daily. Fresh water must be always accessible. If the mother has inadequate food and water supplies, milk production will decrease and the young will not thrive.

During the first few days postpartum, the dam will spend almost all of her time with the litter. She might be reluctant to allow people to handle the young. The number of visitors should be kept to a minimum for the first three days, but the dam and the litter should not be completely isolated. Some dams will not voluntarily leave their litters; constipation and urine retention can result. Bitches should be taken for short walks several times a day; queens should be offered fresh litter pans, and the kittens should be removed for 30 to 60 minutes if necessary.

By Day 3, most dams are relaxed and comfortable with motherhood and with human visitors. We believe that puppies and kittens should be handled daily from this time on in order to promote socialization with people. Socializing with adults and young of the same species also is vital. Normal social development depends on proper companionship for orphaned litters and for litters of one.

Characteristics of Normal Newborns

Neonatal puppies and kittens should be plump, firm, pink, and healthy in appearance. The size and coat color of an individual puppy or kitten can differ significantly from its littermates. Neonates breathe 15 to 35 times per minute. Heart rate is greater than 200 beats/min until they are two weeks old. Normal rectal temperature for newborn puppies and kittens is 96° to 97° F. Body temperature gradually increases to 100° F by seven days of age. For the first week, rectal temperature should be between 96° and 100° F. A chilled puppy or kitten less than seven days old should not be warmed to 100° to 102° F, normal adult rectal temperature. Occasional twitching during sleep is characteristic of normal, well-fed puppies and kittens.

Normal birth weight for kittens is 100 ± 10 g (100 g = 0.22 pounds = 3.5 ounces). The minimum weight gain expected for a kitten is 7 to 10 g/day. By six weeks of age, kittens should weigh at least 500 g (approximately 1 pound). Normal birth weights for puppies depend on the breed. Suggested minimum birth weights are as follows: Pomeranian, 120 to 400 g; beagle, 240 to 260 g; greyhound, 450 to 525 g; and Great Dane, 500 to 750 g. A puppy should gain 5% to 10% of its birth weight per day; the birth weight is doubled by 10 to 12 days.

Puppies and kittens with lower than normal birth weights are weaker than their littermates, often are ineffective nursers, and have higher death rates. Some normal neonates do not nurse well during the first 24 hours; however, they should learn quickly and begin gaining weight by the second day. Chances for survival are poor if a neonate loses more than 10% of its birth weight.

The eyes and ears of puppies and kittens are closed at birth but will open at approximately 12 to 14 days of age. The exact day that they open varies between littermates and between individuals. Although the ear canals are closed, newborn puppies and kittens can hear. When the eyes open, the iris is usually a gray-blue color that gradually changes to the normal adult color by four to six weeks of age. Even though the eyes open at approximately two weeks, vision is very poor. The visual system continues to develop until three to four weeks of age.

Newborn puppies and kittens cannot stand or walk. They make swimming movements with their legs and slide along on the abdomen. Neonates move their heads from side to side seeking a nipple. During the first four days of life, the flexor muscles are stronger than the extensor muscles. Healthy puppies and kittens therefore will curl their bodies and limbs inward. A healthy, warm puppy will rest on its front or side with the neck extended (Figure 2).

Reflexes are very slow at birth. Puppies and kittens can balance and straighten their heads from birth, but because they are weak they are slow to do so. By seven days of age, they actively struggle to correct body posture. Although newborn animals can feel pain, their withdrawal reflexes are slow. For this reason, burns are common when poorly controlled heating pads or heat lamps are used.

Puppies and kittens can use their front legs to stand and walk at one to two weeks of age. Shortly thereafter, the rear legs also can support the body. Walking begins at approximately 16 days of age. By 21 days, puppies and kittens walk with a steady gait. They are usually very curious at this stage and become lost easily. The whelping or queening box helps keep them safely confined.

Touching around the mouth stimulates a suckling reflex in normal neonates. Tactile stimulation of the anus and the genitalia will cause defecation and urination. This stimulation, necessary to induce elimination until 16 to 18 days of age, is provided by the dam by licking. Once a puppy or kitten begins to walk, it can usually defecate and urinate voluntarily; at this stage it will begin to soil the box. Bedding therefore will need to be changed more frequently, often several times daily for large litters. The natural instinct to eliminate away from the nest is the first sign that paper training can occur. Providing a designated waste area away from the nest will hasten paper training.

Neonatal Care

A normal, healthy dam will provide all the necessary neonatal care when a clean, warm, dry environment is available. The role of the owner and the technician in neonatal care is to provide the optimal environment and to recognize abnormalities in the dam and the newborn. Signs of illness should be checked promptly. Illness in newborn animals usually progresses rapidly; the younger the animal, the faster the progression. Hopeless deterioration can occur within a matter of hours in neonatal diseases. A wait-and-see approach to illness, often sensible in mature animals, usually results in death during the first week of life.

When the dam has finished her initial cleaning, each neonate should be systematically weighed and examined. The skin should be pink, with no bruises or tears. The fur should be clean and shiny. The umbilical cord should be clean and dry, with no evidence of herniation. Breathing should be regular and comfortable. The gums and the tongue should be pink; the head should be of normal size and shape. There should be no swelling or discharge from the eyes or the ears. All limbs and digits should be present,

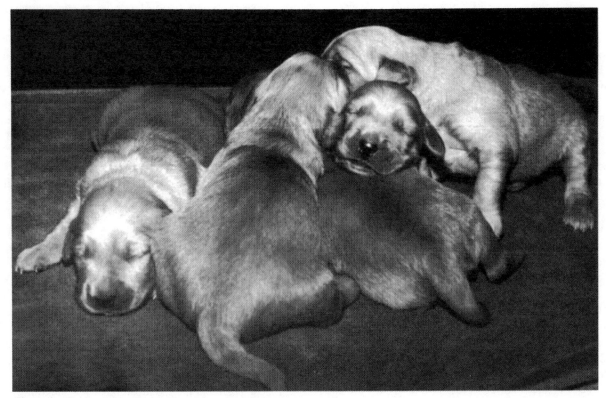

Figure 2—Golden retriever puppies resting comfortably.

with proper proportions and freely movable joints; there should be good muscle tone and muscle activity. The chest and the abdomen should be symmetric and round. The tail, the anus, and the genitalia should be present and normal.

The dam and the neonates should be examined and handled daily. In particular, the dam's food and water intake and urine and fecal output should be noted. Any significant change in the normal pattern justifies further evaluation. The mammary glands should be examined for evidence of increased redness, pain, sore or misshapen nipples, or abnormal milk. Certain dog breed standards require dewclaw removal or tail docking; these surgeries are usually done at three to five days of age, depending on the size and health of the puppy.

By five to seven weeks, the dam's milk and her patience are usually exhausted; the young must begin to eat solid food. We recommend that solid food be introduced at three to four weeks to ensure a gradual, comfortable transition from milk for all concerned. High-quality dry food intended for puppies and kittens should be mixed with water to a gruellike consistency. Initially, puppies and kittens will walk, sit, fall, and play in the food; but they quickly learn that solid food is best eaten. The diet must be nutritionally balanced and complete; diets marketed by reputable pet food manufacturers are preferable. The manufacturer's recommendations for food preparation should be followed. Puppy and kitten diets are not the same and should not be interchanged. The dam should be removed while the puppies or kittens are eating because she might

compete for the food and injure the young. Homemade formulas are unlikely to be nutritionally balanced and complete.

Common Signs of Illness

During the first week of life, it is normal for littermates to sleep in piles. Older puppies and kittens observed to be inactive and piled on top of each other usually are too cold. If they are not touching the dam or each other, littermates might be too hot; however, rejection by the dam can be an important sign of illness. If puppies are panting or if the gums and skin are red, the animals are definitely too hot. A dry, lackluster, rough haircoat can be a sign of illness or maternal neglect in neonates. Puppies and kittens that cry for periods longer than 20 minutes are probably not well. They may be cold, hungry, neglected, or ill. Decreased activity might be the only sign of illness. Decreased muscle tone, causing a limp or flat appearance, is a grave sign. Labored breathing and gums that are pale, gray, or bluish—rather than pink—also are serious.

Common Causes of Illness

Because a normal dam provides all of the necessities of neonatal survival (warmth, food, and sanitation), anything affecting her health will affect the neonates. Ill, neglected puppies or kittens are often the first sign of illness in the dam. If one neonate is ill, the entire litter and the dam should be carefully examined.

Hypothermia (low body temperature) is a common cause

of neonatal death. The importance of a proper environment and adequate maternal care for the regulation of neonatal body temperature has been discussed. As body temperature begins to fall, newborn puppies and kittens usually cry. With continued hypothermia, crying stops, activity and muscle tone decrease, and the neonates become limp. Respiratory rate and heart rate drop rapidly as temperature falls. Dams will usually cull cold puppies or kittens as if they were already dead. Hypothermic puppies and kittens nonetheless may be saved if they are recognized early.

Feeling the neonate's skin is not an accurate way of estimating body temperature; puppies or kittens can feel warm to the touch and yet have subnormal rectal temperatures. Neonates that are actually cold to the touch usually are profoundly hypothermic. Chilled (hypothermic) neonates should be warmed until the rectal temperature is 97° to 100° F (not higher). This warming is achieved by wrapping the patient in a blanket and surrounding it with hot-water bottles or hot-water blankets or by the cautious use of a heat lamp. Warming must not be fast or hot enough to burn the skin.

As chilled puppies or kittens warm, they become more active. When they are warm, the dam will accept them again. Barring additional problems, they should thrive. If they have not warmed after one to two hours, they are unlikely to do so and usually die. The cause of hypothermia must be determined and corrected. The owner or technician should check for drafts, damp bedding, and maternal neglect, as discussed.

Hypoglycemia, or low blood sugar, is another common cause of neonatal mortality. Glucose (sugar) is the body's major source of energy. Because neonates have few energy reserves, they must eat frequently to maintain normal blood sugar. Anything that alters the quality or quantity of the dam's milk can cause hypoglycemia in the young.

Hypothermia often results in hypoglycemia. The enzymes that digest milk into glucose cannot function at low temperatures. Also, the movement of food through the digestive tract is delayed. Thus, even if a chilled puppy or kitten has a stomach full of milk, the energy in the milk is unavailable. Sugar solutions should be used to treat hypoglycemia. Glucose is preferable to milk or colostrum because it can be absorbed directly into the blood without digestion. Honey, corn syrup, or sugar-water (two parts sugar to one part water) can be used. Hypoglycemic neonates should be checked for hypothermia, and hypothermic neonates should be checked for hypoglycemia. Mother's milk should be reinstituted when the hypoglycemia and hypothermia have been corrected.

Trauma is a common cause of death in puppies and kittens. In one colony, trauma caused 37% of puppy deaths. Some neonates are accidentally crushed by the dam. Others are cannibalized. Some are wounded by dams that bite the umbilical cord too close to the abdominal wall or that puncture the neonate's body while carrying it. Bite wounds and cannibalism are most common with dams that are anx-

ious or frightened. The technician should strive to provide a stress-free environment to minimize further neonatal mortality. Dams demonstrating such behavior for one or more litters should be culled from breeding programs. Because maternal behavior is inherited, aggressive behavior toward neonates is considered to be a serious fault. A dam's persistent aggression toward additional litters justifies her removal from the breeding program.

Stillbirths, anatomic abnormalities, and low birth weights accounted for more than 50% of kitten deaths in one colony. If dams producing dead, small, or deformed offspring are intended for repeated breeding, the cause of the abnormality should be investigated in an attempt to prevent the problem in future pregnancies. If the cause is hereditary, future litters probably will be affected.

Infections, which cause illness and death in puppies and kittens, are acquired from the dam or from the environment. Common infections (bacterial, viral, and parasitic) can be prevented by proper sanitation and hygiene, proper vaccination, and deworming of the dam. Good sanitation and hygiene are important in dogs and cats of all ages and stages of life. Vaccination and deworming should be a routine part of prebreeding care. Very young and very old animals are usually the first to suffer from poor environment.

The physical appearance of an ill or dead puppy or kitten does not necessarily indicate the cause of death. For example, hypothermia, hypoglycemia, and many infections make newborns weak and less active. A neonate that is close to death is likely to be limp and hypothermic regardless of the cause. Unexplained deaths should be investigated by necropsy performed by a veterinarian. The results can help determine how to treat or protect the littermates and the dam, how to protect the remainder of the colony, and how to prevent recurrence in future litters of the dam.

Summary

The goal of neonatal care in puppies and kittens is to maximize the health and well-being of newborns. This is best accomplished by assuring optimal maternal health, providing a proper environment, and recognizing problems early. Neonatal health problems must be corrected quickly because deterioration is usually rapid in the young. The cause of a problem is determined most expediently by prompt examination of the affected neonate, its dam and littermates, and its environment. Examination of the patient only is insufficient.

BIBLIOGRAPHY

Lawler DF (ed): Pediatrics. *Vet Clin North Am [Small Anim Pract]* 17(3), 1987.
Lawler DF, Bebiak DM: Nutrition and management of reproduction in the cat. *Vet Clin North Am [Small Anim Pract]* 16:495–520, 1986.
Lawler DF, Monti KL: Morbidity and mortality in neonatal kittens. *Am J Vet Res* 45:1455–1460, 1984.
Mosier JE (ed): Canine Pediatrics. *Vet Clin North Am* 8(1), 1978.

Management of Canine Acute Pancreatitis

An understanding of canine acute pancreatitis enables the technician to provide vital support to the patient; such support can positively affect the patient's immediate and long-term prognosis for survival.

Sheila Grosdidier, LVT
Hill's
Topeka, Kansas

Canine acute pancreatitis (CAP) is frequently frustrating for the clinician. The complex nature of the disease also often presents management challenges to the technical support team. A confirmed diagnosis of pancreatitis can be made only through biopsy; information must therefore be gathered, however slowly, before confirmation of acute pancreatitis can be made and a course of treatment can be determined. Biochemical profiles, urinalysis, pancreatic enzyme assays, radiographs, and electrocardiograms assist the clinician and provide information that can determine ongoing medical treatment and clinical management. An understanding of canine acute pancreatitis enables the technician to provide vital support to the patient; such support can positively affect the patient's immediate and long-term prognosis for survival.

UNDERSTANDING THE DISEASE

The major function of the pancreas is to secrete digestive (exocrine) and hormonal (endocrine) enzymes. A normal pancreas is shown in Figure 1. Pancreatitis results when these enzymes are re-

Originally published in Volume 13, Number 1, January/February 1992

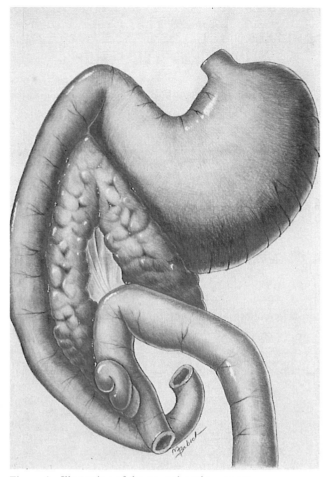

Figure 1—Illustration of the normal canine pancreas.

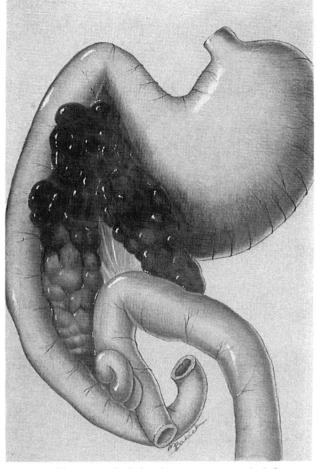

Figure 2—Illustration depicting the severe pancreatic inflammation that occurs in cases of canine acute pancreatitis.

leased into the parenchyma and interstitial fluid and result in necrosis and inflammation[1] (Figure 2). There are two types of pancreatitis, which vary in severity. The edematous interstitial form of pancreatitis is more mild than necrotic hemorrhagic pancreatitis, which is far more severe and damaging. The sequela of both types of disease, however, can permanently alter the effectiveness of the endocrine and/or exocrine functions of the pancreas and result in diabetes mellitus, exocrine pancreatic insufficiency, or chronic pancreatitis.[2] The occurrence of these two types of canine acute pancreatitis also accounts for the diversity of clinical signs in the patient. Tissue autolysis caused by pancreatic enzymes affects the severity of signs as well as the degree of the pain the animal is experiencing (see Signs of Canine Acute Pancreatitis).

Canine acute pancreatitis is estimated to account for 1% to 2% of all cases of dogs presented to veterinarians, thereby making it the most common pancreatic disease.[2] The most commonly affected pets are sedentary and somewhat obese miniature schnauzers, dachsunds, or Shetland sheepdogs[2] (see Factors That Can Precipitate Pancreatitis).

LABORATORY FINDINGS

Laboratory findings in cases of canine acute pancreatitis can be nonspecific and may indicate other diseases. Results of the biochemical profile, complete blood count (CBC), urinalysis, and electrocardiogram as well as radiographic findings are used to establish the primary diagnosis and to evaluate the health status of the patient.

Leukocytosis with a left shift is commonly seen. The total white blood cell count (WBC) indicates the degree of necrosis and severity of tissue damage. The microhematocrit is an effective screening device to check for hyperlipidemia, icterus, dehydration, and buffy coat. (The buffy coat is the light stratum made up mostly of white blood cells of the blood clot, which occurs when the sample is centrifuged. Platelets are the topcoat; the following layers, in order, are lymphocytes and monocytes, granulocytes, and reticulocytes.) Anemia is present on rare occasions; however, the pathophysiology of this phenomenon is unknown.[1] The presence of a nonregenerative left shift suggests toxemia, shock, or overwhelming infection.[3] This finding is serious and indicates a severe progression of the

Signs of Canine Acute Pancreatitis

Vomiting	Dehydration
Diarrhea	Respiratory distress
Patient assumes	Cardiac arrhythmia
"prayer" position	Leukocytosis
Pain in the right	Elevated liver enzymes
cranial abdomen	Hyperglycemia
Depression	Hypercholesterolemia
Anorexia	Hyperlipidemia
Elevated temperature	Azotemia
Icterus	Hypertriglyceridemia
Ascites	Bleeding disorders

Signs may occur in various combinations and to varying degrees.

Factors That Can Precipitate Pancreatitis

Drugs: *isoniazid, corticosteroids, chlorpromazine, sulfasalazine*

Infection

Cushing's disease

Trauma (hit by car)

Thoracolumbar surgery

Hypercalcemia (high supplementation)

Uremia

Ischemia

Heredity

High-fat diet (well above energy requirements, especially treats)

Infections agents: *herpesvirus, picornavirus, parvovirus*

---

disease; if a nonregenerative left shift is present, the prognosis for survival is poor.

Biochemical Profiles

Exposure of the liver to toxic properties transported by means of the portal system of the pancreas produces an increase in liver enzymes.[4] An increase in bilirubin resulting in icterus is sometimes seen in the serum or on physical examination.[4] Azotemia can be seen in dehydrated animals.[5] Elevated lipase and amylase enzymes can also indicate impaired renal function; renal failure must therefore be ruled out. Serum values of amylase and lipase increased two to three times the normal level more strongly indicate canine acute pancreatitis than renal failure.[2]

Hyperglycemia as a result of stress can be present. Increased amounts of fat in the blood, which can result in lipemic serum and can (in turn) alter the results of serum enzyme assays, are often seen in cases of acute pancreatitis. (Valid results can be obtained by sending the samples to laboratories skilled in reducing lipid content in a sample through manipulation.) Moderately lowered calcium levels are not of major importance because the active iodized portion of the calcium usually is normal.[2]

Urinalysis

Renal failure can be ruled out through urinalysis and biochemical profile; the diagnosis of pancreatitis can thus be substantiated. Urinalysis is inexpensive and should be included in the diagnostic process. In addition, the hydration status of the patient throughout treatment can be determined using urinalysis.

Pancreatic Enzyme Assays

A significant increase in pancreatic enzymes, lipase, and/or amylase can provide the most accurate means of diagnosing clinical pancreatitis. Although catalytic and saccharogenic assays may be used,[3] the pancreatic enzyme assay is the most accurate because it is species specific and the values are less likely to be altered by the presence of other enzymes.[3] It is commonly believed that parallel increases in lipase and amylase are seen in diagnosing canine acute pancreatitis; however, amounts can vary and still be revealing (lipase can be significantly increased without increased amylase or vice versa). An increased level of lipase, however, is more reliable than a comparably increased level of amylase.[6] In addition, as a result of depleted storage of enzymes in the pancreas (which subsequently diminishes their amount in peripheral circulation), a normal enzyme serum value can be noted in dogs with canine acute pancreatitis.[6] Lipase can also be elevated as much as fivefold as a result of dexamethasone therapy without resulting in clinical pancreatitis.[6]

Radiographs

Although they are not singularly diagnostic, radiographs can assist in providing a tentative diagnosis. Ventrodorsal and lateral abdominal radiographs with a survey of the thorax are the most useful. Increased density and diminished contrast coupled with granularity of the right cranial abdomen are regularly seen in cases of canine acute pancreatitis. This is sometimes called a ground glass appearance.[7] Ventral displacement of the descending duodenum with a static gas pattern in the transverse colon often coincides with the ground glass appearance on the radiograph.

Electrocardiograms

Because cardiac arrhythmia occurs in canine acute pancreatitis, the cardiac health of the patient must be evaluated. The most common abnormal patterns in dogs with canine acute pancreatitis are preventricular contractions and ventricular tachycardia.[2] Arrhythmia must be closely monitored and may require intensive therapy.

TREATMENT AND MANAGEMENT OF ACUTE PANCREATITIS: THE TECHNICIAN'S ROLE

Canine acute pancreatitis is life-threatening and unpredictable. If the animal has a chance to survive, vital supportive care is essential; however, the patient may succumb to the disease even if provided with meticulous care.[8] The main objective of treatment and management of canine acute pancreatitis is to alleviate clinical signs while providing supportive therapy to the critically ill patient in a manner that allows the pancreas to return (as much as possible) to normal function. As with any severe illness, the best approach is determined by assessing the situation and managing the most life-threatening signs first and then systematically approaching each of the other signs. As soon as the clinician has assessed the course of treatment, the technician must assume the challenge of administering the supportive care in a manner that results in the least stress for the patient. A technician who completely understands the treatment and monitors the patient closely is the one who is best prepared to recognize subtle changes in the animal's condition.

Imagine that the patient is adrift on the ocean in a very leaky boat. Which leak should be sealed first? What can be done to keep the boat from sinking before the patching process is complete? In cases of canine acute pancreatitis, the first item that should be taken care of is hydration. If the animal is to recover, hydration must be maintained through use of intravenous normal saline solutions that maintain fluid replacement. The technician should be alert and attentive during such therapy, and the patient should be closely monitored for hypokalemia.[5] Low serum potassium can cause weakness, ataxia, and cardiac arrhythmia. Most intravenous solutions have 4 mEq/L of potassium. If replacement therapy is necessary, the technician must not ex-

ceed 0.5 mEq/kg/hr.[5] Excessive administration of potassium may result in cardiotoxicity and death.[9] In cases of canine acute pancreatitis, treatment of metabolic acidosis may also be indicated. Metabolic acidosis is commonly treated by administration of lactated Ringer's solution; if necessary, bicarbonate may be added.[5] Animals that evidently are azotemic often regain normal pH balance as soon as their hydration status has improved.[5]

To diminish production of pancreatic enzymes and to prevent their entrance into the digestive tract, the patient should be given nil per os (NPO) for at least 24 to 36 hours after the last documented episode of vomiting. Administration of antibiotics is necessary to control bacteria, which thrive in the environment of necrotizing tissue. These bacteria often are gram-negative enteric and anaerobic organisms.[10] Under normal circumstances, populations of bacteria are controlled within the gastrointestinal tract with the movement of digesting materials and the integrity of intact tissue.[9]

The pain involved in canine acute pancreatitis is dramatic. To expedite recovery and reduce the stress associated with pain, many patients require analgesia.[9] The drug of choice is meperidine hydrochloride because it has sedative properties that enable the patient to rest more comfortably.[9] The technician, however, must monitor the animal's individual response to the medication to determine if the dose being administered is appropriate. Meperidine hydrochloride is contraindicated in the presence of hepatic or renal disease.[9]

The technician should carefully monitor blood and urine glucose for the presence of diabetes mellitus. Although hyperglycemia from stress is frequently present, blood levels above 200 mg/dl suggest further pancreatic damage.[5] The patient also should be monitored for the development of disseminated intravascular coagulation (DIC), which results from the release of tissue thromboplastin from necrotic tissue.[1] Disseminated intravascular coagulation can be diagnosed using a coagulation profile, including platelet count, prothrombin time, partial thromboplastin time, and fibrin degradation products. The use of a prohibitive agent (e.g., heparin) should be considered as a preventive measure.[11]

The clinician can evaluate the integrity of the pancreas during recovery by monitoring lipase and amylase levels. Chemistry profiles are routinely performed to determine liver damage, acute renal failure, or obstruction to the bile duct that has resulted from pancreatic edema.[10] Plasma electrolytes, which can be deranged by canine acute pancreatitis or as a result of aggressive fluid therapy, must also be evaluated.[5]

Episodes of vomiting must be closely monitored to determine when the patient can begin oral intake of food and water. Oral intake of food and water can begin after the patient has gone nil per os for 24 to 36 hours with no incidents of vomiting. In the next 12 to 24 hours, water may be given. I have found that providing ice cubes periodically for the first 12 hours is an effective way to begin giving water because the patient is unable to ingest the water too rapidly and the ice cubes diminish the likelihood of vomiting.

Food should be withheld until no incidents of vomiting have occurred for 18 to 24 hours. After this time, small amounts of a highly digestible, fat-restricted diet should be offered. The patient should initially be offered a small portion of diet to lessen the chances of vomiting. On the first day, only 1/3 of the usual caloric intake should be given (the patient should continue to be offered small amounts of water). On the second day, the patient can be given 2/3 of the usual total caloric intake; on the third day, the patient may be allowed a normal amount of calories. At this time, dividing total caloric intake into four to six meals a day also diminishes the likelihood of vomiting. The patient should remain on intravenous fluids until water intake returns to normal, which usually occurs at approximately the same time that caloric intake reaches two thirds of the normal level. If vomiting recurs at any time during this process, all oral intake of food should be discontinued and begun again in 12 hours.

The technician's ability to understand and anticipate the nursing needs of the pancreatitis patient completely can increase the chances of survival and allow the animal to live a modified (but normal) life. Methods used by the technician during the patient's hospital stay directly influence future dietary management and health of the patient.

THE TECHNICIAN AS TEACHER

Information provided by the technician to the pet owner directly affects the care that the animal receives at home. The technician must have a complete understanding of the disorder and be ready to answer the client's questions. The time that the technician spends in studying the disease is well spent.

Although controversial, oral pancreatic enzymes prescribed by the veterinarian are sometimes administered after canine acute pancreatitis as a form of maintenance therapy to decrease the work load of the pancreas. In humans, administering pancreatic enzymes has been shown to lessen pain.[12] The technician must be prepared to justify the use of these agents to clients.

The client must be aware that any supplements to the diet can result in relapse of acute pancreatitis. Increased dietary protein stimulates cholecystokinin (CCK) release that, in turn, overstimulates the pancreatic exocrine glands and results in pancreatic inflammation and destruction.[8] The technician must emphasize to clients that there is no nutritional justification for sedentary and/or obese dogs to ingest high-fat treats or be fed a high-fat diet. This point should especially be addressed to clients who feed these treats, meat scraps, or bacon grease. It is worth mentioning that although dogs are carnivorous, they are not true carnivores because they lack the ability to eliminate large amounts of fat from their systems without possible adverse effects.[13] Chronic relapses result in loss of functioning cells.[14]

Diseases that are secondary to canine acute pancreatitis can be significant and serious. Dogs with the disorder often return with diabetes mellitus, pancreatic exocrine insufficiency, and less often, secondary pyelonephritis resulting from septicemia.[15] Onset of pancreatic exocrine insufficiency indicates that 90% of functional exocrine tissue has been compromised.[14] The client should be informed of the signs associated with such problems and be encouraged to contact the veterinary clinic with any concerns. The dietary management of canine acute pancreatitis plays an important role in the long-term functioning of patients with this disease condition. Long-term dietary therapy is important to discuss with the owner during convalescence and at home. The patient must be observed carefully. Are there risk factors that could potentiate recurrence? If the animal is overweight, a weight-reduction program should begin after the initial convalescent period of approximately two weeks. A diet that has increased fiber, is low in fat, and is nutritionally balanced for weight loss is indicated. The described diet possesses the nutritional qualities necessary for dietary management of pancreatitis as well as for weight reduction. Fiber regulates fat absorption from the intestinal tract and provides satiety, which is important for dogs that have problems with hyperlipidemia in association with canine acute pancreatitis. Some research has indicated that hyperlipidemia contributes to onset of canine acute pancreatitis.[15]

THE TECHNICIAN AS COUNSELOR

Effective counseling of the client can play an integral role in the long-term management of cases of canine acute pancreatitis. Effective communication with the client can be developed during the animal's hospitalization. When it is shared with a client on an ongoing basis rather than just at the animal's discharge, information is more easily assimilated and remembered. When technicians help clients understand that their pets have a serious illness and must be on a restricted diet, these clients will be less likely to continue to feed high-fat foods and are more likely to adhere to the prescribed diet. Clients should understand that the care and food provided to their pets contribute to the long- and short-term prognosis for survival of their pets.

Counseling should be carried out in a manner that encourages client participation and cooperation. Clients must be provided with specific information that will assist them in preventing a recurrence and should be reminded that any high-calorie, high-fat treats that have been given to the dog in the past must be discontinued. Treats can be harmful because the additional fat and protein contained in them can result in a relapse of pancreatitis and/or detract from the nutritional completeness of the prescribed diet. If pet owners insist on "treating" their pets, an alternative recipe can be prepared from the diet itself (see Dog Treat Recipe). If the veterinarian has prescribed any specific medication, that technician must fully explain the use of such medication to the client.

Clients must be reminded that they are as much a member of the support team as the veterinarian and technician and that canine acute pancreatitis is a disease that requires lifelong cooperation between the veterinary staff and the client. The condition should be discussed with the client before the pet is ready to be discharged. If they are counseled before their pets are discharged, clients are more likely to pay attention to what is being said instead of being distracted by their pets from which they have been separated. If possible, clients should be shown pictures to illustrate key points and should be given written instructions that can be taken home and reviewed later.

Technicians should make a follow-up call in five days. In addition to being asked about the dog's condition, clients should be encouraged to discuss their part of the supportive care to ensure that they fully understand their role in the support program. The technician should reiterate the information that has already been given to the client; the client should also be reminded that a team effort ensures that the pet is receiving the highest quality care available. Clients must be encouraged to consult the veterinary team at any time in the future if they have any questions or concerns.

CONCLUSION

Canine acute pancreatitis is an unpredictable and serious disease that can result in death. Although there are times when even the most meticulous care cannot change the outcome, excellent medical management and long-term dietary supervision can frequently affect the patient's short- and long-term prognosis for survival. Not only do they

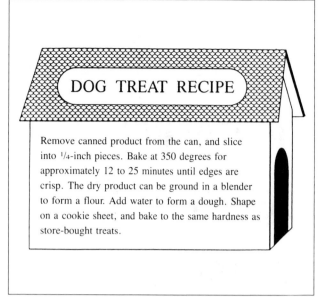

DOG TREAT RECIPE

Remove canned product from the can, and slice into ¼-inch pieces. Bake at 350 degrees for approximately 12 to 25 minutes until edges are crisp. The dry product can be ground in a blender to form a flour. Add water to form a dough. Shape on a cookie sheet, and bake to the same hardness as store-bought treats.

play a critical role in the management of canine acute pancreatitis during the time the patient is in the hospital, technicians can be invaluable to clients in teaching and counseling them on this life-threatening disease.

REFERENCES

1. Williams DA: Exocrine pancreatic disease, in Ettinger SJ (ed): *Textbook of Veterinary Internal Medicine.* Philadelphia, WB Saunders Co, 1989, pp 1528–1554.
2. Drazner FH: Diseases of the canine and feline pancreas. *Proc 52nd Annu AAHA Meet*: 293–301, 1985.
3. Coles EM: *Veterinary Clinical Pathology*, ed 3. Philadelphia, WB Saunders Co, 1980, pp 230–231.
4. Schaer M: The diagnosis and treatment of acute pancreatitis in the dog and cat. *Proc 54th Annu AAHA Meet*: 308–310, 1987.
5. Kirk RW, Bistner SI: Clinical procedures, in *Veterinary Procedures and Emergency Treatment*, ed 3. Philadelphia, WB Saunders Co, 1981, pp 573–596.
6. Williams DA: Pancreatitis—Recent findings. *Proc 7th Annu ACVIM Vet Forum*: 787–790, 1989.
7. Williams DA: Pancreatitis. *Proc 55th Annu AAHA Meet*: 136–137, 1988.
8. Leib MS: Acute pancreatitis: An inconsistent entity—Atypical case presentations. *Proc 7th Annu ACVIM Vet Forum*: 115–118, 1989.
9. Weber AJ, et al: *Veterinary Pharmaceuticals and Biologicals*, ed 5. Lenexa, KS, Veterinary Medicine Publishing Co, 1986, p 547.
10. Lewis LD, Morris ML, Hand MS: *Small Animal Clinical Nutrition*, ed 3. Topeka, KS, Mark Morris Associates, 1987, pp 7/17–7/22.
11. Williams DA: Exocrine pancreatic pathobiology. *Proc 55th Annu AAHA Meet*: 252–255, 1988.
12. Williams DA: Acute pancreatitis. *Proc 55th Annu AAHA Meet*: 256–258, 1988.
13. Hilton J: Do high fat dog foods predispose dogs to pancreatitis? *Can Vet J* 29:885–886, 1988.
14. Stock-Damage C, Bouchet P, Dentinger A, et al: Effect of dietary fiber supplementation of the exocrine pancreas of the dog. *Am J Clin Nutr* 38:843–849, 1983.
15. Pidgeon G: Exocrine pancreatic disease in the dog and cat. *Comp Anim Pract*: 67–71, 1987.

Emergency Medicine: CPR Techniques

Timing and patient selection are critical in the performance of cardiopulmonary resuscitation; the length of arrest is a significant prognostic factor.

Melani Poundstone, DVM
TenderCare Veterinary Medical Center
Greenwood Village, Colorado

Cardiopulmonary arrest is a sudden cessation of ventilation and effective circulation that requires emergency intervention in order to prevent death. The technique used to reverse cardiopulmonary arrest is referred to as cardiopulmonary resuscitation (CPR). The resuscitation techniques used on small animals are largely derived from those used on humans. Recent modifications have improved the techniques used in small animal medicine.

The purpose of this article is to familiarize technicians with current resuscitative techniques. Cardiopulmonary resuscitation has been subdivided into four phases: readiness and prevention, recognition and basic cardiac life support, advanced cardiac life support, and post-resuscitative care.[1,2]

FIRST PHASE: READINESS AND PREVENTION

Readiness

Readiness and prevention is probably the most important phase in cardiopulmonary resuscitation. Seconds can mean the difference in saving an animal's life; being prepared to handle an emergency

Originally published in Volume 13, Number 5, June 1992

can save precious time. Preparation requires setting up an area to handle emergencies and having needed items close at hand. An area in the hospital should be designated for emergencies only. The selected area should be readily accessible and well lighted. It should include an adjustable table, an oxygen supply, electrical outlets, and the equipment needed to handle an emergency. All items must be kept in one area and easily available.

A crash cart can be used for this purpose. The cart contains drugs, syringes, endotracheal tubes, and other essential materials (see the Readiness Checklist). Emergency drugs should be labeled clearly so they are easily identifiable, and syringes should have preplaced needles. A bag of isotonic fluids is hung and ready for use. The area should be checked and restocked daily.

Being ready to handle an emergency requires more than just being prepared. All staff members who will handle emergencies must receive additional training and practice. In-house seminars and mock drills improve response time and patient treatment. Each member should be evaluated after a drill, and methods of improvement should be discussed. A code word is established to alert staff members of an emergency so that each individual arrives quickly at the designated area. Staff should receive designated assignments—one member intubates while another connects the electrocardiograph machine, and so on. Research into the effectiveness of cardiopulmonary resuscitation demonstrates that patient survival rates increase from 5% to 20% when a readiness program is instituted.[1]

Prevention

Although clinics are prepared to handle patients in cardiopulmonary arrest, prevention is the primary objective. Prevention of arrest applies to hospitalized patients, which can be closely monitored. Clinical signs of impending cardiopulmonary arrest include a change in respiration, a weak or irregular pulse, pale or cyanotic mucous membranes, and hypothermia.[3,4] Recognizing and correcting these signs early may prevent cardiac arrest.

SECOND PHASE: RECOGNITION AND BASIC LIFE SUPPORT
Recognition

The technician is usually the first to assess an animal either by a telephone conversation or at the clinic. When assessing a patient's condition over the phone, the first priority is to determine the nature of the problem. This is difficult if the client is upset; it may be necessary to calm the client. If the animal needs veterinary attention, the technician can give the client advice that will help the animal before transportation to the hospital (e.g., application

---

Readiness Checklist

- Well-lighted room with a table to work on
- Clippers
- Crash cart equipped with:
    - Emergency drugs (expiration dates checked)
    - Endotracheal tubes of various sizes (checked for leaks)
    - Tracheostomy tubes of various sizes
    - Oxygen masks
    - Resuscitator bag
    - Oxygen tank with pressure gauges (if wall oxygen unavailable)
    - Tie gauze and syringe for inflating endotracheal cuff
    - Syringes with preplaced needles
    - Assorted spinal needles
    - Laryngoscope
    - Sponge forceps
    - Aspiration device and suction tips
    - Intravenous catheters (peripheral and central) of various sizes
    - Intravenous fluids (a bag of lactated Ringer's solution set up and lightly pressurized)
    - Defibrillator paddles and electrocardiographic paste
- Electrocardiograph machine
- Defibrillator
- Doppler blood-flow detector and cuffs

---

of pressure bandages or placing the animal on a backboard). If the patient's situation is critical, the client should be directed to the closest clinic that offers emergency care. It is advisable to know the locations and telephone numbers of nearby clinics.

Any animal admitted in an emergency situation must be evaluated immediately, and its condition must be prioritized. Triage is the art of classifying patients based on the need for emergency care.

Triage is typically composed of four classifications.[5] Class I patients have life-threatening injuries and need immediate medical attention. This category comprises animals that are unconscious or are in respiratory distress, arrest, or hypovolemic shock. Patients in class II have adequate respiratory function but may progress to class I if they do not receive medical attention within one hour; most trauma patients are in this category. Class III patients have medical conditions, such as open fractures, that require treatment within a few hours. Class IV patients have less serious conditions but must receive medical treatment within 24 hours.[5]

Evaluation of a patient must be rapid, systematic, and complete. Initial assessment on arrival involves evaluation of mentation, respiration, mucous membrane color, pulse rate and quality, ambulation, and temperature. The patient should be assessed for active bleeding and open fractures. An abnormality that is detected during the assessment of one area must be corrected before moving to the next area. If cardiopulmonary arrest is diagnosed (by the presence of respiratory apnea, cyanotic mucous membranes, an undetectable pulse, and dilated pupils), resuscitation is begun.

Basic Life Support Techniques

The major objective of cardiopulmonary resuscitation is to supply adequate oxygen to the brain and heart until advanced life support techniques can restore normal cardiopulmonary function. The ABCs used in human medicine apply to small animals, but some of the methodology must be adapted.[1-7]

Airway

If a patient is presented with respiratory apnea or difficulty breathing, the first step in cardiopulmonary resuscitation is to secure an airway. The pharynx must be cleared of obstructions (vomitus, mucus, blood, or foreign bodies) so that resuscitative efforts are effective and an endotracheal tube can be placed. Vomitus and mucus can be cleared by hand, by inverting the patient, or by a suction device. Some foreign bodies may need to be removed with a sponge forceps. If an endotracheal tube cannot be placed because of a laryngeal obstruction (e.g., an unremovable foreign body or trauma), a tracheostomy must be performed.

Breathing

Once an airway is established, the next step in resuscitation is to breathe for the patient. Artificial ventilation can be performed by breathing into the mouth or nose of a patient, by using a rebreathing bag and room air, or by supplying oxygen. If an endotracheal tube is not available, mouth-to-mouth or mouth-to-nose resuscitation is necessary. The resuscitator's mouth must cover the patient's nostrils and mouth to achieve effective ventilation. In large dogs, the commissures of the mouth can be pinched to limit loss of air.

The American Heart Association recommends 20 ventilations per minute. This ventilatory rate does not take into account that the respiratory rates of dogs and cats are normally higher than those of humans. Previous recommendations included an initial four ventilations that did not allow

the patient to expire fully. Failure to allow full expiration during the initial ventilations causes a prolonged positive end expiratory pressure to be sustained; this may stop a weakly beating heart.[1]

In one-rescuer cardiopulmonary resuscitation, the current recommendation is to provide an initial two full breaths (1 to 1.5 seconds each) and then to ventilate every two seconds thereafter.[1,3] In two-rescuer cardiopulmonary resuscitation, it is recommended that simultaneous compression and ventilation be performed after the initial two ventilations have been provided.

The amount of inspired oxygen obtained from room air (21%) or from expired air ventilations (16% to 17%) is not enough to prevent hypoxemia in arrest patients.[4] In order to reduce the amount of hypoxemia and metabolic acidosis that occurs, positive-pressure ventilations should be performed with 100% oxygen.[1,3,4]

Circulation

If a pulse or heartbeat cannot be detected, external cardiac compressions should be initiated. The goal of cardiac compression is to maintain adequate blood flow to the brain and heart. The cardiac pump and thoracic pump are the mechanisms involved in the generation of blood flow.[1,3,8] The most important mechanism of blood-flow generation, especially in large dogs, is the thoracic pump.

The thoracic pump relies on compression of the thoracic cavity and generation of intrathoracic pressure to maintain blood flow. Factors that influence the effectiveness of the thoracic pump include the position of the patient, ventilations, airway pressure, and abdominal wall movement during compressions.[1,8] To increase intrathoracic pressure effectively, it is recommended that patients that weigh more than seven kilograms be placed in dorsal recumbency and have cardiac compressions performed over the distal third of the sternum.[3] Patients that weigh less than seven kilograms should be placed in lateral recumbency, and cardiac compressions should be performed over the fourth and fifth intercostal spaces.[3]

Intrathoracic pressure also can be increased by ventilating with airway pressures between 80 to 100 mm Hg and performing cardiac compression during peak inspiration.[1,8] During cardiac compressions, abdominal wall movement should be restricted to improve the generation of intrathoracic pressure.

Abdominal wrapping or interposed rhythmic abdominal compressions have increased survival rates and neurologic recovery by increasing venous return to the heart.[1,3] A compression rate of 60 to 120 per minute is currently recommended in small animals. In one-rescuer cardiopulmonary resuscitation, two ventilations are given for every 10 to 15 compressions. In two-rescuer resuscitation, simultaneous ventilations and compressions are recommended to increase intrathoracic pressure. With three rescuers available, cranial abdominal compressions can be administered between thoracic compressions.

THIRD PHASE: ADVANCED LIFE SUPPORT TECHNIQUES

Advanced life support techniques include diagnosis, the use of emergency drugs or defibrillation and open-heart massage, and the rapid infusion of fluids. In order to assist the veterinarian effectively, it is necessary for the technician to understand the procedures to be performed.

Diagnosis

During the course of resuscitation, the patient should be connected to an electrocardiograph (ECG) machine. Electrocardiogram recordings common with cardiac arrest include ventricular fibrillation, ventricular tachycardia, ventricular asystole, electromechanical dissociation (EMD), and bradycardia. If not treated quickly, ventricular tachycardia can lead to ventricular fibrillation and ventricular asystole. Electromechanical dissociation occurs when the heart has electrical activity but is not contracting. A patient with the condition may have a normal or nearly normal complex on the electrocardiogram but lacks a palpable pulse.[1] It is thus important that pulses be checked periodically during the performance of cardiopulmonary resuscitation.

Emergency Drugs

If time allows, doses of emergency drugs should be precalculated for class I and II patients. Because most emergency patients enter the hospital in cardiopulmonary arrest, emergency drug doses should be calculated per 10 pounds of body weight and posted so that the doses can be easily read (Figure 1). Common emergency drugs are atropine, dexamethasone sodium phosphate, epinephrine, furosemide, lidocaine, and sodium bicarbonate.

Atropine should be administered in the presence of sinus bradycardia or ventricular asystole. Dexamethasone sodium phosphate is used to treat shock and is an effective treatment for electromechanical dissociation.[1] Epinephrine is used to treat ventricular asystole and electromechanical dissociation. The recommended dose for epinephrine has been increased from 0.01 to 0.02 mg/kg to 0.1 to 0.2 mg/kg. The higher dose has been demonstrated to be more effective in increasing cerebral blood flow.[1]

Furosemide is a loop diuretic that is used to treat pulmonary and cerebral edema. Lidocaine is used to treat premature ventricular contractions and ventricular tachycardia. The use of sodium bicarbonate has changed over the years. Bicarbonate has been demonstrated to decrease oxygen delivery to the tissue, induce paradoxic cellular acidosis, and decrease myocardial function. It is currently recommended that the drug be administered only during prolonged cardiopulmonary resuscitation or in cases of confirmed metabolic acidosis.[1,3] Immediate electrocardioversion (defibrillation) is the preferred treatment in patients with ventricular fibrillation.

Routes used to administer emergency drugs include intracardiac, central or peripheral intravenous, endotracheal, and intraosseous. Intracardiac administration of emergency drugs was common but is no longer recommended.[1,3] This route makes it possible to lacerate a coronary vessel or to inject a drug into the myocardium and thus cause ventricular arrhythmia. Another disadvantage is that closed-chest cardiopulmonary resuscitation must be stopped in order to administer the drug.

Studies have demonstrated that a central venous catheter is the best route for administering emergency drugs.[1] A central catheter may not be in place when cardiopulmonary arrest occurs, and placement after arrest is difficult. Cardiac levels of drugs administered by the peripheral route are low because of the vasoconstriction that occurs during cardiopulmonary arrest. Drugs should be administered through a peripheral vein only if other routes are inaccessible. If a central vein cannot be catheterized, the next best method is the endotracheal route.

If an endotracheal tube is in place, the endotracheal route can be used to administer atropine, epinephrine, and lidocaine.[1,3,4] Sodium bicarbonate should not be given by the endotracheal route because the agent can cause pulmonary atelectasis.[3] Studies indicate that this method is effective in achieving rapid, high blood concentrations (as when administering drugs through a central catheter).[1] Recommendations concerning this route include administering twice the normal dose, diluting the drug with 3 to 10 milliliters of sterile saline or sterile water, and giving several positive-pressure ventilations after instillation of the drug.[1,3]

The intraosseous route also can be used to administer emergency drugs. All emergency drugs, as well as large volumes of fluid, can be given by this route. An advantage of the intraosseous route is that the medullary cavity does not collapse in shock states; placement of a catheter thus is easier than in a central or peripheral vein.

If external cardiac compressions and administration of appropriate drugs produce no response within one to two

EMERGENCY DRUGS	10 POUNDS	20 POUNDS	40 POUNDS	60 POUNDS	80 POUNDS	100 POUNDS
EPINEPHRINE (concentration 1:1000) Dose: 0.1 mg/lb intravenously 　　　0.2 mg/lb endotracheally, diluted 　　　　in 3–10 ml sterile saline or water. Repeat at five min intervals	1.0 cc 2.0 cc	2.0 cc 4.0 cc	4.0 cc 8.0 cc	6.0 cc 12.0 cc	8.0 cc 16.0 cc	10.0 cc 20.0 cc
ATROPINE (concentration 0.5 mg/ml) Dose: 0.02 mg/lb intravenously 　　　1 cc/10 lb endotracheally, diluted 　　　　in 3–10 ml sterile saline or water. Repeat at five min intervals	0.4 cc 1.0 cc	0.8 cc 2.0 cc	1.6 cc 4.0 cc	2.4 cc 6.0 cc	3.2 cc 8.0 cc	4.0 cc 10.0 cc
LIDOCAINE (2%) (concentration 20 mg/ml) Dose: 2–4 mg/kg intravenously in dogs 　　　0.5 mg/kg intravenously in cats 　　　8 mg/kg endotracheally, diluted 　　　　in 3–10 ml sterile saline or water.	1.0 cc 0.1 cc 2.0 cc	2.0 cc 0.2 cc 4.0 cc	4.0 cc 8.0 cc	6.0 cc 12.0 cc	8.0 cc 16.0 cc	10.0 cc 20.0 cc
SODIUM BICARBONATE (concentration 　　1 mEq/ml) Dose: 0.25 mEq/lb intravenously Give one half over 10 minute period	2.5 cc	5.0 cc	10.0 cc	15.0 cc	20.0 cc	25.0 cc
MANNITOL (20%) (concentration 200 mg/ml) Dose: 0.13 g/lb intravenously Give over 10 minute period	6.5 cc	13.0 cc	26.0 cc	39.0 cc	52.0 cc	65.0 cc
EMETIC DRUGS 　Morphine (dogs only) 15 mg/ml Dose: 0.5–1 mg/lb intramuscularly 　Xylazine (cats only) 20 mg/ml Dose: 0.2 mg/lb intramuscularly						

Figure 1—An emergency drug chart.

minutes, it is necessary for the veterinarian to perform open cardiac massage. Open-chest massage requires an emergency thoracotomy.[1,8] Items needed for a thoracotomy are a scalpel blade, Mayo scissors, and a Balfour abdominal retractor or rib spreader. With open-heart massage, it is recommended that the patient's ventilation be timed with every second or third cardiac compression.[1]

Fluids

The rapid infusion of fluids is often used to increase blood volume during cardiopulmonary resuscitation. Studies demonstrate that the infusion of fluids in patients that do not exhibit volume depletion before arrest can impair nutrient delivery to the brain and heart.[1,3,4] Rapid fluid administration thus should only be used in patients with cardiopulmonary arrest caused by volume depletion.

Fluids that contain glucose should not be used for volume replacement. Glucose is an energy substrate and in excessive amounts leads to the production of superoxide radicals and neuronal lactic acid. The use of glucose in fluids has been associated with neuronal damage and deterioration of previous neurologic signs.[1]

FOURTH PHASE: POSTRESUSCITATIVE CARE

It is relatively common for a patient to rearrest in the postresuscitative period.[3,4] Close monitoring of the respiratory pattern, electrocardiogram, body temperature, blood pressure, and pulse quality is necessary to prevent subsequent arrests. Other potential problems are acute renal failure, sepsis, neurologic damage, and disseminated intravascular coagulation.[9] Urine production and neurologic status should be carefully monitored. The patient's electrolytes, packed cell volume, total protein, and acid–base status also should be checked periodically.

Patients in the postresuscitative period should receive oxygen. Methods of delivery that can be used in dogs and cats include mask, nasal, intratracheal, or cage oxygen.[10] During this period, extensive diagnostic testing can be performed if the cause of the arrest has not been determined. Treatment of the underlying problem may prevent another arrest.

CONCLUSION

Timing and patient selection are critical in successful cardiopulmonary resuscitation. Studies demonstrate that the length of arrest is an important prognostic factor of success. At Colorado State University, most successful resuscitations involved patients that required oxygen therapy only and did not have cardiac involvement.[3,4]

Cardiopulmonary resuscitation in terminally ill patients is generally unsuccessful. If a patient has an irreversible disease, a staff member at the clinic should talk to the owner regarding the condition of the pet and whether resuscitation should be performed in the event of an arrest. If a patient presents in cardiopulmonary arrest, resuscitation should be begun while a staff member advises the owner of the cost involved in resuscitating the pet. Cardiopulmonary resuscitation should be performed only if a life-threatening disease is reversible or if the arrest was unexpected.

■

REFERENCES

1. Crowe DT: Cardiopulmonary resuscitation in the dog: A review and proposed new guidelines. Part II. *Semin Vet Med Surg [Small Anim]* 3(4):328–348, 1988.
2. Robello CD, Crowe DT: Cardiopulmonary resuscitation: Current recommendations. *Vet Clin North Am [Small Anim Pract]* 19(6):1127–1149, 1989.
3. Wingfield WE, Henik RA: Cardiopulmonary arrest and resuscitation, in Ettinger SJ (ed): *Textbook of Veterinary Internal Medicine.* Philadelphia, WB Saunders Co, 1989, pp 171–180.
4. Henik RA, Wingfield WE: Cardiopulmonary resuscitation in cats. *Semin Vet Med Surg [Small Anim]* 3(3):185–192, 1988.
5. Crowe DT: Handling the critical patient: Getting past the initial crisis. *Vet Med* 84(1):33–53, 1989.
6. Haskins SC: Monitoring the critically ill patient. *Vet Clin North Am [Small Anim Pract]* 19(6):1059–1077, 1989.
7. Wingfield WE, Henik RA: Treatment priorities in cases of multiple trauma. *Semin Vet Med Surg [Small Anim]* 3(3):193–201, 1988.
8. Crowe DT: Cardiopulmonary resuscitation in the dog: A review and proposed new guidelines. Part I. *Semin Vet Med Surg [Small Anim]* 3(4):321–327, 1988.
9. Murtaugh RJ: Emergency medicine, in Ettinger SJ (ed): *Textbook of Veterinary Internal Medicine.* Philadelphia, WB Saunders Co, 1989, pp 209–216.
10. Pascoe PJ: Oxygen and ventilatory support for the critical patient. *Semin Vet Med Surg [Small Anim]* 3(3):202–209, 1988.